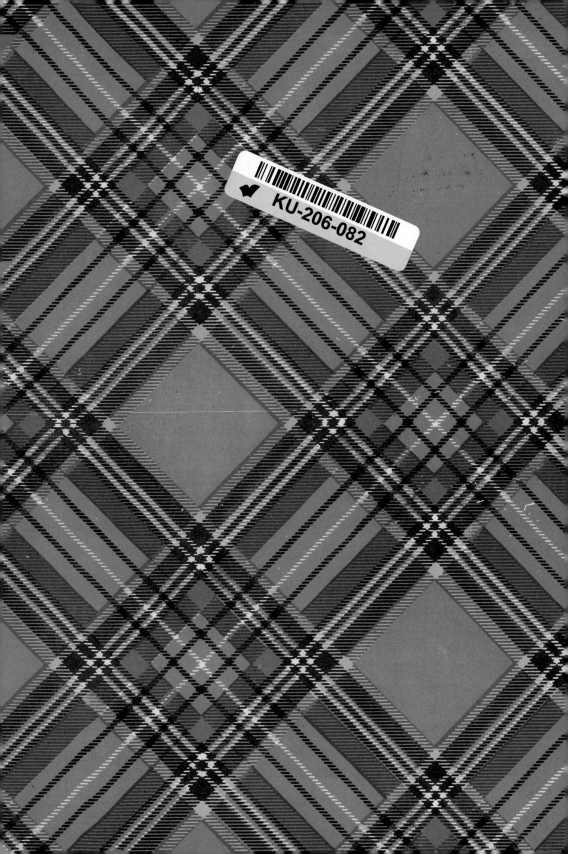

A

RESEARCH STUDIES

IN

MEDICAL HISTORY

No. 4

HISTORY

OF

SCOTTISH MEDICINE

TO 1860

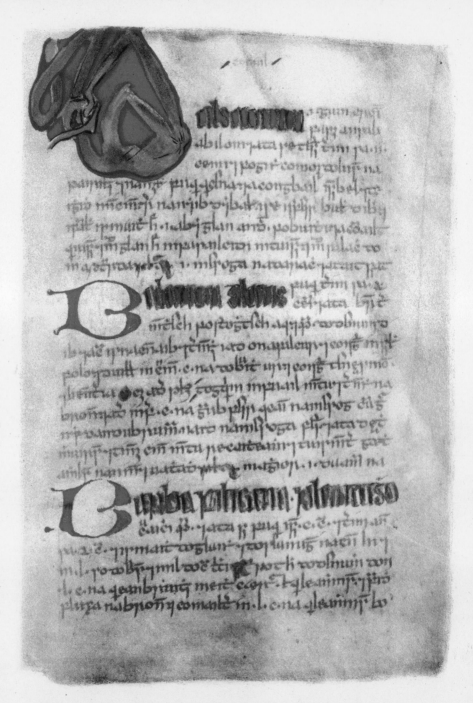

GAELIC MEDICAL MS. DATING FROM A SHORT TIME AFTER 1400 A.D.

This MS. belonged at one time to John Beaton. It deals with Materia Medica, the substances being mentioned in alphabetical order. This page treats of Balsamum, Balanon and Barba. (*See page* 22)

(Reproduced from page 39 *of Gaelic Medical MS. III in the National Library, Edinburgh)*

HISTORY

OF

SCOTTISH MEDICINE

TO 1860

BY

JOHN D. COMRIE

M.A., B.SC., M.D., F.R.C.P.

Lecturer on Practice of Medicine in the School of Medicine of the Royal Colleges at Edinburgh
and on History of Medicine in the University of Edinburgh; President, History of Medicine Section,
British Medical Association Meeting, 1927; late Consulting Physician to the Forces in North Russia.

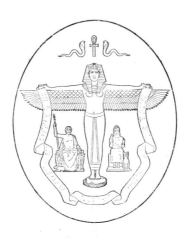

Published for

THE WELLCOME HISTORICAL MEDICAL MUSEUM

54A, WIGMORE STREET, LONDON, W.

by

BAILLIÈRE, TINDALL & COX

7 & 8, HENRIETTA STREET, COVENT GARDEN

LONDON

COPYRIGHT   1927   PRINTED IN ENGLAND

Printed in England for

The Wellcome Historical Medical Museum, 54ª, Wigmore Street, London, England

(The Wellcome Foundation Ltd.)

PREFACE

THIS volume, dealing with the History of Medicine in Scotland up to 1860, is issued by the Wellcome Historical Medical Museum on the occasion of the inauguration of a Section for History of Medicine at the Meeting of the British Medical Association at Edinburgh in July, 1927.

Several of the Universities, Medical Corporations and large Hospitals have from time to time issued accounts of their individual histories; but, up to the present, there has been no work dealing with Scottish medicine as a whole, although medicine in Scotland presents characteristic features. I have tried to show the influence which various educational and philanthropic institutions, as well as persons distinguished in Scottish medicine, have exerted upon one another, and on the development of medical knowledge.

Part of the material set down here has been already included in papers contributed to the *Edinburgh Medical Journal* and *British Medical Journal*, or read at the International Congresses of Medical History in London and Geneva.

It is hoped that the book may appeal to the increasing number of persons who, at the present day, take an interest in the history of the medical profession, and that it may also prove valuable to those who wish to make further research in this direction. It has been possible to offer only a limited amount of information in the compass of this small volume, but great care has been taken to give references to other works, which may be consulted by those desiring to pursue the subject.

There are various reasons for ending this section of medical history about the year 1860, which is beyond the memory of most people now alive. The Medical Act of 1858 was then coming into general operation, and had abolished apprenticeship and many of the privileges of the medical corporations; the University of Aberdeen was formed from the two Colleges of that city in 1860 ; and the other provisions of the Scottish Universities Act came into operation about the same time.   Finally, the introduction of new surgical principles in relation to Pasteur's earlier discoveries followed a few years after Lister became Professor of Surgery at Glasgow in 1860.

I desire to acknowledge my indebtedness to many persons who have helped in the preparation of the book.   My gratitude for indicating sources of information is due to Mr. T. H. Graham, Librarian to the Royal College of Physicians at Edinburgh, who has also been good enough to read the proofs ; and to Mr. F. C. Nicholson, Librarian of the University of Edinburgh. For reading the chapter dealing with the Aberdeen Medical School, I have to thank Mr. G. M. Fraser, Librarian of the Public Library at Aberdeen, and for reading the chapters on the Glasgow Medical School, Dr. John F. Fergus.

The Panel of the Altar-piece from Trinity Church, Edinburgh, is reproduced by gracious permission of His Majesty the King.

For kindness in providing other illustrations, I must especially thank Mr. T. C. F. Brotchie, Superintendent of the Glasgow Art Galleries ; Mr. Stanley Cursiter, Keeper of the Scottish National Portrait Gallery ; Mr. A. J. H. Edwards, Assistant Keeper of the Scottish National Museum of Antiquities ; Mr. Charles B. Boog Watson ; the Rt. Hon. Lord Torphichen ; Major C. H. Scott Plummer ; Fleet-Surgeon W. E. Home, R.N. ; Professor G. Lovell Gulland ; Mr. D. M. Greig, F.R.C.S. ; the Royal Faculty of Physicians and Surgeons of Glasgow ; the University of Edinburgh ; H.M. Office of Works ; the Secretary of St. Andrews University ; the Treasurer of Dumfries and Galloway Royal Infirmary ; the Town Clerk of the City of Edinburgh ; the Librarian of the Scottish National Library ; and Messrs. A. and C. Black.

I am greatly indebted to my secretary, Miss M. S. Cairns, for the careful manner in which she has read the proofs and verified the references.

Finally, I have to thank those connected with the Wellcome Historical Medical Museum, especially Mr. L. W. G. Malcolm, M.Sc., F.R.S.E., Conservator of the Museum, for the great amount of labour they have expended in seeing the book through the press.

J. D. C.

25, Manor Place,
    Edinburgh.
        July, 1927.

CONTENTS

LIST OF ILLUSTRATIONS

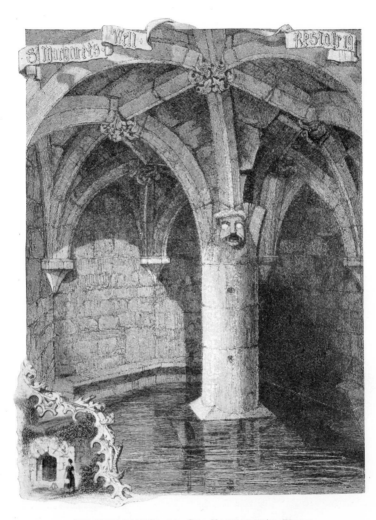

ST. TRIDUANA'S OR ST. MARGARET'S WELL

The well-house was removed about 1860 from its original site at Restalrig to its present position south of Holyrood, where it covers another sainted spring, known as St. David's or the Rood Well

CHAPTER 1

EARLY MEDICINE IN SCOTLAND

I N primitive times, when Scotland consisted of a number of isolated lake-villages and hill townships, separated by bog and dense forest, the healing art was presumably no further developed than the practice of such simple remedies and applications as experience would show to be generally useful.

When Christianity was introduced about the 6th century, the more learned of the Culdee missionaries, in addition to a knowledge of Christian doctrine, may have possessed some acquaintance with the medical lore of the ancients, which was to be found among manuscripts in the libraries of the wealthier religious houses of other countries. Legends of the early Saints indicate that some of their influence was due to their powers of healing, although in the popular estimation, these powers are usually credited with a supernatural or miraculous origin.

Numerous wells with miraculous powers of healing were associated with the names of various Saints. Of these, one of the most famous was the Well of St. Triduana, at Restalrig, near Edinburgh. St. Triduana was a recluse of the primitive church, whose tomb after her death became a shrine for pilgrims afflicted with eye diseases. In early life, her beauty had attracted a Pictish chief from whom she fled, and, being pursued by his emissaries, she plucked out her eyes and sent them to him impaled upon a thorn, as they had been the cause of his unwelcome attentions.

For many centuries the Well at Restalrig, afterwards called St. Margaret's Well, was the resort of those who, in the words of Sir David Lindsay, went to " St. Trid well to mend their ene." So hard does tradition die that even now (1927) people with eye disorders frequently come with bottles to collect the water, despite the fact that the ancient well-house has been removed to another spring about a mile distant, close to Holyrood.

Various celebrated amulets were also used for mediæval treatment, chiefly by administering to a sick person water in which the relic had been immersed. St. Columba himself is recorded in Adamnan's 7th century Life of the Saint as having used this method of treatment with a stone that he had blessed.

One of the most celebrated of these charms was the Lee Penny, a small red stone set in a silver coin, said to have been brought from the Holy Land by Sir Simon Lockhart, of Lee, and celebrated as "The Talisman," in Sir Walter Scott's novel of that name. This charm was used by drinking of, or bathing with, the water in which it had been dipped three times. Balls of rock crystal, one known as the "stone of the standard," possessed by

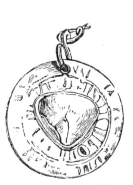
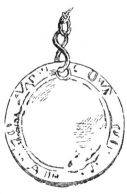

THE LEE PENNY

the Chief of the clan Donnachie, another known as the stone of Ardvoirlich, in the possession of the family of that name, and others belonging to the families of Campbell of Glenlyon, Baird of Auchmeddan, and others, have been used in a similar manner from very early times.

At the shrine of St. Fillan (an 8th century abbot and recluse), near Tyndrum, a form of treatment was used, especially for lunacy, which resembled the procedure in the temples of Asklepios. The mentally afflicted person, after being dipped in a sacred pool, was bound and laid on the floor of the church or in a stone coffin overnight, the bronze bell of St. Fillan, a sacred relic, being placed beside him or on his head. If in the morning he was found free from his bonds, recovery from the madness was likely to take place. Those who recovered sometimes related visions that had appeared to them in the night.[1]

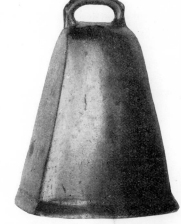

THE BELL OF ST. FILLAN
(Preserved in the Royal Scottish Museum of Antiquities)

Some of these magical methods of healing, however, had long antedated Christianity, for Pliny[2] speaks of ceremonies which the wizards and physicians of the Druids practised in Britain. Many of these have doubtless come down in the medical folk-lore still to be found in country places and recorded in the popular medical

---

[1] Anderson : " Scotland in Early Christian Times," Edinburgh, 1881.
[2] Pliny : " Natural History," Book XXX., para. 4.

works of the 18th century, including the sacrifice of different animals for various maladies, the administration of blood, bile and excrements as remedies, the wearing of coral necklaces, purification by dew and by fire at the feast of Beltane in May, etc.

With the advent of the Norman civilisation, which came to Scotland in the end of the 11th and the beginning of the 12th centuries under Queen Margaret, and especially David I., schools and religious houses were established and a much greater knowledge of ancient learning, including that of medicine, became available. Intercourse between the north of Scotland and the Baltic countries, and between the southern part of the kingdom and the Low Countries and France, speedily sprang up, and this led to a further diffusion of knowledge and to the introduction of new habits and modes of thought in Scotland.

The 13th century was one of great prosperity in southern Scotland. The Angles of Northumbria had been driven out and peace had reigned in Lothian for 200 years. The Norsemen had been expelled from the Scottish mainland. On the east coast, Berwick, reputed the chief port in Britain before the 14th century, was at the height of its prosperity, and in the west, Glasgow Cathedral, to-day the finest ecclesiastical building in Scotland, was then rising under Bishop Jocelyn's hand. The beautiful Abbeys of Jedburgh, Kelso, Melrose, Dryburgh, Newbattle and Holyrood had been founded as centres of light and learning by David I. during the 12th century. Here, amid the pleasant vales and woods of Tweedside and Lothian, peaceful Norman settlers had introduced art and learning without the strife from which England then suffered under Richard, John and Henry III. To the people in the south and east of Scotland, learning had become a matter of desire, and grammar schools existed in all the towns of any size. An acquaintance with Latin was widespread, and many manuscripts of Greek and Roman learning were accessible in the monasteries. To Scotland came monks from England, France and distant Italy, and many Scotsmen went abroad, bent upon commercial enterprise, the acquisition of learning or the gaining of fame and standing in the martial service of foreign princes.

Each monastery possessed, in addition to its library containing copies or Latin translations of ancient medical books, a physic garden, where simples were cultivated. The kind of herbs used by the monks in preparing remedies may be learned from the list of those grown in the 9th century at the monastery of St. Gall. This celebrated monastery was established at the cell of an Irish hermit of that name who lived in the 7th century. The medicinal plants were rose, bean, savory, costus, hedge mustard, cumin, fennel, lybisticum, lily, sage, rue, gladiola, pennyroyal, mint, rosemary and fenugreek.[1]

---

[1] Keller: " Bauriss des Klosters St. Gallen vom Jahre 830," Zurich, 1844.

Most of the monasteries also possessed hospitia, situated sometimes at the monastery itself, sometimes on a route used by pilgrims and travellers. In these hospitia, monks specially skilled in medicine cared for sick or wounded travellers, and for persons of the district who required medical attention. An example of such a hospitium in Scotland is still to be seen in the few ruined remains of Soutra Aisle, situated on the road from Edinburgh to Kelso and Dryburgh Abbeys, which was founded by Malcolm IV. in 1164, for the care of travellers and pilgrims proceeding to these shrines.

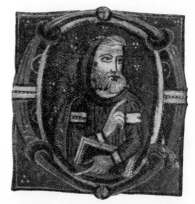

As an example of a Scot who journeyed to the Continent and attained a reputation as a scholar and a doctor in foreign parts Michael Scot[1] may be mentioned. He was born on the Scottish borders about the year 1175 and died about the year 1232, after his return to his native country. He affords a good example of the learned churchmen who practised medicine at a time when learning of this kind was necessarily restricted to churchmen, because the means of deriving a knowledge of medicine were to be found solely in the libraries of the religious houses, or of

PORTRAIT OF MICHAEL SCOT
(From Bodleian MS., "De Physionomiæ")

princes. During his life abroad, between the years 1200 and 1208, Scot had acted as tutor to Frederick, King of Sicily and later Emperor of Germany, a prince famous for his talents and for his encouragement of learning.

As a marriage present to Frederick, Scot composed for him his " Liber Physionomiæ," a guide in the knowledge of men, intended to be useful to a pupil about to pass from his charge into the stormy life of European politics.[2] This work aims at giving a description of the character, peculiarities and diseases of men which can be gained from their outward appearances. The subject was an important branch of the knowledge of medical men in the Middle Ages, as is indicated in the Charter of the Edinburgh Surgeons and Barbers, who were expected to know the " nature and complexion of every member humanis bodie, and als thatt he knaw in quhilk member the signe hes domination for the tyme." The book attained a great popularity in manuscript, and, after the introduction of printing, no fewer than 18 editions appeared between 1477 and 1660. Part of the work is influenced by Aristotle's " History of Animals," part is taken from the " Liber ad Mansorem " of Rhazes, but the greater portion is apparently from Scot's own observation. Of the three books, into which it is divided, the first deals with

---

[1] *See* Wood Brown : " Life and Legend of Michael Scot," Edinburgh, 1897.
[2] Comrie : " Michael Scot : A 13th century Scientist and Physician," *Edinburgh Medical Journal*, July, 1920.

the mysteries of birth and generation, the second expounds the evidences of the different complexions as revealed in various parts of the body or by dreams, and the third explains what signs of the inward character can be read in each of the bodily members.

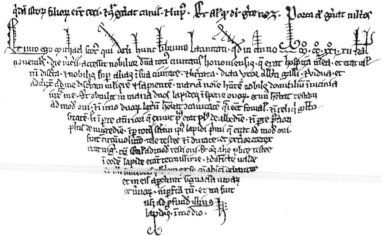

Michael Scot was also celebrated as a translator of Aristotle, as a writer on alchemy and as a contributor to what was then an important science—that of astronomy and astrology. His eminence as a writer is testified by Vincent of Beauvais, Albertus Magnus and Roger Bacon. The enactments of Frederick II., regarding the practice of medicine in Italy and Germany, had an important influence in standardising medicine and in confirming the social status of its practitioners so far as these countries were concerned, and the inception of these regulations is probably correctly attributed to his tutor, Michael Scot.[1] Scot is also stated by de Renzi to have been one of the early teachers in the mediæval medical school of Salerno.[2]

As a practising physician, Scot enjoyed a great reputation, being specially celebrated for his treatment of leprosy, gout and dropsy. One of his consultations on a case of calculus is still preserved in the margin of a manuscript in the Library of Gonville and Caius College.[3] One of his pills, known as " Pilulæ Magistri Michaelis Scoti,"[4] is noted by a 13th century copyist as effective to relieve headache, purge the humours wonderfully,

---

[1] Huillard-Brehollis : " Diplomatic History of Frederick II." Paris, 1851.
[2] De Renzi : " Collect. Salern," i., p. 292.
[3] *Catalogue of Gonville and Caius College,* 109 (i., 3).
[4] British Museum : Additional MSS. 24068 (22), fol. 97.

produce joyfulness, brighten the intellect, improve the vision, sharpen hearing, preserve youth and retard baldness. These pills were composed of aloes, rhubarb and nine fruits and flowers made into a confection, and might fairly be described as excellent after-dinner pills.

Scot had gained even in Italy a reputation as a seer of the future and magician, so that Dante placed him in the Inferno along with other soothsayers as

> " That other, round the loins
> So slender of his shape, was Michael Scot,
> Practised in every slight of magic wile." [1]

It was natural, therefore, that on his return to the Scottish Lowlands, in his later years, an ignorant peasantry regarded him as a wizard, whose alleged association with the devil is indicated by several striking features of the landscape in the Scottish borders :—

> " A wizard of such dreaded fame,
> That when, in Salamanca's cave,
> Him listed his magic wand to wave,
> The bells would ring in Notre Dame." [2]

An important phase of early Scottish medicine is found in the Gaelic medical manuscripts which are preserved in some of the libraries of Ireland and Scotland.[3] The Gaelic medical literature comprises over twenty manuscripts preserved in the Advocates' (National) Library at Edinburgh, one in the Library of the Scottish Antiquarian Society, one in the Library of the University of Edinburgh, two in the British Museum, and several in private collections. They all possess this feature in common, that their substance is mainly of foreign origin, being translations made from Latin. Several of them are translations of medical treatises from the early Greek physicians and philosophers, and others from compilers of the Arabian school ; several of them are taken from authoritative treatises issued from the great mediæval medical schools of Salerno and Montpellier. They were prepared for or by Gaelic physicians attached to the great nobles of the north of Scotland, and the oldest dated manuscript which could be found by Professor Mackinnon[3] bore the date of 1403, although this authority admits that some of the undated translations may be earlier in origin. The greater number, however, date from the 16th century. They include such subjects as an abstract of Galen's anatomy, anatomical descriptions taken from Galen, Avicenna, Lanfranc and Guy de Chauliac, chapters on wounds, attributed to John of Vigo, and frequent paragraphs devoted to blood-letting, with the veins appropriate to be opened and the proper seasons and days for the operation.

---

[1] Dante : " Inferno," XX, 115-117. (Cary's Translation).
[2] Scott : " Lay of the Last Minstrel," Canto ii., 13.
[3] Mackinnon : Report, 17th International Congress of Medicine, Section XXIII. London, 1913, p. 401. See also " A Descriptive Catalogue of Gaelic Medical Manuscripts in the Advocates' Library, Edinburgh, and elsewhere in Scotland," by Donald Mackinnon, M.A., Edinburgh, 1912. Also George Mackay, M.D., " Ancient Gaelic Medical Manuscripts," in *Caledonian Medical Journal*, October, 1904.

The classification of diseases in some of the larger manuscripts is full and elaborate, as well as the remedies prescribed for each disease. Questions of climate, diet, nursing and kindred topics are largely discussed, and in one manuscript a chapter is devoted to the appropriate method of weighing and measuring drugs. Various cases are also included, and several theories believed to influence the health of the individual, such as the elements, the planets and the doctrine of the humours, are subjects of frequent and

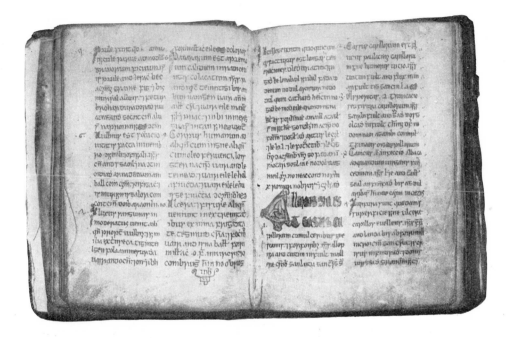

GAELIC MEDICAL MS. OF THE 15TH CENTURY
(Preserved in University of Edinburgh Library)

lengthy exposition and discussion. The margins of the manuscripts are frequently covered with notes, which have probably been added by the possessors of the manuscripts, dealing with the weather during the various months and the foods and drinks most suitable in each.

These manuscripts mainly belonged to two families, who practised medicine in the Highlands of Scotland for several centuries. The first of these bears the name of MacBheathadh, which means the " son of life," a very happy name for a physician. The name later came to be written in Latin, Betonus or Beaton, and in its modern form MacBeth. Several of these physicians were well-known men, such as Fergus McBetha, or Fergus the Fair, who was attached to Donald,

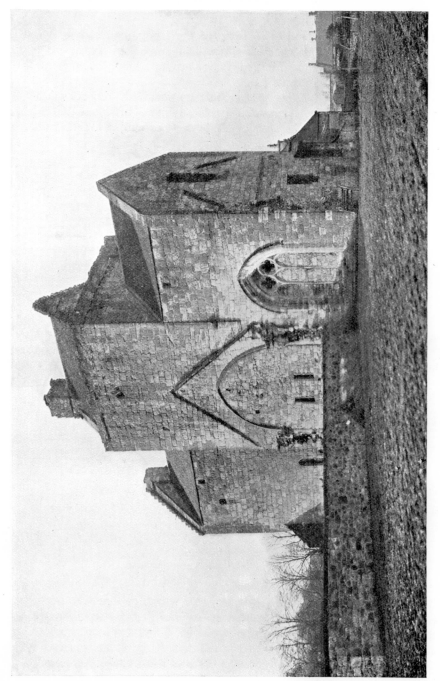

PRIORY OF TORPHICHEN, as it appears at the present day

(Photo by H. M. Office of Works)

Lord of the Isles, defeated at the battle of Harlaw in 1411. Another settled in Islay in the days of Robert the Bruce, and is said to have obtained so great a reputation that he was summoned to the bedside of the King of Scotland and effected a cure when the court physicians had failed. One of his descendants, Farquhar, who is described as *Medicus Regis*, obtained an important grant of property, in 1386, from Alexander Stewart, the Wolf of Badenoch.

The other hereditary medical family was that of the McConachers of Lorn, of whom there are records as early as 1530. One of these, Duncan McConacher, with the help of friends, made a copy of Bernard Gordon's " Lilium Medicinæ," in 1596–1597, and commenced in 1598 a treatise which was to be an epitome of the teaching of Avicenna. Duncan was the possessor of a copy of a treatise on materia medica, preserved in the Advocates' (National) Library, containing references to 312 articles. This is the most complete copy of a treatise, which is repeated several times among the Gaelic medical manuscripts, and upon which the Gaelic physicians placed great value. Other copies of it are to be found in the British Museum, the Advocates' Library, etc.[1] A later descendant, Donald O'Conacher, seems to have been so celebrated as a physician that, in 1639, he was brought for a consultation to the town of Irvine.

An important example of the care which religious institutions exercised over the physical well-being of the community is still to be seen in the Priory of Torphichen, established by the Knights of the Order of St. John of Jerusalem, with the consent of David I., in the year 1124.[2] A hospitium had been established at Jerusalem as a pious foundation by the merchants of Amalfi some time before 1048, for the purpose of giving shelter to pilgrims arriving at the Holy City.

With the appearance of the Crusaders at Jerusalem in 1099, the character of the fraternity of serving brothers, spending their lives in devoted attention to the sick and destitute among the pilgrims, changed. They now took the very important step of undertaking in addition to their charitable work, the protection of pilgrims both in Palestine and in their journeys to and from it. This introduced a military element into their duties, and in 1099, under the mastership of Raymond de Puy, their title was changed to that of the Knights Hospitallers of the Order of St. John of Jerusalem, whose uniform consisted of a red surcoat with a plain white cross. The cross sometimes takes the form of a Maltese cross and sometimes, as at Torphichen, has a double crosspiece. The Order was made up of three classes—knights of noble birth, who carried arms; priests or chaplains, who performed religious ceremonies; and serving brothers, who attended the sick and relieved the pilgrims.

---

[1] For accounts of this treatise on materia medica, *see* paper by Sir Norman Moore in Vol. XI. *Bartholomew Hospital Reports;* also extracts by Dr. H. C. Gillies, *Caledonian Medical Journal,* Vol. VIII., pp. 102, 143.

[2] Beatson : " The Knights Hospitallers in Scotland," Glasgow, 1903.

The Order gradually came to hold much property in different countries, and it was divided into national corps, known as provinces or langues. Over every langue, such as that of England, presided a Grand Prior, under whom were placed Preceptors or Commanders, governing the different houses or commanderies in the province. A Preceptory, or Priory, served as a home for aged Knights and as a recruiting station for aspirants to the Order. It is presumable that the Priory at Torphichen was an offshoot of the English langue, which had been established in 1100 A.D. and later developed into a wealthy monastery at Clerkenwell, in London, of which the gate still remains. In a dispute between the Scottish Hospitallers and the Abbot and Canons of Holyrood, between 1210 and 1214, the settlement was sealed by the Chapter of the House of the Hospitallers in London, showing that Scotland was nominally at least under the English langue.[1] Nevertheless, many of the Scottish recruits served in the various langues of France. The toughness of the young Scottish knights is attested by the fact that one of them, Thomas Elliot, who was hanged at Hexham early in the 14th century, was found to be alive when the body was removed for burial, so that he was granted a free pardon and allowed to depart abroad.[2]

The Priory at Torphichen stands some five miles south of Linlithgow, an important Royal residence of the mediæval Scottish kings, in a hollow among the hills, where it was protected by a surrounding morass from attack. Although at the present day shorn of its outer defences, it still presents a combination of a religious and military edifice.

Here, in the 13th century, the Knights and their followers continued to exercise a beneficent influence over the surrounding district, and here a " Sanctuary," wherein no man might be seized or harmed, extended for one mile in every direction round the building. The grounds of the Preceptory were a Scotch acre in extent, enclosed by a moat, and a portion of them was known as " the Knights' Garden," in which medicinal herbs were cultivated. Donations and land were freely bestowed upon it by several of the Scottish kings, and at one time it is said to have held possessions in eight of the counties of Scotland and to have had a large revenue. The Scottish property of the Knights Templars was transferred to it in 1312 A.D. on the suppression of the latter Order.

The head of the Hospital in Scotland, from 1291 to 1298, was Alexander de Welles, an Englishman, who swore fealty to Edward I., in 1296, and fell at the battle of Falkirk fighting on the English side in July, 1298.[3] Before the battle, the Priory had been used as headquarters by William Wallace, and

---

[1] " Charters of Holyrood " (Bannatyne Club), p. 36.
[2] Edwards : " Transactions of Scottish Ecclesiological Society," 1906–1909, Vol. II.
[3] M'Call : " History of the Parish of Mid-Calder," Edinburgh, 1894, p. 252.

here, in March, 1298, he signed the only charter issued by him as Guardian of the Kingdom of Scotland in the name of King John Balliol.

One of the most distinguished patients to whom help was rendered at the Priory was Edward I. Being severely injured by a kick from his horse on the night before the battle of Falkirk, he was conveyed to Torphichen, and there carefully tended and restored to health. The fact that Edward was conveyed some eight miles for medical treatment is a testimony to the high estimation in which the skill of those at the Preceptory was held, for Edward was accompanied by no less than seven medical men of his own, including a King's physician with two juniors (valetti), a King's surgeon and two assistants (socii) and a simple surgeon. The King's physician and surgeon were of high standing, receiving the pay of Knights (2s. daily).[1] This serves to indicate the important social and military standing of surgeons who accompanied the armies of the 13th century.

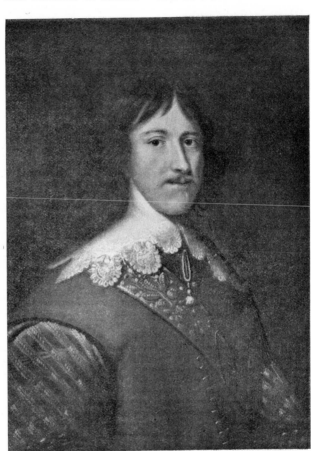

SIR JAMES SANDILANDS
Last Preceptor of Torphichen and First Lord Torphichen
(From a portrait in the possession of the Rt. Hon. Lord Torphichen)

A service like that rendered by the Good Lord James Douglas to King Robert Bruce was presumably rendered by a Scottish Knight of the Hospital to James I., whose heart was removed from his body and carried on a pilgrimage to the east. From the Exchequer Rolls of Scotland it appears that, in 1443, a Knight of

---

[1] Smart: *British Medical Journal*, 1873, Vol. I.

St. John returned from Rhodes bringing back the heart of King James, which it had not been found possible to deposit in Jerusalem. This Knight received £91 for his travelling expenses.[1]

The age at which a novice might enrol among the Knights of the Hospital was sixteen, and he took up residence in the Preceptory at the age of twenty, after which he underwent three years' of active service and two years' residence in the Preceptory, learning the duties of office. After this, he was appointed Commander of some subsidiary station, and presumably managed the property of the Hospital in some outlying district, and thereafter he was eligible for promotion to a more important position.[2] During the 15th and 16th centuries, the Knights of the Hospital, established first at Rhodes and later at Malta, carried on unceasing warfare with the Turks and the pirates of the Southern Mediterranean shore. Here many of the Scottish Knights took part in the great adventure of this bulwark between the Christian countries and the invading Moslem hosts and fleets.

The last four Preceptors at Torphichen were Sir William Knollis, who was Treasurer of Scotland, Sir George Dundas, Sir Walter Lindsay, and Sir James Sandilands. Of Lindsay, who was Preceptor from 1533 to 1547, at the end of an adventurous life, his contemporary Pitscottie says :—

" . . . ane nobill and potent lord nameit Schir Walter Lyndsay knycht of Torfeichin and lord of S. Johnne, who was weill besene and practissit in weiris baitht in Itallie and had fouchin oft tymeis against the Turkis in defence of the Christieane men in companie witht the lord of the Rodis *(Rhodes)*, and thair he was maid knycht for walliezand *(valiant)* actis and thairefter come in Scottland and seruit our king. . ."[3]

This sagacious old warrior was in command of the Scottish vanguard at the battle of Haddenrig, near Jedburgh, in 1542, when an English army of 10,000 men was defeated.

Sir James Sandilands, like his father, was a personal friend of John Knox and of the Reformation. Although he had been presented to the Preceptorship of Torphichen by the Pope in 1547, he threw in his lot with the Reformers, and, in 1563, resigned the Preceptorship, when the possessions of the Hospital of St. John in Scotland were made into a temporal barony carrying with them the title of Lord Torphichen, which he assumed. The present Lord Torphichen is descended from him. Those of the brethren of the Hospital who remained attached to the Roman Catholic religion left Scotland with David Seton, who was made Roman Catholic Preceptor, and died in Germany in 1591.[4]

---

[1] " Exchequer Rolls of Scotland," Vol. V., pp. xliv., 156, 179.
[2] Porter : " The Knights of Malta," London, 1884, p. 320.
[3] Lindesay : " Historie and Cronicles of Scotland," Edinburgh, Vol. I., Chap. xxxvi. p. 396.
[4] Bedford and Holbeche   " The Order of the Hospital of St. John of Jerusalem," London, 1902, p. 67.

CHAPTER II

EARLY SCOTTISH HOSPITALS AND REGULATIONS
FOR ISOLATION

IT has already been mentioned that the early hospitals were connected with religious foundations, and that those who carried out the treatment of the sick in them were at first clerics. It should be remembered that the nature of a mediæval hospital and the diseases treated there were different from those found in hospitals as they exist at the present day.

In the first place, hospitals were not generally intended for the treatment of acute disease. For one thing, means of transport was difficult, and a patient suffering from such a disease as acute pneumonia could not be transported to hospital on horseback unless it happened that he took ill at the very gate of a monastery.

In the second place, the early stages of chronic disease were not recognised. Thus, there was no means of diagnosing valvular disease of the heart, as such, before the end of the 18th century, and persons suffering from this condition would not be regarded as subjects for treatment until their condition was so advanced that the case might be classed as one of " dropsy." Similarly, diseases of the kidneys could hardly be recognised with exactness before Bright's treatise of 1827. If it be true that syphilis did not occur, in a severe form at least, before 1494, many diseases such as locomotor ataxia, general paralysis and several other nervous conditions, must have been non-existent in the Middle Ages. Speaking generally, therefore, only persons who had been so disabled as to be quite unfit for work and active life formed the class from which hospital patients were drawn in mediæval times.

Virchow has shown that after the edict of Pope Innocent III., early in the 13th century, directing the foundation of hospitals in all Sees, some 150 hospitals of the Holy Spirit were founded in Germany alone.[1] To this period belongs the founding or re-organisation of several great hospitals in London, and, at this time, numerous hospitals appear to have been founded in Scotland also.

At the time of the Reformation, the following hospitals were in existence in Scotland, having come down from a much earlier period. One of the oldest hospitals in this country was that of Soltray or Soutra, in Midlothian, sixteen miles south of Edinburgh, on the road leading to Kelso and England. This hospital more nearly fulfilled the conditions of a modern hospital than many others, because, being situated on an important route, it gave aid to travellers,

---

[1] Virchow : " Gesammelte Abhandlungen aus dem Gebiete der Oeffentlichen Medizin," Berlin, 1879, Vol. II. p. 24.

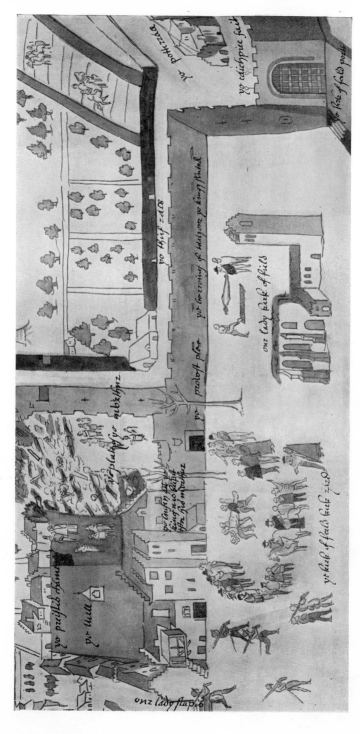

KIRK O' FIELD

Sketch made 10th February, 1567, for Queen Elizabeth, showing the surroundings of Darnley's murder. In the foreground is the ruined church of St. Mary de Campis; behind are buildings, including the Hospital of St. Mary, used by the Duke of Châtelherault, and, fifteen years later, taken over for the Town's College. The city-wall crosses the picture, with an angle opposite the Potterrow.

(Original in H.M. State Paper Office)

pilgrims and persons of the district who were urgently in need of medical assistance.

The hospital had been founded by Malcolm IV., in 1164, for the relief of pilgrims and poor and sickly people. In the neighbourhood was a well dedicated to the Holy Trinity, which was much frequented by sick and diseased persons because of its reputed curative properties. The hospital is mentioned several times during

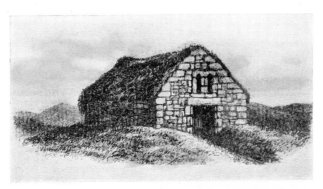

SOUTRA AISLE
A present-day remnant of Soutra Hospital

the 13th century, but, apparently having become less necessary at a later date, the parish and church of Soutra were annexed to Trinity College, in Edinburgh, where a hospital was founded by Mary of Gueldres, following on a Bull of Pope Pius II. in 1460. Remnants of Soutra hospital, in a district which is now moorland, are still visible. On some lands belonging to this hospital at St. Leonards, near Edinburgh, Robert Ballantine, Abbot of Holyrood, founded a hospital for seven distressed people.

There were also in Edinburgh at the time of the Reformation a hospital in Bell's Wynd, known as the Maison Dieu, and another in St. Mary's Wynd, for which the Town Council, in 1575, authorised the taking of a collection in St. Giles's Church. There is a reference to this hospital in 1500, and it was re-roofed in 1508, but the deed of foundation appears to have been lost in 1583, when the Town Council authorised Baillie Michael Chisholm to search for it.[1]

A hospital is also mentioned in connection with the Church of St. Mary de Campis, popularly known as the Kirk o' Field, which was one of the buildings burned by the English in 1544; so that in this year the religious community, not having means to rebuild it, sold the hospital to James, Earl of Arran, who built on it a lodging that afterwards was used as the College of Edinburgh. The University of Edinburgh now stands upon this site.

---

[1] "Extracts from the Records of the Burgh of Edinburgh, 1573–1589," pp. 39 and 314; and Extracts 1403–1528, pp. 79 and 117.

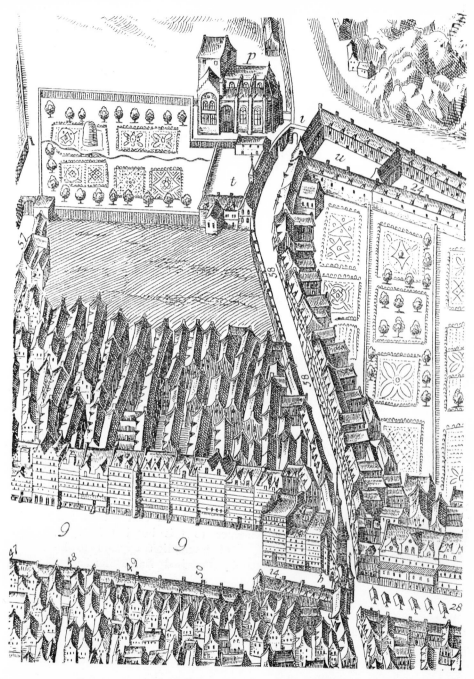

TRINITY COLLEGE, CHURCH AND HOSPITAL, EDINBURGH

From Gordon of Rothemay's Plan of Edinburgh in 1647

9, High Street; 14, John Knox's house; 28, Canongate, with fleshers' stands; 47, Dickson's Close; 48, Blackfriars' Close; 49, Todrig's Close; 50, Gray's Close; 57, Halkerston's Wynd; 58, Leith Wynd; 24, the Correction House, formerly Hospital of Our Lady; p, Trinity Church; t, *Trinity Hospital*; i, Leith Wynd Port; u, Paul's Work; h, Netherbow Port. The garden, later used (from 1676) as the Botanic Garden, is seen adjoining Trinity Church and Hospital

A very important Edinburgh hospital was the Trinity Hospital, founded at the instigation of Queen Mary of Gueldres, in memory of her husband, James II. The funds of several religious houses, including those of the Hospital of Soutra, were appropriated for the purpose of founding Trinity Hospital and its collegiate church,[1] and numerous references to it occur in the Town Council minutes of the following century. On 21st June, 1578, a minute of the Town Council refers to the reorganisation in the hospital of Trinity College, where twelve furnished beds were now made ready for " pepill seiklie and vnabill to laubour for thair leving." These people were called " bedesmen," " bedrels," " betherells," or " beadles." They were given an allowance for food and clothing, and they had been obliged, prior to the Reformation, to carry out the duties, so far as they were able, of attendance on religious services twice daily, and of praying for the soul of the founder. In the minute of this date, nine persons were admitted. It is not specified what were their diseases, except in the case of Dauid Forester, who was a blind man. Of the nine, Jhonne Thomesoun retained his place only for about six weeks, being ejected on 2nd August, 1578, because he was proved to be " ane drunkard." On 9th August, Bessy Jhonnstoun, a widow, was added to the company, being a " pure impotent bedrell." Many gifts to the hospital are recorded in the following years, and, in 1581 and 1584, the roof and windows were repaired.[2] The hospital continued its beneficent work for the sick and impotent up to the 19th century, and although the buildings disappeared to make way for the railway in 1845, its revenues are still employed by the Town Council in giving valued grants to aged and sick persons of the city.

Another hospital in Edinburgh, of almost equal age with Trinity Hospital, was established by Thomas Spence, Bishop of Aberdeen, in the year 1479. It was situated on the opposite side of Leith Wynd from Trinity Hospital, was designed for the reception and maintenance of twelve men, and was known as the Hospital of Our Lady. Subsequently it received revenues from other benefactors, including a chapel dedicated to St. Paul. The Town Council of Edinburgh became proprietors of this charity under a grant by Queen Mary, and in a minute of 15th June, 1582, they refer to it as the " hospitall of Sanct Pawles Work, callit our Lady Hospitall," and lay down an elaborate set of rules for the master of the hospital and the bedesmen. The latter were to be " na papistes, bot of the trew religioun." They were to be " not defylit with blame of ony notable vyce, bot of guid fame and conversatioun," and persons who would have exercised themselves in some honest trade if " seiknes, aige or impotencie " had not prevented them.[3]

This hospital, however, appears to have passed into desuetude, and in 1619 the buildings, having become ruinous, were reconstructed under the name

---

[1] " Charters Relating to the City of Edinburgh, 1143–1540," Scottish Burgh Records Society, Edinburgh, 1871, pp. 84–119.
[2] " Extracts from the Records of the Burgh of Edinburgh, 1573–1589," pp. 77, 80, 81, 553, 208, 211 and 328.
[3] " Extracts from the Records of the Burgh of Edinburgh, 1573–1589," pp. 564–567.

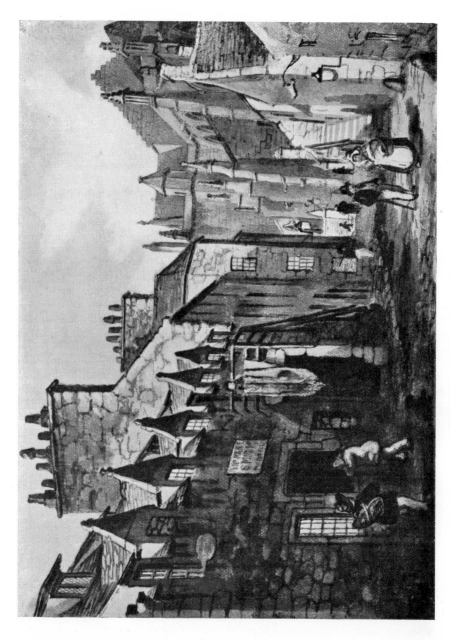

HOSPITAL OF OUR LADY, EDINBURGH

The Hospital is on the left, with Trinity College Church in the background

(From a sketch by Sir Daniel Wilson, in the Library of the University of Edinburgh)

of Paul's Work, to receive boys and girls who should be taught a trade; and, finally, the Town Council converted it into a House of Correction. In 1650, this hospital was used for the soldiers of General Leslie's army wounded in the repulse of Oliver Cromwell, when he attacked Edinburgh.

A hospital existed in connection with the Convent of St. Catherine of Siena, inhabited by Dominican nuns, a short distance south of Edinburgh, in a district which has come to be called, by corruption, " Sciennes." The hospital, which was presumably originally a place for the reception of the neighbouring sick, appears to have reverted after the Reformation to the possession of the Town Council. After some trouble with a neighbouring proprietor, Henry Kincaid, who also claimed the buildings, the Magistrates took possession in 1575 and used it as an isolation hospital for persons suffering from the plague, which had been prevalent in Edinburgh.[1]

Still another Edinburgh hospital which, however, was founded shortly before the Reformation, was the Hospital of the Magdalen Chapel in the Cowgate, founded by Michael Makquhen and Janet Rynd, his wife, in 1537, for seven bedesmen. This Hospital lasted for some 115 years. Its Chapel still stands.

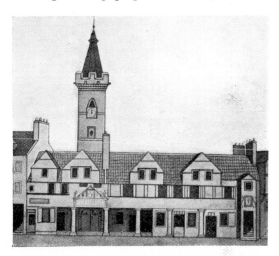

HOSPITAL OF ST. MARY MAGDALEN WITH ITS CHAPEL
(From a sketch of 1816)

Other hospitals in the southeast of Scotland, which were in existence in the 13th century— a fact established by their Superior having taken an oath of fealty to Edward I. in 1296—were Ballincrief, in the county of Edinburgh, dedicated to St. Cuthbert ; St. Germains, at Setoun, in the county of Haddington (the property of this hospital passed later to the support of Marischal College, Aberdeen) ; a hospital at Lauder, and another at Ligertwood in Berwickshire ; and the Maison Dieu in the vanished town of Roxburgh. The hospital of St. Mary Magdalen, at Rutherford in Roxburghshire, founded by King Robert III. in 1396, had in its charter the curious provision that if it should be destroyed by an English invasion, it was to be rebuilt in the same place. The hospital of St. Mary Magdalen, in Linlithgow, belonged to the religious order of Lazarites, and is mentioned in the year 1426, when Robert de Lynton was nominated to the post

---

[1] "Extracts from the Records of the Burgh of Edinburgh, 1573-1589," pp. 30, 37 and 38.

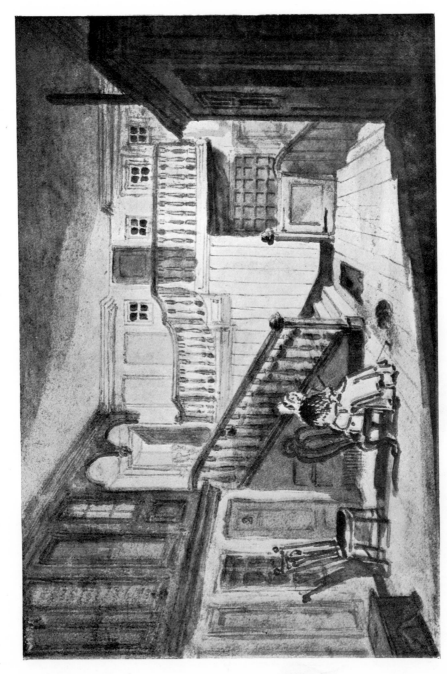

INTERIOR OF TRINITY HOSPITAL, EDINBURGH

As it appeared early in the 19th century, showing the mediæval arrangements

(From a sketch by Sir Daniel Wilson, preserved in the Library of the University of Edinburgh)

of master by Queen Jean, wife of James I. A hospital at Ednam, dedicated to St. Laurence, received a charter from King James I. in 1426.

Glasgow was early furnished with a hospital of St. Nicholas, founded by Master Michael Fleming, and endowed by Bishop Muirhead in the 15th century, after whom it was sometimes called the Bishop's Hospital.[1] In this hospital there existed the unusual provision of waiting maids to attend the sick.[2] In Aberdeen, a hospital was founded by Bishop Gavin Dunbar, in 1531, for the maintenance of twelve poor men. In the shire of Aberdeen, there were also hospitals at Kincardine-O'Neil, at Newburgh, where the hospital had been founded by Alexander, Earl of Buchan, in the reign of King Alexander III., and at Turriff, where another hospital had been founded by Alexander, Earl of Buchan, for twelve men.

At Stirling, a hospital of St. James stood at the end of the bridge (*see page* 38), having been granted to the Canons of Cambuskenneth serving God there, by King Robert III., in March, 1403. The Chapel attached to the Hospital, along with a Chapel to St. Roche, was destroyed at the Reformation, but a reference to the Hospital as still existing is found as late as 1709.[3] In the town the Hospital of Spittals stood in St. Mary's Wynd, having been founded by Robert Spittal, tailor to King James IV. The Hospital of Suggeden was situated in Perthshire on the river Tay, in the year 1296, when its Superior swore fealty to King Edward I.

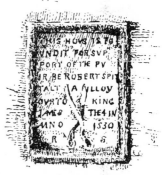

FOUNDATION STONE
of Hospital founded at Stirling in 1530 by Robert Spittal, tailor to King James IV.

In the north of Scotland, the See of Moray had two hospitals, that of St. Nicolas, founded by Walterus de Moravia, near the bridge over the Spey, and the hospital at Rothfan, for seven leprous persons, founded in 1226. In Brechin, Forfarshire, a Maison Dieu was founded before 1477. At Lanark, a Hospital of St. Leonards had existed before 1393, and, two miles east of Peebles, at Chapel Yards,[4] a hospital of St. Leonards received a charter from King James I., in the year 1427. There were also a hospital of the Holy Trinity at Houston, a hospital attached to the monastery of Holywood, which had been founded by Archibald the Grim, Earl of Douglas, in the reign of Robert II., and a hospital at Sanquhar, which is mentioned as a new erection in the year 1296.[5] Chalmers mentions the names of several in other places.[6]

---

[1] M'Ure: "History of Glasgow, 1830," p. 22.
[2] "Chartulary of Paisley," p. 297; and Keith: Op. cit., p. 475.
[3] J. S. Fleming: "The Old Ludgings of Stirling," Stirling, 1897.
[4] Chalmers: "Caledonia," Vol. II, p. 943.
[5] Right Rev. Robert Keith: "An Historical Catalogue of the Scottish Bishops down to the year 1688," Edinburgh, 1824, pp. 474–480.
[6] Chalmers: "Caledonia," London, 1807.

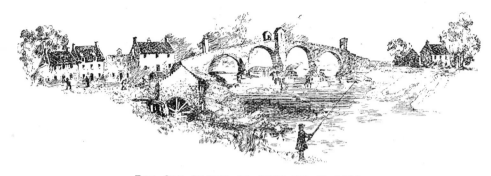

THE OLD BRIDGE OF STIRLING IN 1700

Showing the HOSPITAL OF ST. JAMES at the end of the bridge behind the mill and ruins of one of
the two Chapels which previously stood there

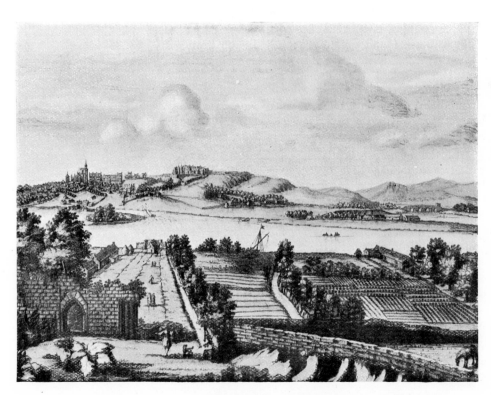

STIRLING, FROM CAMBUSKENNETH ABBEY, ABOUT 1680

Showing the considerable distance separating the Town from the Bridge, with its Hospital and Chapels
(From the engraving by Slezer)

Hospitals must have existed in connection with the settlements of the Knights Hospitallers. Of these the Preceptory at Torphichen has been mentioned, where the site of a hospitium is still pointed out. There was another Preceptory at Kirkstyle, in the Parish of Ruthwell, where several tombstones are to be seen in the churchyard bearing the insignia of this celebrated fraternity,[1] and still another at Balantrodach in Midlothian. In regard to houses belonging to the Hospitallers at Linlithgow and Glasgow, Beatson suggests that these were used as Hospitals for the sick.[2]

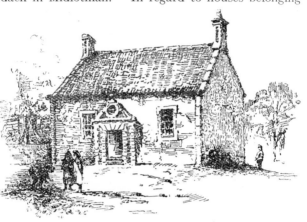

NETHER HOSPITAL AT STIRLING

Illustrating the type of small hospital erected in the 17th and 18th centuries for sick paupers

Before the Reformation, the 13th century hospitals were, in some places, falling into disuse, and in other places their funds were being misappropriated, so that the support of their inmates became impossible. This had become very noticeable by the year 1548, and at a Provincial Council, Holden by the Prelates and Clergy of the realm of Scotland, at Edinburgh, in 1549, a resolution was passed anent the condition and repair of hospitals. Every ordinary was enjoined to make diligent inquiry throughout his diocese regarding the foundations of hospitals. If the charters and instruments could be found, he was to consider to what extent these places were dilapidated, who were their present possessors, and how the funds had been misappropriated. Masters of works of every monastery were enjoined to visit every year places attached to monasteries and churches for the repair of dilapidations.

Little attention appears to have been paid to this, and at another Provincial Council, held at Edinburgh, in January, 1552, the above visitation was ordered to be put into effect before the next Michaelmas, and a report made to Commissaries General so that suitable remedies could be provided.[3]

These orders, however, came too late, for the Reformation was at hand, and along with the possessions of other religious houses, the revenues of most of the hospitals were re-appropriated, usually for educational purposes, or simply for the benefit of neighbouring proprietors.

---

[1] Chalmers : " Caledonia," Vol. III, p. 154.
[2] Beatson : " The Knights Hospitallers in Scotland," Glasgow, 1903, p. 26.
[3] " Statutes of the Scottish Church, 1225–1559," Patrick, Pub. of Scottish Hist. Soc., pp. 119 and 139

The manner in which a hospital gradually disappeared is well exemplified by the experience of St. Thomas's Hospital at Edinburgh which had been founded in 1541, in the reign of James V., by George Creighton, Bishop of Dunkeld.   The building was in the Burgh of Canongate, close to the Water-gate, and the patronage of the hospital was vested by the founder in himself and his heirs.   It was natural that the heirs should not be interested in hospital work, and, in 1617, an arrangement was reached between David Creighton, the patron at the time, and the bedesmen of the hospital, that Creighton should retain the endowments while the bedesmen and chaplains were allowed to sell the hospital buildings to the Magistrates of the Canongate. The Magistrates established here a hospital for the poor of the burgh, and, in 1634, sold the patronage of the hospital to the Kirk Session for the same purpose.   In the words of Arnot : " Its revenues were, by degrees, entirely embezzled."   In 1747, the building was converted into coach-houses, and, becoming ruinous, was pulled down in the year 1778.[1]

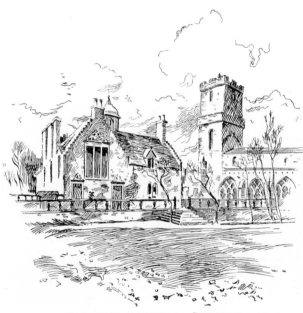

COWANE'S HOSPITAL, STIRLING

After the Reformation there was practically no new foundation of hospitals in Scotland until the voluntary hospital movement, which took place in the 18th century.   In some places the Kirk Session of various parishes established temporary hospitals for the reception of sick paupers. The most notable exception was the establishment by John Cowane, a merchant in Stirling, who died in 1637, and left funds to endow a hospital, to be called " Cowane's Hospital," for twelve decayed members of the Stirling Guildry.   This foundation was on the pre-Reformation plan of taking in sick and decayed persons for the remainder of their lives, but it proved quite unsuited to modern habits and ideas, and accordingly, about 1852, the hospital ceased to exist as such, the rooms for the patients were converted into a hall, and the endowments were used to provide grants for sick and decayed persons in their own

---

[1] Arnot : " History of Edinburgh," 1779, p. 249.

homes.[1]   A similar arrangement was made in regard to the endowments of various hospitals in Scotland, such as the Trinity Hospital in Edinburgh, and Spittal's Hospital in Stirling.   The word " hospital " in Scotland also came to be used in the 17th and 18th centuries to indicate educational foundations, such as schools for boys.

Very clear pictures of true leprosy are given in three mediæval treatises : one in the " Lilium Medicinæ," by Bernard Gordon, who is traditionally reputed to have been a Scotsman, and who taught at Montpellier between 1285 and 1307 ; one by Gilbert, the Englishman, whose " Compendium Medicinæ" was published in 1510 ; and a third by Guy de Chauliac, who wrote his treatise on surgery about 1363. Nevertheless, the diagnosis of leprosy was probably made somewhat recklessly, and no doubt in the Middle Ages persons with other skin diseases were sometimes segregated as lepers.   Among the definitely admitted Scottish lepers, the most distinguished was King Robert the Bruce.[2]

The earliest leper house founded in England, so far as is known, was the Hospital of St. Peter and St. Leonard, at York, founded in 936 A.D. by King Athelstane, which provided for 206 bedesmen.   Another was endowed at Canterbury by Lanfranc, the first Norman Archbishop of that See.   Others were founded later at Westminster, South-wark, Highgate, and other places in London, and there were numerous other hospitals throughout England.[3] Sir James Y. Simpson collected references to over 100 leper estab-lishments in this country.[4]

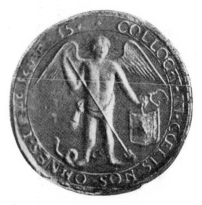

SEAL OF LINLITHGOW LEPER HOUSE

The following law regarding lepers was enacted by the Scottish Parliament in the 12th century, and it shows incidentally that the burghs of Berwick, Roxburgh, Edinburgh and Stirling were then provided with leper hospitals outside the towns :—

" Gif [if] ony that duellis in the kyngis burgh or was borne in it be fallyn in lepyr that is callit mysal gif that he hafe gudis of his awne thruch the quhilk [which] he may be sustenyt and cled he sal be put in the spytaile [hospital] of the burgh.   And gif he has nocht of his awne the burges of that toune sal ger [cause] be gadderyt amangis thaim a collec to the valure of xx s. of the quhilk he may be sustenyt and cled.   And it is to wyt [to be known] that mysal men sal nocht entre in the toune gangande [going] fra dur [door] to dur bot anerly [only] to pas the he [high] way thruch the toune and thai sal sit

[1] Shearer : " Stirling, Historical and Descriptive," Stirling, 1897, p. 65.
[2] " Chronicon de Lanercost " (Bannatyne Club), p. 259 ;   also Sir J. Y. Simpson : " Archæological Essays," Vol. II., pp. 113–115.
[3] Charles Creighton, M.A., M.D.: " History of Epidemics in Britain," Cambridge, 1891, Vol. I., p. 86.
[4] Simpson : Op. cit., p. 19.

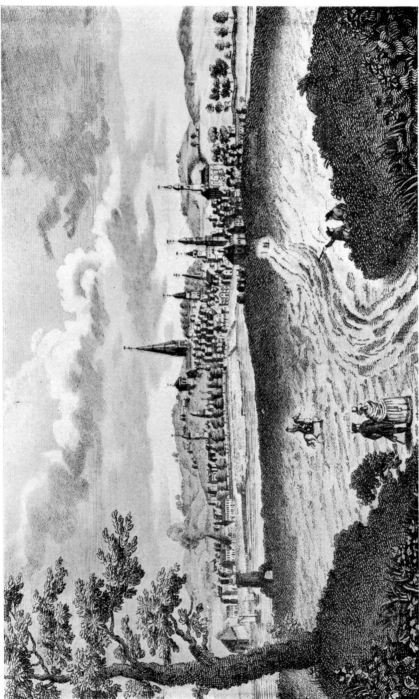

GLASGOW

(*Engraving by T. Grainger, circa 1760*)

Although crude in execution and draughtsmanship and sadly lacking in perspective, this plate contains much of interest to the student of the past. It shows Glasgow as little more than a village glorified by a Cathedral and the campanilli of many churches. Interesting to students of the story of healing is the little group of quaint houses on the south bank of the River Clyde. The country road leading from those houses to the very foreground of the picture is now the busy but somewhat sordid Main Street of Gorbals. To medical men the interesting point is, that these houses occupy the supposed site of the one-time famous Leper Hospital—known as St. Ninian's Hospital—erected about 1350 by the "Lady of Lochow", at the south bridge end of "The Auld Brig" of Glasgow—erected by Bishop Rae in 1350, and taken down finally in 1850.

at the toune end and thar ask almous at [*alms from*] furth passand men and ingangand. And mar attour na man sal tak on hand ony mysal man in his house to herbery na reste wythin the burgh on payn of a full forfalt [*forfeit*].[1]

In the Forest Laws of Scotland, at an early date, when wild beasts were found dead or wounded, the flesh was to be sent to the house of the leper men if any such happened to be situated near by.[2]   Another Act provided that flesh of pork or salmon, found to be corrupt in the markets and accordingly seized, was to be sent to the lepers.[3]

In the Parliament of James I., which met at Perth on 1st March, 1427, very definite enactments were made in regard to the lepers.   Persons afflicted by this disease were not to enter any burgh except on Mondays, Wednesdays and Fridays, between 10 and 2 o'clock ; when a market fell on any of these days, they were to delay till the following day ; lepers were to beg only at their own hospitals or at the town gate, and in other places outside burghs ; bishops, officials and deans were enjoined to enquire, at the visitations to every parish church, whether there were any lepers in the parish, and to notify these to the bishop if they were clerks, or to the King if they were laymen.[4]

As regards Scotland, the richest foundation for lepers was at Kingcase, near Prestwick, in Ayrshire, which was endowed by King Robert Bruce with lands and contained a hospital of eight beds.   Various leper houses were built by the rich Abbeys of Tweedside, such as the Hospital of Aldcambus, in Berwickshire, founded in the reign of William the Lion, and Aldnestun, in Lauderdale.   A hospital at Rothfan, connected with the cathedral at Elgin, which was endowed in 1226, and existed before that time, had accommodation for seven lepers, a chaplain and a servant.

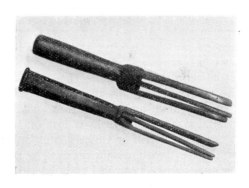

LEPER CLAPPERS
Intended to give warning of the approach of a Leper

Most of the Scottish leper houses appear, however, to have been refuges in which the lepers supported themselves by begging in the neighbouring towns.   Such a hospital was that at the Gorbals of Glasgow, founded about 1350.   This had been established by Marjory   Stuart,   Lady   Lochow.[5]

From the hospital on the south bank of the river, the lepers were permitted under certain strongent conditions, to enter the town for the purpose of asking

---

[1] Laws of the four burghs (Berwick, Roxburgh, Edinburgh and Stirling), confirmed by King David I.   "Acts of the Scottish Parliament (1124–1423)."   Vol. I., p. 344, cap. 58.
[2] "Acts of the Scottish Parliament," Vol. I., p. 692.
[3] Op. cit., Vol. I., p. 729.
[4] Op. cit., Vol. II, p. 16, cap. 8.
[5] M'Ure : "History of Glasgow," 1830, p. 52.

alms.   To give warning of their approach, they were provided with clappers, and were obliged to wear a cloth over the mouth and face, because of an idea that the infection rested chiefly in the breath.   The number of lepers was not great.   A report had to be presented to the Town Council every Michaelmas as to the number admitted to the hospital during the year, and this usually amounted to about four or five.   In the latter part of 1605, there were seven lepers in the hospital.[1]

In Edinburgh, a Leper Hospital was founded by the Town Council.   In 1584, they enquired into " the estait and ordour of the awld fundatioun of the lipper hous besyde Dyngwall,"[2] which was the name of the residence of the Provost of Trinity College, and stood on part of the ground now occupied by the London and North-Eastern Railway Station.   Apparently this was not found in a satisfactory condition, for, in 1589, an Act was passed by the Magistrates to build a leper-house at Greenside, and, in 1591, five lepers of the city were consigned to this hospital.[3]   Two of the wives of the lepers voluntarily shut themselves up in the hospital along with their diseased husbands.   Very severe regulations were made by the Magistrates to prevent those affected by leprosy from mixing with the citizens of Edinburgh. The lepers were commanded to remain within the walls of the hospital night and day, and to have the door shut after sunset, under pain of death.   That this might not be deemed an empty threat, a gallows was erected on the gable of the hospital for the immediate execution of offenders.[4]

This leper hospital appears gradually to have fallen into disrepair.   It is mentioned in a charter given to the city by Charles I. in 1636, but in 1652 the Magistrates ordered it to be demolished, and its material used for other purposes.   The suburb of Liberton owes its name to a conversion of the term leper-town.   The district is mentioned in old charters of the reign of David I., who died in 1153, as in the foundation charter of Holyrood, where its mill and chapel are mentioned, but the date at which a leper hospital was founded here is lost in obscurity.   A well in the neighbourhood, at the Priest's Hill or Grace Mount, was specially celebrated in the Middle Ages for the treatment of skin diseases, because of the mineral oil which floated on the surface of the water, and this was in all probability used specially by the lepers of Liberton.

In 1528, the Town Council of Edinburgh published an edict dealing with lepers, as follows :—

22 JANUARY, 1528
" The quhilk day, the baillies and counsale statutes and ordanis that [blank] Wilsoun, tailyeour, and all vtheris suspect of lipper within this towne devoyde thame of the samyn

---

[1] Cleland : " Statistical Facts," 1837, p. 22; also " Extracts from the Records of the Burgh of Glasgow, 1573–1642," p. 238.
[2] " Extracts from the Records of the Burgh of Edinburgh, 1573–1589," p. 352.
[3] " Manuscript Records of the Town Council," Vol. IX., pp. 9, 12 and 123.
[4] Arnot : Op. cit., p. 258.

within xv dayes, and gif the said [*blank*] Wilsoun will allege that he hes nocht na sic seiknes that he caus the medicinaris to purge him be thair aythis in the meanetyme ; and als chairges all maner of lipper folkis that ar in lugeis and hospitales about this towne that thai convers nocht amang clene folks nother in kirk merkat or vther wayes bot hald thame be thame selffis in quyet vnder the payne of banissing the towne." [1]

In Aberdeen, a Leper Hospital, which had existed before 1363, is mentioned and figured by Gordon as standing in the 17th century half-way between the Gallowgate Port and Old Aberdeen.

" Such as goe out at the Gallowgate Port toward Old Aberdeen, halff way almost, may see the place wher of old stood the lepers hospitall, called the Seick Hous, hard by the waye syd, to which ther was a chappell adjoyned, dedicated to St. Anna, quhome the papists account patronesse of the leapers. The citizens licencit one Mr. Alexander Gallaway, then person of Kinkell, for to build that chappell anno 1519." [2]

In the beginning of the 18th century, the remains of the hospital and grounds were sold, though its burial ground is still left. The money was made over to the fund for the proposed lunatic asylum. [3]

Leprosy appears to have prevailed in Scotland after its disappearance from England, and it gradually retreated northwards. The last native leper in Great Britain was an inhabitant of the Shetland Isles, and died at Edinburgh in 1798.

The disease known at the present day as syphilis is generally believed to have broken out for the first time in Europe, about the year 1494, among the people in Naples, and among the troops of Charles VIII. of France, who were besieging that city. The earliest notices of it appear between 1492, when Columbus discovered the New World, and 1494, when this outbreak occurred. It is generally believed that the followers of Columbus either imported this disease to Europe for the first time, or, what is more probable, that they introduced a variety of the disease due to a New World strain of the causal organism, which then spread in an almost epidemic form. The disease was known by a variety of names, such as gor, gore, grandgore, grantgore and glengore, as well as the French sickness and sickness of Naples. The word " grandgore " was used by Rabelais in 1532. The word " syphilis " was introduced in 1530 by Fracastoro, in the title of his Latin poem, in which the chief character bears this name.

By 1497 and 1498 there are numerous references to the incidence of the disease in different parts of Europe. Those which concern us here are especially regulations promulgated by the Town Councils of Aberdeen and Edinburgh, with the object of checking its spread. The regulation in regard to Aberdeen is dated 21st April, 1497, and is the earliest notice of this kind in Britain. It runs as follows :—

---

[1] " Extracts from the Records of the Burgh of Edinburgh, 1403–1528," p. 232.
[2] Gordon of Rothemay : " Abredoniae Utriusque Descriptio," Spalding Club, 1842, p. 19.
[3] Simpson : " Archaeological Essays," Vol. II., p. 13.

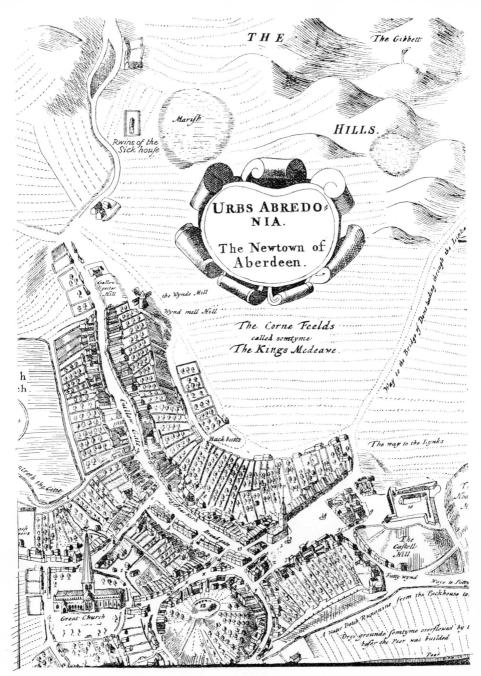

The following labels appear within the map:

THE

The Gibbett

HILLS.

Marish

Rwins of the Sick house

URBS ABREDO-NIA.

The Newtown of Aberdeen.

Gallow geiter Hill

the Wynds Mill

Wynd mill Hill

The Corne Feelds
called somtyme
The Kings Medeawe.

Way to the Bridge of Done leding through the Linkes

Back butts

The way to the Lynks

Galow

Great Church

The Castell Hill

Futty wynd

Waye to Futty

A water Ditch Runinne from the Packhouse to.

Drue grounde somtyme overflowed by t
befor the Peer was builded

Peer

MAP OF ABERDEEN IN 1661
By Gordon of Rothemay
Showing the site of the Leper Hospital (*Rwins of the Sick house*) on the road leading to Old Aberdeen

" The said day, it was statut and ordanit be the alderman and consale for the eschevin [*avoidance*] of the infirmitey cumm out of Franche and strang partis, that all licht weman be chargit and ordanit to decist fra thar vicis and syne of venerie, and al thair buthis and houssis skalit [*emptied*], and thai to pas and wirk for thar sustentacioun, vnder the payne of ane key of het yrne one thar chekis, and banysene of the toune." [1]

A few years later, in 1507, the Aberdeen Town Council passed several statutes connected with the public health, and one of these dealt with the segregation in their own houses of persons infected with the " strange seiknes of Nappillis," while another forbade folks infected with this sickness to appear at the common flesh-house or to hold converse with fleshers, bakers, brewers and " ladinaris," for the safety of the town.[2]

It is interesting to note that the Town Council of Aberdeen appear to have clearly discerned the method in which this disease was usually spread, at a time when Continental authorities were still in the dark as to its origin.

The Town Council of Edinburgh, apparently acting under instructions from King James IV., issued a stringent and celebrated regulation on 22nd September, 1497, through which segregation was to be still more effectively carried out by banishing all those sick of this disease, together with those who professed to cure it, to the Island of Inchkeith. Unfortunately, these restrictions, both in Aberdeen and Edinburgh, although well-designed, appear to have been ineffective. The regulation in Edinburgh was as follows :—

" It is our Soueraine Lordis will, and the command of the lordis of his counsale send to the provest and baillies within this burgh, that this proclamatioun follow and be put till executioun for the eschewing [*avoidance*] of the greit appearand dainger of the infectioun of his liegis fra this contagius seiknes callit the grandgor, and the greit vther skayth [*damage*] that may occure to his legeis and inhabitouris within this burgh, that is to say: We charge straitlie and commandis be the authoritie aboue writtin, that all maner of personis, being within the fredome of this burgh, quhilkis [*who*] ar infectit or hes bene infectit vncurit with this said contagious plage callit the grandgor, devoyd red [*leave clear*] and pas furth of this toun and compeir [*assemble*] vpoun the sandis of Leith at x houris befoir none, and thair sall thai haue and fynd botis reddie in the havin ordanit to thame be the officeris of this burgh reddely furneist with victuallis to have thame to the Inche [*Inchkeith*], and thair to remane quhill God prouyde for thair health ; and that all vther personis the quhilkis takis vpoun thame to hale the said contagious infirmitie, and takis the cure thairof, that thay devoyd and pas with thame, sua that nane of thir personis quhilkis takis sic cure vpoun thame vse the samyn cure within this burgh in presens [*at present*] nor peirt [*appear*] ony maner of way ; and quha sa beis fundin infectit and nocht passand to the Inche as said is be Monounday at the sone ganging to [*sunset*], and in lykwayis the saidis personis that takis the said cure of sanitie vpoun thame gif [*if*] thai will vse the samyn, thai and ilk [*each*] of thame salbe [*shall be*] brynt [*branded*] on the cheik with the marking irne that thai may be kennit in tyme to cum, and thairefter gif ony of thame remainis that tha salbe banist but [*without*] favouris." [3]

[1] " Extracts from the Council Register of the Burgh of Aberdeen," 1398–1570, p. 425.
[2] " Extracts from the Council Register of the Burgh of Aberdeen, 1398–1570," Spalding Club, 1844, p. 437.
[3] " Extracts from the Records of the Burgh of Edinburgh," 1403–1528, pp. 71 and 72.

That these regulations were not merely formal, and that the profession to cure this disease was treated as a grave responsibility, is made clear by the following notice regarding Thomas Lyn, a burgess of Edinburgh, under whose treatment Sir Lancelote Patonsoun had died :—

18 JANUARY, 1509

" Respitt made to Thomas Lyn, burges of Edinburgh, for ye slauchtir of vmquhile [*deceased*] Schir Lancelote Patonsoun, Chapellain, quhilk happinnit be negligent cure and medicine yat ye said Thomas tuk one him to cure and hele ye said vmquhile Schir Lancelote of ye infirmite of ye grantgor, yat he was infekkit with.   To endure for xix zeris.   (Subscriptum per dominum Regem, apud Edinburghe)." [1]

The disease seems to have made its first appearance all over Scotland, as appears from the following five notices in the Treasurer's accounts, indicating that King James IV. had distributed alms to persons afflicted by the disease at Linlithgow, Stirling, Glasgow and Dalry :—

2 OCTOBER, 1497

" Item to thaim that hed the grantgor at Linlithquho...   ...   viijd."

21 FEBRUARY, 1498

" Item, that samyn day at the tounne end of Strivelin to the seke folk in the grantgore   ...   .   ijs."

22 FEBRUARY 1498

" Item, the xxij day of Februar giffin to the seke folk in the grangore at the tounn end of Glasgo   ...   .   ijs."

APRIL, 1498

". . . . seke folk in grangor in Lithgw as the King com in the toune...   ijs. viijd." [2]

1 SEPTEMBER, 1497

" Item, to a woman with ye grantgore thair (at St. John's Kirk of Dalrye, when the King was on a Pilgrimage to ' Quhithirne ') ...   ...   iijs. vjd." [3]

It is very probable that these moneys were given to patients who had submitted themselves to different forms of treatment tried upon them by the King himself.

The disease was apparently looked upon with great detestation, for, in 1591, a year of great activity against witches, one of the charges against Ewfame Mackalzane was that she had bewitched Marie Sandelandis and dissuaded her from marrying Joseph Dowglas, of Punfrastoune, alleging that he had the glengore himself.   For this, along with twenty-seven other charges, she was taken to the " Castel-hill of Edinburghe and thair bund to ane staik and brunt in assis, quick, to the death."   This was the severest sentence ever pronounced by the Court, for, in ordinary cases of witchcraft, the culprit was previously strangled at the stake before being burned.[4]

---

[1] Robert Pitcairn : " Criminal Trials in Scotland," Vol. I, Part I, p. 110.
[2] Sir J. Y. Simpson, Bt. : " Archæological Essays," Vol. II, Edinburgh, 1872, p. 310.
[3] Robert Pitcairn : " Criminal Trials in Scotland," Vol. I, Part I, p. 117.
[4] Robert Pitcairn : " Criminal Trials in Scotland," Vol. I, Part II, pp. 252 and 257.

Numerous references to the disease occur in the contemporary poems of Sir David Lyndsay and William Dunbar.

Although the disease was present in Glasgow in 1497, the Town Council do not seem to have become seriously alarmed about it until the year 1600, when, on 17th April, the Kirk Session consulted as to how the infection of the glengore within the city might be removed : " Some sent to the Council to deplore the infection that's in this city by the Glengore, and some to convene again in the Blackfriars Kirk anent it, and the whole chirurgeons and professors of medicine to be present.   So much was given to a man for bigging a lodge without the Stable Green Port to the women that hath the glengore."[1]   A minute of 3rd May, a fortnight later, continues : " The provest, bailleis and counsale hes appoyntit Weddinsdye nixt, eftir the preiching, to convein thameselffis for taking tryall of the inhabitantis anent the greit suspicioune of sindry persones infectit with the glengoir, quhilk, gif it be nocht preventit, will endanger the haill towne, and hes ordanit the haill chyrurgianes to be warnit to that effect to compeir in the Grayefreir Kirk and qu'haever beis warnit (and comes nocht) to pay fyve li. of vnlaw."[2] The town's surgeon, Mr. Peter Lowe, had, four years earlier, written a book on the disease which he had called " The Spanish Sicknes."   Possibly his large experience in treating " Spaniards and French, both men and women, of divers temperatures, who had often been treated both in Spain, Lowe Countries and Fraunce," and whom, he says, he had cured " by the help of God and my confection," may have had some effect, if not in staying the disease, in robbing it of some of its terrors.[3]

[1] " Glasgow Ancient and Modern," I, p. 131.
[2] " Extracts from the Records of the Burgh of Glasgow, 1573–1642," p. 206.
[3] " Memorials of the Faculty of Physicians and Surgeons of Glasgow." Maclehose, Glasgow, 1896, p. 15.

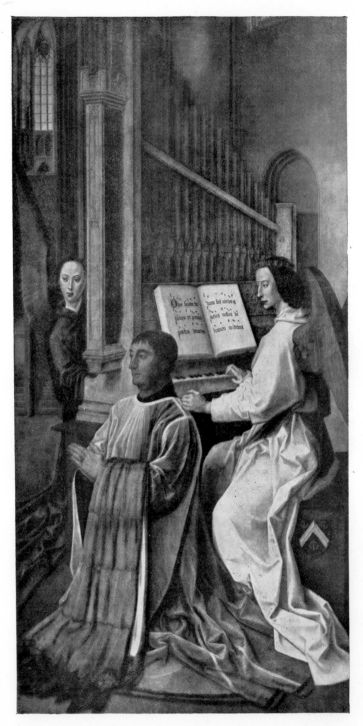

CHAPTER III

MEDICAL RENAISSANCE IN THE TIME OF JAMES IV.

DURING the 15th century the Town Council of Edinburgh appears to have become very much exercised about the health of the city and its cleansing, with the result that many minutes appear in the records of the burgh during the latter half of this century and the early 16th century, containing regulations for the prevention of the spread of infectious diseases.

An objectionable practice of the inhabitants of the city in early times appears to have been the keeping of swine, which were allowed to wander freely in the streets and pick up what they could. In 1450, it was ordained that all men and women who had " swyne " wandering in the town should remove them out of the town or keep them " in band." If the swine were found loose, they were to be forfeited and their price applied to the building of the Kirk.[1] In 1494, various regulations were laid down in regard to the sale of poultry, geese, flesh and other easily corruptible kinds of food. It is quite in accord with recent legislation that the dealers in poultry, geese and other wild fowl

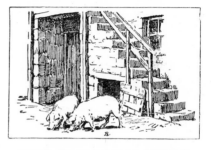

SWINE IN EDINBURGH STREETS

Showing the outside stair, which was a feature of old Scottish houses, with the sty beneath it

were obliged to sell them alive or fresh pulled, and forbidden to "powder" them, while any fleshers " powdering " flesh for preservation were liable to have this confiscated.[2]

With the rise of democracy in the 14th century, guilds of craftsmen came into existence in the towns, forming trades unions with very stringent regulations. In Scotland, as in England, the merchant burgesses of the towns were favoured by the Crown as an offset to the dangerous power of the nobles. Among other guilds, that of the Barbers was in active operation prior to 1451. In that year we find Queen Mary of Gueldres exerting her influence to obtain the entrance of Aitkyne, a barber, presumably attached to the Court, whom she desired to be admitted to the Guild. It is evident, from the following Town Council minute, that Aitkyne, in addition to practising the minor surgery customary to a barber, also acted as an apothecary :—

> " 12th May, 1451. Aitkyne, barbi tonsor, effectus est burgensis ad instantiam domine Regine gratis datur et etiam conceditur sibi [*blank*] gilde pro tempore vite sue et in amplius vt possit vti libertate gilde tempore vite sue, soluendo species et vinum nusquam est sibi successurus post obitum ad libertatem gilde.

---

[1] p. 12, [2] p. 67: "Extracts from the Records of the Burgh of Edinburgh, 1403-1528."

" (Aitkyne, barber, is made burgess at the instance of Our Lady the Queen, without payment, and it is also conceded to him [*blank*] of the guild for the period of his life, and further, that he might use the freedom of the guild for the period of his life, paying spices and wine, and no one shall succeed him in the freedom of the guild after his death)." [1]

An incidental reference in a letter from James IV. to the Town Council, indicates that a house and booth in the Bellhouse of the city had been occupied in the time of his grandsire (James II., 1431–1460) by an apothecary. The letter of 1509 requests that the same house and booth may be assigned to " Maister Stephane, ypothegar, sa that he may be enterit thairintil and vse the samin with his materiall and spisery sa that he may be fundin thair redy to do ws seruice." [2]

We may assume that in making regulations for the betterment of the public health, which were sometimes apparently initiated at the instance of the King, the Town Council took the opinion of those like Aitkyne who had experience qualifying them to give advice.

The apothecaries of the 15th century seem to have practised successfully and unostentatiously, but an indication of the drugs they used and of their general method of practice may be gained from the Gaelic medical manuscripts to which reference has already been made. There seems to have been a tendency to long and imposing prescriptions, which are satirised by Robert Henryson (1430–1506), the Dunfermline poet, in " Sum Practysis of Medecyne." The fact that a well-known and popular poet should consider it worth his while to poke fun at the apothecaries shows that this calling was of good standing, and that his humour would be appreciated by all classes of society. The following remedy for sleeplessness is one of six humorous prescriptions that he gives :—

DIA LONGUM.

Recipe, thre ruggis of the reid ruke,
The gant of ane gray meir, The claik of ane guss,
The dram of ane drekterss, the douk of ane duke,
The gaw of ane grene dow, The leg of ane lowss,
fyve vnce of ane fle wing, the fyn of ane fluke,
With ane sleiffull of slak, that growis in the sluss;
myng all thir in ane mass with the mone cruke.
This vntment is rycht ganand for your awin vss,
With reid nettill seid in strang wesche to steip,
For to bath your ba cod,   ⎫
quhen ye wald nop and nod ;   ⎬ To latt yow to sleip. [3]
Is nocht bettir, be god,   ⎭

King James IV. (1473–1513) was an enlightened monarch, who, despite his faults, did much for the arts and commerce of his country. Among other branches of human activity, his foresight, and perhaps his inquisitiveness, led him

[1] p. 12. " Extracts from the Records of the Burgh of Edinburgh, 1403–1528."
[2] p. 125. " Extracts from the Records of the Burgh of Edinburgh, 1403–1528."
[3] " The Poems of Robert Henryson," Ed. by G. Gregory Smith, Edinburgh, 1908, Vol. III, p. 151.

to take a special interest in medical affairs. A contemporary historian remarks of him : " In the meane tyme this nobill King James the fourt was weill leirnit in the art of mediecein and also ane cuning sorugenar that nane in his realme that wssit [used] that craft bot wald tak his counsall in all proceidingis."[1]   Buchanan also says of him : " He greedily imbibed an ancient custom of the nobility, for he was skilful in curing wounds."   He was also a patron of the dentist's art and, on occasion,

patients suffering from toothache submitted to a trial of his skill at Holyrood and accepted his largesse. His self-confidence as a surgeon possibly led him at times to undertake operations which he could not successfully accomplish.   In his Treasurer's accounts there is an ominous entry :—

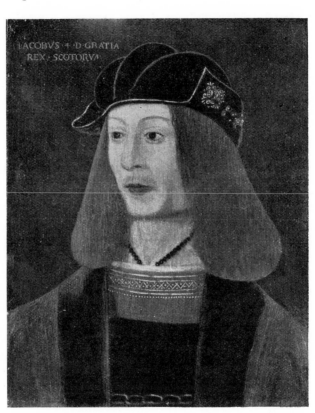

10 April, 1497.   "Item, giffin to ye blind wif yat hed her eyne schorne xiijs."[2]

This very probably refers to an attempt on the part of James to couch cataracts, with an unsuccessful result.   Thirteen shillings does not seem too much compensation to receive for loss of vision.

Lindesay of Pitscottie records a case which illustrates James's curiosity in matters of physiology.   A man child was

KING JAMES IV. (1473-1513)
(Original preserved in the Royal Scottish National Portrait Gallery)

born with two bodies from the waist upwards.   The King caused him to be carefully brought up and taught, and he lived to the age of twenty-eight years. One body, it is said, died long before the other, to the great grief of the survivor.

---

[1] Lindesay of Pitscottie : " Cronicles of Scotland," Edinburgh, Vol. I, p. 235, Book XX, Chap. VII.
[2] Pitcairne : " Criminal Trials in Scotland," Vol. I, Part I, p. 117.

The same historian naively records an experiment in the domain of psychology, which the King carried out in the year 1493 :—

> " And also the King gart [*caused*] tak ane dum woman and put hir in Inchkeytht [*the Island of Inchkeith*] and gaif [*gave*] hir tua zoung bairnes in companie witht hir and gart furnische them of all necessar thingis . . . to knaw quhat langage thir bairnes wald speik quhene [*when*] they come to lauchfull aige. Sum sayis they spak goode hebrew bot as to myself I knaw not."[1]

King James also took a great deal of interest in chemical experiments, and among his letters is one of 1508 thanking a certain James Inglis for books on alchemy, which were handed over to the King.[2] There are numerous items in the Treasurer's accounts for aqua vitæ, flasks, etc., and one entry is for money paid to William Foular, potingair [*apothecary*] for potingary to the King and Queen, distillation of waters, aqua vitæ, and potingary books in English from the 17th day of December, 1506.[3]

The interest taken by the King in the treatment of the new disease " grantgore " is mentioned elsewhere.

In addition to the surgeons who practised in the burghs, there were at this time royal surgeons who had country districts placed under their care, and who were paid by lands or fees from the Crown revenues much in the same way as parish doctors now receive allowances from the local authorities. Thus, Henry Railston had an annual fee of six merks from the rents of Kere Lawmond and Little and Meikle Lupas in Bute during his life, for the surgical art which he rendered at the instance of the King and Queen. Another royal surgeon, John Watson, received £21 1s. 6d. annually, though this was later reduced to £14 1s. At a slightly later date, Robert Kynnaird, the King's surgeon, received £20 annually, which was paid half by the Treasurer and half by the Comptroller, and John Murray, the King's barber (barbitonsor) received £10.[4]

For diseases requiring great skill, it appears that resort was made at this time to Paris. Thus Patrick Panther, the King's Secretary, went there when ill and died of fever ; and Henry Sinclair, Bishop of Ross, went to Paris for a surgical operation.[5] The fee paid to a Scottish surgeon on one occasion is mentioned as thirty-two shillings.[6]

Sir David Lyndsay, of the Mount, in the following reign, has an amusing poem regarding a jousting between James Watson and Jhone Barbour, servitouris to King James V., which is said to have taken place before the King and Queen, at St. Andrews, on a Whit Monday. It is possible that professional rivalry may have induced these two representatives of the medical profession of the day

(*Continued on page* 57)

---

[1] Lindesay of Pitscottie : " Cronicles of Scotland," Vol. I., p. 237.
[2] " Epistolæ Reg. Scot.," Vol. I, p. 119.
[3] G. Gregory Smith : " Days of James IIII," London, 1890, p. 110.
[4] " Exchequer Rolls of Scotland," Vol. XIV, pp. 81, 466 and 467.
[5] " Exchequer Rolls of Scotland," Vol. XIV, Pref. p. cxvi.   [6] Op. cit., p. 362.

SEAL OF CAUSE

GRANTED TO THE GUILD OF SURGEONS AND BARBERS AT EDINBURGH BY THE
MAGISTRATES ON 1ST JULY, 1505, AND CONFIRMED BY KING JAMES IV. ON
13TH OCTOBER, 1506

(From the original preserved in the Records of the Town Council of the City of Edinburgh)

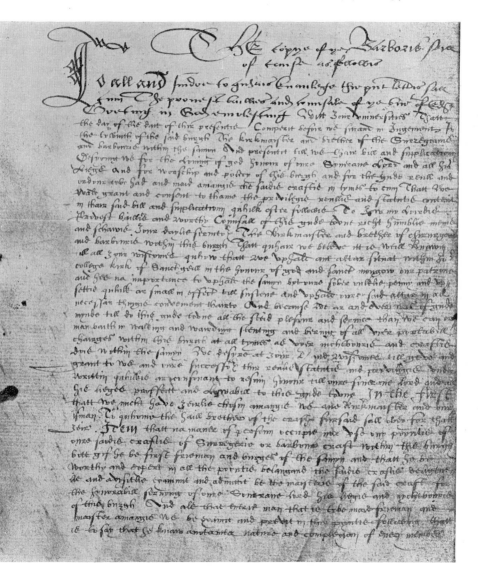

SEAL OF CAUSE (*Page 1*)

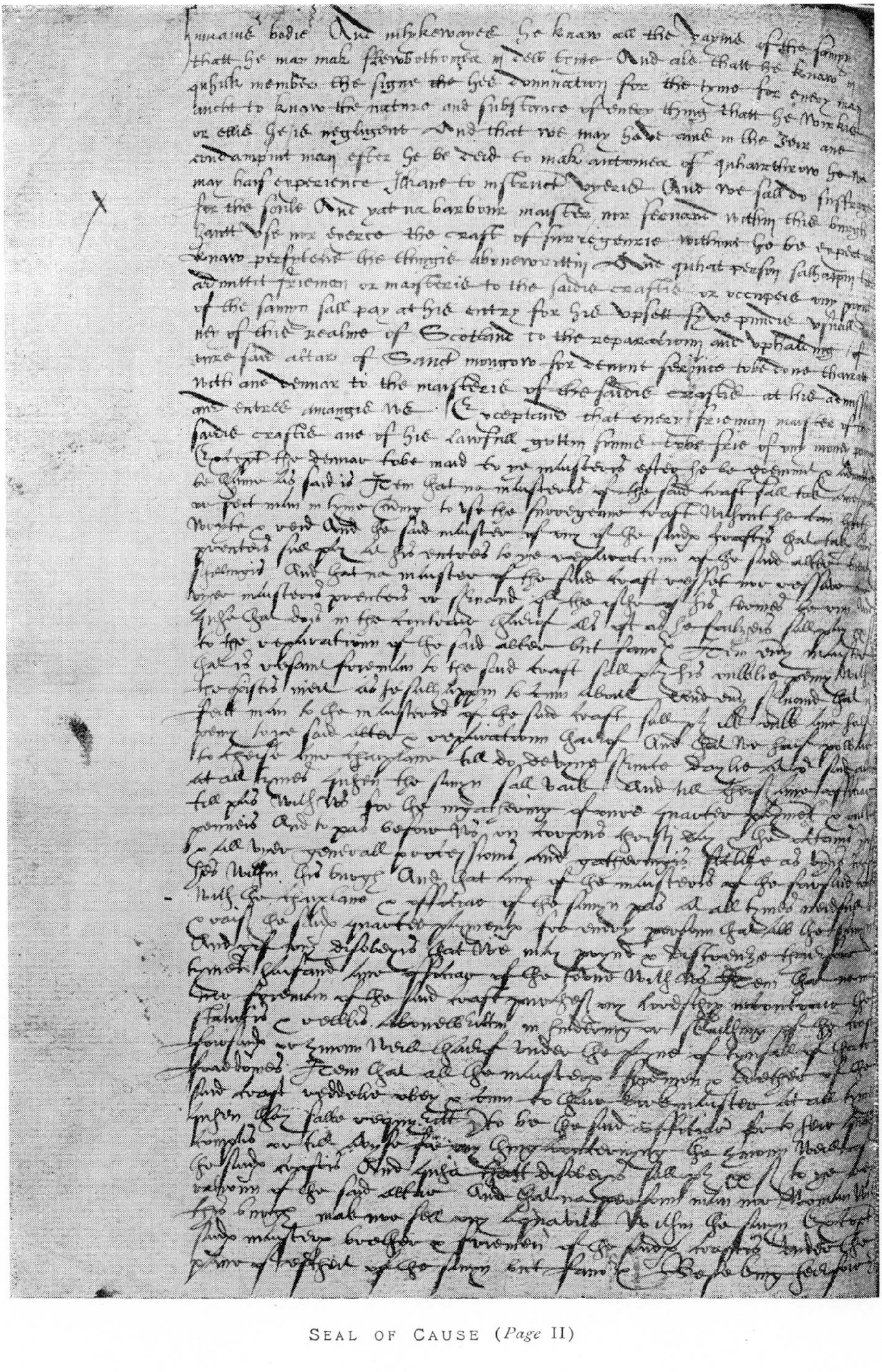

SEAL OF CAUSE (*Page* II)

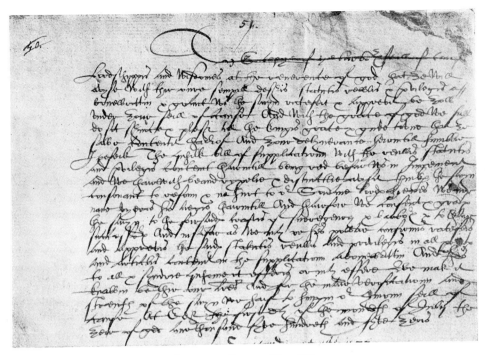

SEAL OF CAUSE (*Page* III)

to engage in combat before the Court. In any case, Lyndsay turns their strife into a ridiculous affair :—

> " James was ane man of greit intelligence,
> Ane medicinar ful of experience ;
> And Johne Barbour, he was ane nobill leche,
> Cruikit carlingis, he wald gar thame get speche."

At the first onslaught with lances, James would have been struck down if John through fierceness had not happened to faint, and, at the same time, John would have suffered severely had not James unfortunately broken his lance among the horses' feet. After the unsuccessful charge with lances, they drew their swords, but each missed his blow at the other, and thereafter they took to boxing-gloves and " dang at utheris facis." Finally, they gave up for weariness without shedding blood. Perhaps in this poem a sly reference may be traced to John Watson, who was one of the royal surgeons, and Thomas Leche, a well-known surgeon of the time.[1]

The Seal of Cause, granted by the Town Council to the surgeons and barbers in the year 1505, was probably given at the instance of King James IV., and in

---

[1] Sir David Lyndsay's Works: Ed. by Laing, Edinburgh, 1879, Vol. I, p 125.

any case it was confirmed by him in the following year.   This document has important contemporary relations.   Public dissections had been carried out in most of the Universities in the 14th and 15th centuries (Venice from 1368), but this was the first enactment on the subject in Britain, preceding even the law of Henry VIII. in 1540, by which four bodies of executed criminals were granted to the surgeons and barbers of London.   In the latter year, too, Henry VIII. granted to the surgeons and barbers of London privileges very similar to those granted by James IV. to the Edinburgh company in 1506.

In the larger Scottish towns, as in other countries, barbers practised minor surgery.   As we have seen, there is a reference as early as 1451 to Barbers in a Guild at Edinburgh.   By the year 1505, when various craftsmen were applying to the Town Council for charters, the barbers, together with the surgeons in the city, united to apply to the Provost, Baillies and Council of the Burgh for recognition of the two callings joined in a single guild.

It is evident from the application, in which two crafts are mentioned throughout, that along with barbers there existed at this time a superior calling of surgeons.   The surgeons presumably were too few in number to form a guild of their own, and thus united with the barbers just as at Florence, in the previous century, the physicians had included in their guild artists and literary men, who contributed much to the fame and standing of the guild.   The two crafts had for some time maintained an altar, dedicated to St. Mungo, in the Church of St. Giles.   This was supported by the entrance charges to the guild and a weekly subscription of one penny.   The petition asked that their yearly election of a churchmaster and oversman (in later years called the Deacon) should be recognised by the Town Council; that the Guild should have the sole right of practising the crafts of the surgeon and barber within the burgh, and that they should have the right to examine everyone presenting himself for entrance to the Guild in his knowledge of anatomy, complexion of the body, position of the veins, domination of the signs of the zodiac, and ability to read and write.   They also petitioned for the body of a criminal to anatomise once in the year.   The entrance fee was to be five pounds, together with a dinner by the candidate to the already-existing masters of the craft. The Guild was also to have a chaplain to perform daily services before their altar and an officer to collect the dues and precede them in processions.   Another privilege craved was that the members of the crafts should have the sole right to manufacture and sell aqua vitæ within the burgh.[1]   These petitions were granted by the Town Council at Edinburgh on the 1st of July, 1505, and were ratified in the following year by King James IV.

---

[1] This was not so great a privilege in days when the national drink of Scotland was " aill," as it might now appear, but if the monopoly to make and sell whisky in Edinburgh had not been allowed to lapse, the Royal College of Surgeons would to-day be one of the wealthiest corporations in the country.

The books available at this time for the study of anatomy were small compendiums, like those of Mondino of Bologna and Henri de Mondeville of Paris and Montpellier, and it is quite probable that copies of these had been brought to Scotland.

Vesalius, whose "De Fabrica Humani Corporis" (1543) is regarded as the commencement of anatomical renaissance, was not born till 1514, and the desire for anatomical study in Edinburgh is, therefore, independent or influenced from Continental sources, and is a proof of the high aspirations of the 15th century medicine in Scotland. The Seal of Cause runs as follows in the "Records of the Town Council":—

1 JULY, 1505

SEAL OF CAUSE TO BARBERS

"To all and sindrie to quhais knaulege thir present letteris sall cum, the prouest baillies and counsale of the burgh of Edinburgh, greiting in God euirlesting: Witt [know] your vniuersities thatt the day of the dait of thir presentis comperit befoir me, sittand in jugement in the Tolbuith of the said burgh, the kirkmaister and brether of the Sueregianis and Barbouris within the samyn, and presentit till me thair bill and supplicatioun desyring ws for the louing of God, honour of oure Souerane Lord and all his liegis, and for worschip and policy of this burgh, and for the gude reull and ordour to be had and maid amangis the saidis craftis in tymes to cum, thatt we wald grant and consent to thame the privilegis reullis and statutis contenit in thair said bill and supplicatioun quhilk efter follows:

"To yow my loirdis provest baillies and worthy counsall of this gude tovne, richt humblie meins and schawis your daylie servitouris the kirkmaister and brether of Chirurgeonis and Barbouris within this burgh, that quhair [where] we beleve itt is weill knawen till all your wisdomis quhow thatt we vphald ane altar situat within your College Kirk of Sanct Geill in the honour of God and Sanct Mongow our patrone, and hes na importance to vphald the samyn bot oure sober oulklie [weekly] penny and vpsettis [entrance fees], quhilk ar small in effect till sustene and vphald oure said altar in all necessar thingis convenient thairto, and because we ar and ever was of gude mynde till do this gude tovne all the steid plesour and seruice than we can or may, baith in walking and wairding stenting [assessing] and bering of all vther portabill chairges within this burgh at all tymes, as vther nichtbouris and craftis dois within the samyn, we desyre at your lordship and wisdomes till [to] geve and grant to ws and oure successouris thir reulis statutis and previlegis vndir written, quhilkis [which] ar consonant to resoun, honour till oure Souerane Lord and all his lieges, proffeitt and lowabill to this gude tovne: In the first, that we micht have yeirlie chosin amangis ws ane kirkmaister and ourisman [overman] to quhome the haill brether of the craftis foirsaid sall obey for thatt yeir: Item, that na maner of persoun occupie nor vse ony poyntis of our saidis craftis of Surregenie or Barbour craft within this burgh bott gif [unless] he be first frieman and burges of the saymn, and thatt he be worthy and expert in all the poyntis belangand the saidis craftis diligentlie and avysitlie examinit and admittit be the maisters of the said craft for the honorabill seruying of oure Souerane Lord his liegis and nychtbouris of this burgh, and als [also] that euerie man that is to be maid freman and maister amangis ws be examit and previt in thir poyntis following, thatt is to say, that he knaw anotamell [anatomy], nature and complexion of euery member humanis bodie, and inlykewayes he knaw all the vaynis of the samyn, thatt he may mak flewbothomell [phlebotomy] in dew tyme, and als thatt he knaw in quhilk [which] member the signe hes domination for the tyme, for euery man aucht to knaw the nature and substance of euery thing thatt he werkis, or ellis he is negligent ; and that we may have anis [*once*] in the yeir ane condampnit man efter he be deid to mak antomell of, quhairthraw we may haif experience, ilk ane to instrict vtheris, and we sall do suffrage for the soule ; and that na barbour, maister nor seruand, within this burgh hantt [*practise*] vse nor exerce the craft of Surregenrie without he be expert and knaw perfytelie the thingis abouewritten : and quhat person sal happin to be admittit frieman or maisteris to the saidis craftis, or occupeis ony poynt of the samyn, sall pay at his entry for his vpsett [*entrance fee*] fyve pundis vsuall money of this realme of Scotland to the reparatioun and vphalding of oure said altar of Sanct Mongow for deuyne [*divine*] seruice to be done thairatt, with ane dennar to the maisteris of the saidis craftis at his admissioun and entres amangis ws ; exceptand that euery frieman maister of the saidis craftis ane of his lawful gottin sonnis to be frie of ony money payment, except the dennar to be maid to the maisteris efter he be exeminit and admitted be thame as said is : Item, that na maisteris of the said craft sall tak ane prenteis or feit [*hired*] man in tyme cuming to vse the Surregeane craft without he can baithe wryte and reid, and the said maister of ony of the saidis craftis that takis ane prenteis sall pay at his entres to the reparatioun of the said alter tuenty schillingis ; and that na maister of the said craft resset [*steal away*] nor ressave [*receive*] ane vther maisteris prenteis or seruand quhill [*till*] the ische [*end*] of his termes be run, and quha that dois in the contrair thairof, as oft as he failyies, sall pay xx s. to the reparatioun of the said alter but [*without*] fauvouris.   Item, euery maister that is resauit frieman to the said craft sall pay his oulklie penny with the priestis meit as he sall happen to cum about, and euery seruand that is feitt [*hired*] man to the maisteris of the said craft sall pay ilk oulk [*week*] ane half-peny to the said alter and reparatioun thairof ; and that we haif powar to cheise [*choose*] ane chaiplane till do devyne seruice daylie at our said alter at all tymes quhen the samyn sall vaik [*be vacant*], and till cheis ane officiar till pas with ws for the ingathering of oure quarter payment and oulklie pennies, and to pass befoir ws on Corpus Christy day and the octauis thairof, and all vther generall processionis and gatheringis, siclike as vtheris craftis hes within this burgh ; and that ane of the maisteris of the foirsaid craftis, with the chaiplane and officiar of the samyn, pas at all tymes neidfull lift [*collect*] and rais the saidis quarter paymentis fra euery persoun that aw the samyn, and gif ony dissobeyis that we may poynd [*seize*] and distrenye [*distrain*] thairfoir all tymes haifand ane officiar of the tovne with us :   Item, that na man nor freman of the said craft purches ony lordschip incontrair [*contrary to*] the statutis and rewlis aboue written, in hindering or skaithing [*damaging*] of the craftis foirsaidis or commoun weill thairof, vnder the payne of tynsall [*loss*] of thair friedomes.   Item, that all the maisteris friemen and brether of the said craft reddelie obey and cum to thair kirkmaister at all tymes quhen thay sal be requyritt thairto be the said officiar for to heir quarter comptis [*accounts*], or till avyse for ony thing concernyng the commoun weill of the saidis craftis, and quha thatt disobeyis sall pay xx s. to the reparatioun of the said altar ; and that na persoun man nor woman within this burgh mak nor sell ony aquavite within the samyn except the saidis maisteris brether and friemen of the saidis craftis vnder the pane of escheit of the samyn but fauouris.   Beseking heirfoir your lordschippis and wisdomes at the reuerence of God that ye will avise with thir oure sempill desyris statutis rewlis and privilegis abouewritten, and grant ws the samyn ratefeit and apprevit be yow vnder your seill of cause, and with the grace of God we sall do sic seruice and plesour to the Kingis grace and gude tovne that ye salbe contentit thairof, and your delyuerance heirintill humblie I beseik.

    " The quhilk bill of supplicatioun with the reullis statutis and privilegis contenit thairentill being red befoir ws in jugement, and we thairwith beand ryplie [*fully*] and distinctlie avysit, thinkis the samyn consonant to resoun and na hurt to our Souerane Lordis Hienes, ws, nor nane vtheris his liegis thairintill, and thairfoir we consent and grantis the samyn to the foirsaidis craftis of Surregenry and Barbouris and to thair successouris, and in sa far as we may or hes powar, confirmis ratefeis and apprevis the saidis statutis reullis and privilegis in all poyntis and articlis contenit in the supplicatioun abouewritten; and to all and syndrie quhome it efferis [*concerns*] or may effere we mak it knawin be thir our lettres; and for the mair verificatioun and strenth of the samyn we haif to hungin [*appended*] our commoun seill of cause, at Edinburgh, the first day of the moneth of July the yeir of God ane thousand fyve hundreth and fyve yeris." [1]

After the surgeons and barbers had obtained the Seal of Cause, various enactments were made from time to time confirming or extending the privileges granted by this. It is convenient to summarise these here.[2]

The Seal of Cause was confirmed by James IV. under the Privy Seal at Edinburgh on the 13th October, 1506.

Mary, Queen of Scots, again confirmed this, and exempted the surgeons along with doctors of medicine from bearing armour in raids and wars, as well as from sitting on inquests or assizes in criminal or civil actions. This edict was made at Edinburgh on the 11th of May, 1567.

James VI. again ratified all the privileges and confirmed Queen Mary's letter of exemption on 6th June, 1613.

The Town Council passed an Act forbidding any who had not been duly approved by the surgeons from practising the art of surgery within the burgh, on 10th September, 1641.

An Act of the Scottish Parliament, in favour of the surgeons and barbers of Edinburgh, ratifying all their privileges and giving the Deacon and Masters of the surgeons the power to take and apprehend all persons exercising the surgical art who were not freemen of the craft, and to fine them £20 Scots for contravention, was passed on 17th November, 1641.

An Act of the Town Council, confirming the rights conveyed by the above-mentioned Act of Parliament, mentioning that the apothecaries were not exempt from these, and making an attempt to define the conditions which, naturally, called for the surgeon's art, was passed on 27th June, 1655.

An Act of the Town Council, regulating the practice of apothecaries and surgeon-apothecaries in the burgh of Edinburgh, and reaffirming that no one should be admitted to practise the art of apothecary unless he had been examined by members of this body, was passed on 25th February, 1657. In this pronouncement it is distinctly stated that there is no intention of erecting the apothecaries into a corporation, but that the arrangement is merely made for the improvement of the apothecaries' art and the good of the people.

---

[1] " Extracts from the Records of the Burgh of Edinburgh, 1403–1528," pp. 101–104.
[2] See " Collection of Royal Grants and other Documents relative to the Royal College of Surgeons of Edinburgh," Edinburgh, 1818.

An Act of the Scottish Parliament, in favour of the surgeons and barbers in relation to the art of pharmacy, confirming all previous privileges to this incorporation and joining them with the brotherhood of the surgeon-apothecaries and apothecaries in powers to search out irregular practitioners and fine them, was passed on 22nd August, 1670.

The Scottish Parliament ratified a gift and patent granted by King William and Queen Mary, in favour of the surgeons and surgeon-apothecaries, adjusting some of the differences between them, confirming their privileges and providing that their privileges should be nowise hurtful or prejudicial to the erection of the Royal College of Physicians, and this was passed on 17th July, 1695.

A declaration by the Royal College of Physicians, adjusting differences with the surgeons in Edinburgh regarding the practice of pharmacy by the latter, was made on 22nd July, 1695.

An Act of the Town Council of Edinburgh, in favour of the surgeon-apothecaries and apothecaries mentions on 24th June, 1696, that very few of this old fraternity are now living.

An Act of the Town Council of Edinburgh, in favour of the apothecaries and surgeon-apothecaries on 9th December, 1696, mentions that several persons within the burgh are practising the art of apothecaries and keeping open shops without any warrant, and forbids them to do so until they have made application for an examination by the visitors of the fraternity.

The Charter of Erection of the Guild of Surgeons into a Royal College of Surgeons at Edinburgh, conceding them new privileges, was granted under the Great Seal by George III., on 12th May, 1778.

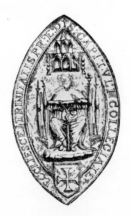

SEAL OF TRINITY HOSPITAL
Before the Reformation

CHAPTER IV

PRACTICE AT EDINBURGH IN THE SIXTEENTH CENTURY

THE surgeons and barbers came into prominence in the year 1505, when, along with various other guilds, they were incorporated under the Seal of Cause from the Town Council, ratified next year by the King. During the following century there are numerous references in the Town Council minutes and other Scottish records to their activities. That the surgeons and barbers were enterprising and patriotic is evidenced by the fact that when an English invasion was threatened in 1558, and the crafts of the burgh were convened in the Tolbooth to provide volunteers for the protection of the town against " our auld inemyes of Ingland," twenty-five members of the Guild of Surgeons and Barbers volunteered for this duty as part of a force of 717 men provided by the various crafts. Their names were as follows : " Jhone Wawchthet, and Edward Wawghthet, his servand (*i.e.*, *apprentice*) ; David Robertsoun, and Thomas Kawpe, servand ; Jhone Weddel ; Patrick Mertene ; Alexander Bruce ; Jhone Libertoun ; Robert Henrysoun, Andro Wyntoun and Gilbert Prymros, his servandis ; Nowye Bruschet, and Thomas Boyes, his servand ; James Lindesay ; Archibald Maw, and Jhone Scot, servand ; Alexander Percy, Thomas Blak, his servand ; Niniane Maw, Jhone Chalmer, his servand ; George Campbell ; Maister Armle, William Gray, his servand ; Maister Babteist, Jhone Pectarne, his servand ; Pate Hardye, Walter Hardye, his sone."[1] There is a note in the Register of the Privy Seal of Scotland, under the date 1542, for disbursements to Anthone Brisset, on account of services to Queen Mary of Guise, and to four surgeons who had apparently taken part in military operations on the borders in that year. This is the first reference to military surgeons in Scotland.

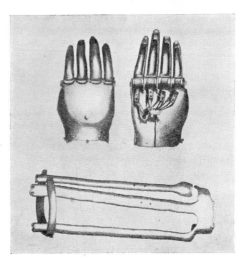

STEEL HAND OF CLEPHANE
(From Sir Walter Scott's " Border Antiquities of England and Scotland")

> *Item*, gevin to Anthone Brisset, Surrurgeane, for laubouris done be him to ye Quenis grace, at this tyme alanerly. . . . . . . xx li.

---

[1] Gairdner : " List of Fellows of the Royal College of Surgeons of Edinburgh, 1581–1873." Edinburgh : 1874, pp. 3 and 4.

Item, to George Leche, William Quhite, George Fothringham and Dauid Robertsoune, Surrurgeanis, passand to ye Bordouris for curing of all personis yat hapnit to be hurt be Inglis menne . . . . . xij li.[1]

The family of Clephane of Carslogie, near Cupar, possessed an iron hand without a thumb, the fingers of which move at the knuckles. It is attached to three flat bars, which were fastened by means of a hoop to the arm just below the elbow. Tradition says that it belonged to a Laird of Carslogie, who received it from a King of Scotland, in consequence of having lost his hand in the service of his country. It is apparently an example of the work of a 16th century Scottish armourer.

In 1557, John Wauchlott, who is described as officer and chirurgeane, received three pounds for curing the leg of James Henderson, injured in a fight with a thief. It appears, therefore, that Wauchlott must have been in the service of the Magistracy.[2] In 1563, Robert Hendersoun, cherurgeane, appears to have been in the service of the town, because a minute of the Council speaks of his great labours and expenses at their command on divers persons hurt within the town. Hendersoun's most notable exploit was said to have been the raising of a dead woman from the grave, when she had lain there two days after having been strangled. He had also dressed the stumps of two false notaries whose hands had been struck off, and he had successfully treated a man and a woman wounded through the body by the sword of a Frenchman. For these surgical exploits he was voted the sum of twenty merks.[3]

The monopoly granted to the surgeons and barbers of making aqua vitæ seems to have been gradually abandoned by them. On 20th March, 1557, Besse Campbell was ordered to " desist and ceis fra ony forther making of aquevite within this burgh in tyme cummyng," or from selling it except on the market day, " conform to the priuilege grantit to the barbouris vnder the seill of caus, without scho be admittit be tham thairto." It would seem, from the latter part of this judgment, as though the surgeons and barbers had been in the habit of leasing or granting to persons outside the craft the privilege of making and selling aqua vitæ. The complete abandonment of the privilege was therefore probably effected gradually.[4]

There are various records of surgeons being consulted in medico-legal cases, and furnishing reports to the Town Council or to the judges. The following is a good example of the form taken by a medico-legal report, dated 27th June, 1569 :—

" Comperit alswa in jugement, in presence of the said Justice-depute, Nowye Buyssat, dekyn of Scherurgianis, and producit this writting following, quhilk bayth the

---

[1] Pitcairne : " Criminal Trials," Vol. I, Part I, p. 325.
[2] p. 16, [3] pp. 165 and 166 : " Extracts from the Records of the Burgh of Edinburgh, 1557–1571."
[4] "Extracts," 1528–1557, p. 262.

parteis foirsaidis desyrit to be insert and registrat in the buikis of Adiornale ; quhairof the tennour followis :—

TESTIMONIAL OF THE CHERURGIANIS

"Apud Edinburt. xxvij⁰. die mensis Junij, Anno Domini millesimo quingentesimo sexagesimo nono. The quhilk day, at sindry tymes befoir, at ye queist and desyre of my Lord Justice Clerk, wes presentit befoir me Nowye Buyssat dekyn, Robert Henrysoune, Patrik Hardy and Alex. Tuedye, cherurgeanis and burgessis of Edinburgh, my breder, ane callit Johnne Farer, quha wes hurte vpoun the left arme, on the elbok, on the arme beneth, and on the hand ; to have our jugementis, quhidder that the said Johnne suld be mutulat or no of the saidis hurtis and woundis than being haill : Eftir lang consultatioune and ernist advysement, we fand the said Johnne nather to be mutulat nor impotent of his arme nor hand ; bot that it wald be daylie better, gif he wald make laubouris vpoune it : And this we testefie be this our hand wrytis and subscriptioune to all and sindry to quhome it efferis, day, zeir and place foirsaidis.

> "Nowy Byssat, Dekin of the Cherurgeanis.
> Robert Henrysoune, wt. my hand.
> Alex. Tuedy, wt. my hand.
> Patk. Hardy, wt. my hand."[1]

By 1563, the surgeons and barbers seem to have been taking means to stop unauthorised people from practising their craft, for in this year the Provost and Council forbade five men and a woman to indulge in " occupeing or vsing of cherurgeanrie or barbour craft " until they should be admitted and made free of the craft.[2]

In addition to furnishing certificates to the Courts, the surgeons were some-times called before the Town Council to give evidence, as in March, 1580, when Jhone Lowsoun, chirurgean, appeared before the Provost and Baillies, and being sworn, gave evidence that Nicoll Haistie, cordiner, was in no danger of his life from a wound given him by Thomas Crawfurd, who therefore was set at liberty upon caution.[3]

At the same Court, seven surgeons appeared, viz., Robert Henrysoun, Howie Brussat, Henry Blyth, Gilbert Primrose, James Lyndsay, James Craig and Henry Lumisdaill, who gave evidence that they had on various occasions examined Robert Asbowane, who had been wounded one week before by James Dowglas, with his servants and accomplices. As they testified that the said Robert Asbowane was in no danger of his life or of mutilation, the prisoners were set at liberty with a fine of five thousand merks. Four of these surgeons had already appeared two days previously and reported that " they as yit culd geve na resolute ansuer towart the hurting of Robert Asbowane be James Douglas and his complices, bot that he is in danger quhill forther tryell." [4]

It may be assumed, therefore, that Gilbert Primrose, James Lyndsay, and James Craig were regarded as persons of greater weight in the profession, seeing

---

[1] Pitcairn : " Criminal Trials," Vol. I, Part II, p. 7.
[2] " Extracts from the Records of the Burgh of Edinburgh, 1557–1571," p. 155.
[3] "Extracts from the Records of the Burgh of Edinburgh, 1573–89," pp. 152 and 153. [4] Ibid.

E

that they enabled the other four within two days to come to a definite decision in this serious case.   All three were later Deacons of the craft.

In the same year Henry Lumsdaill is noted as having given a certificate that a servant to the Earl of Argyle was in no danger from a wound given him by Jhone Small, who was therefore set at liberty.[1]   In 1581 the same three seniors, Gilbert Primrose, James Craig and James Lyndsay, gave evidence that they had examined the wound of Howsteane Braikinrig, a butterman, who had been wounded by Rychert Miller, and, as they declared that Braikinrig was in no danger of his life, Miller was set free.[2]   Similarly, in 1583, Lyndsay, Lumisdaill, Blyth and Craig certified that James Marioribankis was in no danger to life from a wound in the hand and arm given him by William Blythman, flesher, and his complices, and cautiously added " bot gif he was mutilat culd nocht swa suddanelie declair the sam." [3]

Robert Henrysoun has been mentioned as having been employed several times by the town in medico-legal cases.   In June, 1580, a supplication was made on the part of Thomas Morame, town's officer, who had been hurt in the execution of his office " be sum wikket persounis as yitt vnknawin," because his surgeons, doubting of payment, " ar become slak in thairf cure." He had been thrust through the body and was troubled with inward bleeding.   The Baillies and Council therefore ordained their treasurer to pay Robert Henrysoun and James Lyndsay, chirurgeanes, twenty pounds for Morame's cure, and to pay Adame Diksoun, apothecare, the sum of fifty shillings for the drugs supplied by him.[4]

The surgeons and barbers frequently had to contend with persons invading their craft, and, in 1575, the Provost and Baillies had issued a decree forbidding apothecaries and others who did not belong to the surgeons' guild to exercise any part of their craft.   This had been duly intimated by the bellman of the burgh to Alexander Barclay and Robert Craig, apothecaries, and others.   On 12th April, 1587, the Deacon of the surgeons' craft, James Craig, complained to the Town Council that Archbald Mwdie, an apothecary, had been practising surgery, and in particular he had been " curing and pansing of Mathow Weiche of ane vlcer in his fute " for three weeks past, and daily and hourly applying thereto various local remedies.   For this, Archbald Mwdie was fined forty shillings and forbidden in future to exercise any point of the craft of surgery, under the pain of a similar fine.[5]   On 27th June, 1589, however, Baillie Thomas Fyschear, who was not a surgeon, received twenty shillings from the Council for " mending ane Spayngyart's heid." [6]   In the case of a Baillie, the surgeons' guild probably thought it better not to prosecute.

---

        [1] p. 162, [2] pp. 218 and 219, [3] pp. 286 and 287, [4] pp. 165 and 166, [5] pp. 489 and 490, [6] p. 546: " Extracts from the Records of the Burgh of Edinburgh, 1573–1589."

It must have been somewhat of a blow to the surgeons in Edinburgh when, on 5th February, 1589, Phillop Hislop, one of the regents of the Town's College, who suffered from a malady of the eye and feared he was to lose it, obtained leave of absence from the Town Council to proceed to London, where he was " in howpe to be curet thairof." [1]

Another distinguished surgeon of this period was John Chisholm, doctor of medicine, and surgeon to King James VI., who is believed to have been the operator who preserved the life of the Earl of Morton when he was suffering from strangulated hernia, although the Earl was beheaded nine years later, the first victim of " The Maiden," an instrument which he had invented : " November, 1572, James, erle of Mortoun, regent, lay deidlie seik of rumbussanes (*rupture*), and war nocht he was cuttit he haid lost his lyff." [2]

Another surgeon deserving mention is John Naysmyth, surgeon to King James VI., and for some time chief surgeon to the Scots Guards of the King of France.   He was a companion of King James on the hunt at Falkland when James was enticed to Gowrie House in 1600. [3]

The first specialist in surgery of whom there is a record was apparently trained in France, for, in 1595, the surgeons complained against M. Awin, a French surgeon, for practising the art of surgery in Edinburgh without belonging to the guild.   The Town Council fined him twenty pounds and forbade him under pain of imprisonment to practise surgery except certain special branches, viz., cutting for the stone, curing of ruptures, couching of cataracts, curing the pestilence, and distempers of women occasioned by child-birth. [4]

James Henrysoun (a younger contemporary of Robert Henrysoun), who had been busy as a kind of medical officer of health during the epidemics of plague, was apparently employed by the Town Council, after the disappearance of the plague, as a regular officer to treat the poor of the town, for, in 1589, there is a minute that he is to be paid the " sowm of nyne pund fourty penneis, in compleitt payment of all drogs, implasteris and mendicaments furnist be him in curing of the pure in tymes past, at the townis command, conform to the particulare compt thairof presently schawin." [5]

In addition to the surgeons and barbers, numerous apothecaries, some of whom kept shops for the sale of spices and for prescribing and carrying out medicinal treatment, were to be found in the town.   There were also physicians, who had probably been trained abroad or had even received degrees at foreign Universities, among whom one of the most noteworthy was Gilbert Skeen, who had been

---

[1] p. 536 : "Extracts from the Records of the Burgh of Edinburgh, 1573–1589."
[2] "Diurnal of Occurrents," p. 321.
[3] " List of Fellows of the Royal College of Surgeons of Edinburgh from 1581 to 1873," Edinburgh, 1874, p. 6.
[4] Maitland : " History of Edinburgh," Edinburgh, 1753, pp. 46 and 47. Also " Extracts from the Records of the Burgh of Edinburgh, 1589-1603, p. 136.
[5] " Extracts from the Records of the Burgh of Edinburgh, 1573–1589," p. 535.

EDINBURGH IN 1544 FROM NORTH-EAST OF CALTON HILL

(Sketch made by an engineer with the English Army, for Henry VIII)

Showing the attack of the English troops on the town prior to the burning of the city

Under a, Arthur's Seat and Holyrood Palace; b. Monastery of the Blackfriars; c. Church and Hospital of Kirk o' Field, large group of buildings on the skyline; d. Edinburgh Castle, showing David's Tower; above e, Trinity Church and Hospital, appearing in a gap of the Calton Hill; f f f columns of the English Army.

mediciner in King's College, Aberdeen, and who set up practice in Niddrie Wynd, Edinburgh, in the year 1575.   Another physician practising at the same time was William Cassanate, a Spanish physician, who had been trained at Besançon, in Burgundy, and who is mentioned as the physician of the Archbishop of St. Andrews.

In the year 1551, Cassanate was settled in practice in Edinburgh.   He was then thirty-six years old and had been attached for four years to the household of John Hamilton, Archbishop of St. Andrews.[1]   His patron, the Archbishop, was a prominent actor in some of the most important scenes connected with the troubled political history surrounding Mary, Queen of Scots.   Mary was at this time nine years old.   The Archbishop's brother, James Hamilton, Earl of Arran, was next heir to the throne and Regent of Scotland.   The Earl of Arran had succeeded in getting the Scottish Parliament to agree to a Treaty with England, arranged in 1543, by which Mary should be married to Edward, the son of Henry VIII, when she was eleven years old.

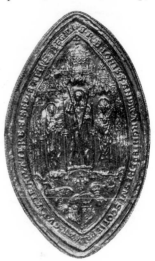

The Scottish barons, however, had declared against this alliance with England, and, as a result of the contention of these two parties, the south of Scotland had been virtually destroyed in two invasions of 1544 and 1547 by the Earl of Hertford. The party in favour of an alliance with England was headed by the Earl of Arran, backed by his brother, Archbishop Hamilton, while the party in favour of an alliance with France was headed by the Queen-Mother, Mary of Lorraine, backed by Cardinal Beaton.

SEAL OF JOHN HAMILTON

In addition to his own ecclesiastical affairs, John Hamilton practically had to manage all that was difficult in the affairs of Scotland from about 1546, when Cardinal Beaton was put to death.   He speaks of himself indeed as being too busy almost to breathe, his health failed from month to month, and at the end of the year 1551, after he had finished his celebrated " Catechism," attacks of asthma, which recurred every eight days and lasted for twenty-four hours, had made him very thin and brought him nearly to the point of death.   Looking around for medical advice, he was counselled by his physician, Cassanate, to seek the help of Jerome Cardan, the famous physician of Milan.

---

[1] See Morley : " Life of Jerome Cardan," London, 1854, Vol. II., Chaps. IV. and V.

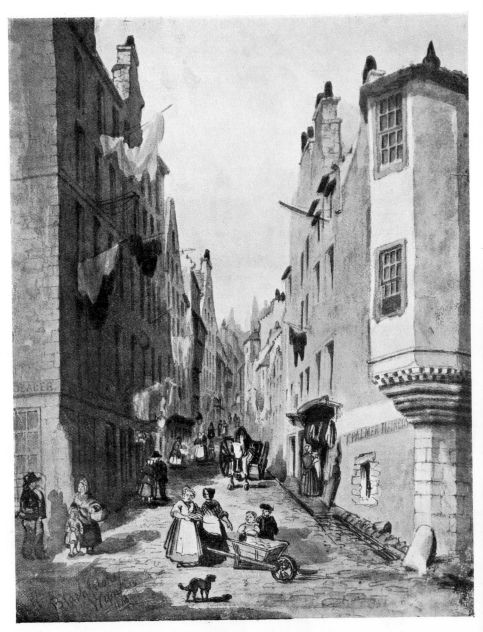

BLACKFRIARS' WYND

Looking from the Cowgate, with the House of the Archbishop of St. Andrews on the right

(From a sketch by Sir Daniel Wilson, preserved in the Library of the University of Edinburgh)

In the end of November, 1551, Cardan received a letter written from Edinburgh two months earlier by Cassanate. As this letter contained matters of great importance, and as it had to be sent across Europe by the hands of a special messenger, and was addressed from one dignified physician to another, Cassanate apparently thought that the occasion warranted a very lengthy literary effort. The letter, as printed in Cardan's works, extends over some sixteen folio pages.[1] It began with a general disquisition on the subject of the formation of friendship, quoting the opinions of Cicero and other writers on the matter. Then followed complimentary references to Cardan's books, especially the books on " Subtilty," which Cassanate had only lately read. Finally, he came to the case of the Archbishop of St. Andrews, which is interesting as giving an idea of theories of pathology in the 16th century.

The Archbishop, he said, had been troubled for ten years with periodic asthma caused by a distillation from the brain into the lungs and associated at first with hoarseness, which had been removed, leaving a bad temperature in the brain. The brain, he continued, was too cold and moist, being nourished with pituitous blood. Whenever the brain became invaded with this matter there was a fresh accession of the asthma due to a flow of the same humour down into the lungs, an accession which agreed almost accurately with the conjunctions and oppositions of the moon. He offered the opinion

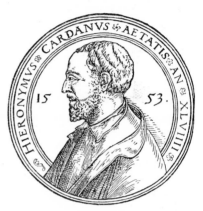

JEROME CARDAN
*(From Frontispiece of his " De Subtilitate,"
edition of 1554)*

that the matter flowing down into the lungs was serous, watery and sweet or insipid, for if it were acrid or salt the lungs would ulcerate and the disease would turn to phthisis. Thin at first, the fluid was expelled by coughing, but part becoming thick, adhered to the lungs, and the consequence was dyspnœa with stertor. Various physical signs, such as the heat of the breath, the character of the pulse, etc., were also given. Cassanate then proceeded that the Archbishop was about to visit Paris and begged Cardan to make an appointment with him in that city, so that they might have the benefit of a consultation. If Cardan could not come to Paris, he might at least travel to Lyons, where the Archbishop would come to meet him.

To this letter, dated 28th September, 1551, Cardan replied that he would go to Paris. On 23rd February, 1552, Cardan set out for Lyons, where he arrived in about three weeks. Here he was met by Cassanate,

---

[1] Cardan : " De Libris Propriis," 1557, pp. 159–175.

bearing a letter of introduction from the Archbishop, written in Latin, speaking of serious, urgent and inevitable business which had detained the Archbishop at home, and extending to Cardan an urgent invitation to come to Edinburgh.   The letter is brief, business-like and so skilful a combination of compliments, with an obvious anxiety on the Archbishop's part to see Cardan, that it appears almost irresistible.   The Archbishop concluded with the words : " Farewell, most learned Cardanus, and visit our Lares to find us not so much of Scythians as you perhaps suppose.—Edinburgh, Feb. 4, 1552." Accompanying the letter were 300 gold crowns as travelling expenses between Lyons and Edinburgh.

The two physicians accordingly set out.   In Paris, Cardan met with the heartiest reception, and saw many noble patients.   He and Cassanate dined with two celebrated physicians of the French king, Jean Fernel, first physician to the French King, and Jacques de la Boë (Sylvius), the Parisian professor of anatomy, in order to discuss the Archbishop's case.   Cardan took great pains not to commit himself.   During the discussion, he listened and said nothing, and, when asked for his opinion, declined to speak before the King's physicians had done so.   Afterwards he abstained from committing himself, because he had not yet seen the case.   Cardan and Cassanate then proceeded to London, and, after resting three days, continued their way to Edinburgh, a journey of twenty-three days from London.   On 29th June, 1552, Cardan personally interviewed his Scottish patient, who resided on the east side of Blackfriars' Wynd, at the corner of the Cowgate.[1]   There had been plenty of time on the journey to discuss the case.   At the Paris dinner-party, Cassanate's opinion in tracing the Archbishop's trouble to a cold brain had been accepted, and it had been recommended that the former treatment should be continued for forty days.   Cardan, however, traced all the evil to a hot brain, and differed with courtesy from his friends in other essential respects.

At the end of forty days the Archbishop became impatient.   He had continued to waste in body and had become restless and dissatisfied.   Cardan then pointed out that he himself had formed another opinion as to the nature of the disease and as to the proper way of attempting its cure.   The natural result was that the Archbishop was indignant with Cassanate and Cassanate with Cardan, but Cardan at all events was in the favourable position that any change he made would likely be for the better.

Cardan now wrote out his whole opinion for the Archbishop at great length.   This is included in a volume of professional opinions subsequently published.[2] Cardan had already discovered that the Archbishop's asthmatic attacks, when he took care of himself, did not occur oftener than every fifteen or twenty days, that he never took the amount of sleep necessary,

---

[1] Maitland : " History of Edinburgh," p 182.
[2] Cardan : " Consilia Medica," Vol. IX., 52nd opinion, pp. 124-148.

that he was a great eater and drinker, that he was irascible, had a skin that exhaled freely, and had become thin.

After his forty days' study of the patient, Cardan's written opinion took the form of a long clinical lecture.   He did not believe with Cassanate that the matter finally expectorated had collected in His Grace's brain during the intervals between attacks, for if so, the operation of the intellect must have been impeded and the matter so collecting would have turned corrupt.   He believed that the thin fluid expectorated was partly serous humour, partly condensed vapour, which descended from the brain into the lungs, not through the cavity of the windpipe, but through its coats, as water soaks through linen.   This thin humour he supposed had been drawn into the brain by the increased rarity of that organ caused by undue heat, for heat made all things rare, and rarefaction in one part of the body, to express the idea roughly, produced suction from another.   The expectorated matter, Cardan thought, was formed from the food.[1]

As a practical application of his theories, Cardan said that the basis of the Archbishop's cure must depend on the use of a food as cold-natured and humid as possible.   The cold-natured food would resist the attraction of the brain, and humidity would obstruct the soaking down of matter from the brain through the coats of the windpipe, thus compelling it to descend by the interior of the channel, from which it could easily be coughed out.   The chief attack by medicine was to be made on the unhealthy temperature of the brain, and with this view the head should be purged, with, of course, previous purgation of the body. Purgation of the head, he explained, might be effected through the palate, the nose or the sutures of the skull.   For procuring a good discharge by the nose he recommended the following prescription : Of milk of a goat or cow, half a pint, of water half a pint, of elaterium two grains ; let this be drawn through the nostrils, when the patient has an empty stomach.[2]

For further purgation of the head, he recommended the application to the shaven head over the coronal suture of an ointment composed of Greek pitch, ship's tar, white mustard, euphorbium and honey of anathardus, sharpened, if desired, by the addition of cantharides.   This ointment, he said, would sometimes fetch out two pints of water in twenty-four hours, although sometimes only three or four ounces.[3]

He advised also the use of the shower bath as recommended by Celsus.   In a well-warmed bedroom, the head was to be washed with hot water containing a few ashes.   Then a pailful of water, cold from the well, was to be dashed upon it suddenly, after which the head was to be rubbed with cool, dry cloths until

---

[1] Cardan reasoned upon principles laid down by Galen. They seem to us now very absurd, but not more absurd perhaps than some physiological theories of 1927 will appear to the medical philosophers of 2000 A.D.

[2] Presumably the patient only took a small part of the pint of fluid at a time ; otherwise, the purgative effects of two grains of elaterium would have been memorable.

[3] This warm nightcap would effectually prevent the Archbishop from any desire for the pleasures of the table for several days.

no trace of moisture remained.　The patient was to remain in the warm room for two hours before going out.　By this habit, said Cardan, the brain is kept in a natural temperature and its substance rendered firm and dense.　He also strongly advised the use of the bath.

He then came to what was perhaps the most important part of the physician's care—to prevent the generation in the body of peccant material.　His Grace should walk in the shade in tranquil weather, and should be careful not to go out in rain or night air.　He should make use of a perfume ball, but the perfume should not include roses, for the scent of roses made some brains warmer.　The Archbishop should not sleep upon feathers but upon unspun silk, for the heating of the spine and vena cava upon a feather bed would cause matter to ascend into the head.　The patient, too, should lie upon his face or side and, as a relief to the digestion, should press the hand upon the stomach.　The pillow should be of dry straw finely chopped or, if His Grace preferred it, might be stuffed with dried seaweed, but not with feathers.　The pillow-case also should be of linen and not of leather, and it should be sprinkled at night with a drying perfume.[1]　The sleep must last for seven to ten hours, and the Archbishop must take the time from business or from his studies.　His hours of business were to be limited to four, and might be from noon to four in the afternoon.

Upon rising, constipation might be corrected by taking a conserve of peaches and sugar of violets, waiting five hours for breakfast and then breakfasting lightly. Breakfast might be replaced by drinking two to four pints of new ass's milk, either in one dose or in several doses.　This would serve to nourish his body and his lungs, allay the excess of heat, be grateful to the palate and help to avert consumption. Special directions were also given for the feeding of the ass which was to supply the milk.

His Grace, on rising, ought to comb his hair with an ivory comb, by which the brain was comforted, to rub his limbs, anoint his spine and chest with oil of sweet almonds, and, after dressing, to walk for a short time in some pleasant spot out of the sun.　Cardan apparently restricted the meals to two in the day, and, discussing whether breakfast or supper should be the chief meal, decided that in every man's case an established custom ought not to be broken.　He then gave a long series of minute directions upon food and cooking.　He prescribed many articles of diet which would be specially suitable for the Archbishop, with the purpose of restoring his bodily weight.　Chief on the list was tortoise or turtle soup.　The whole animal except the shell was to be stewed down with water till it was as nearly as possible dissolved.　The flesh was then to be eaten and the soup to be drunk, no other food or drink being used for about twenty days.

---

[1] The prohibition of feathers and leather is interesting, in view of the modern theory regarding the causation of some cases of asthma by proteins coming from animal materials.

Another thing which Cardan recommended as excellent was soup made from the blood of a young pig and coltsfoot leaves. Two ounces a day of this, taken with a little sugar, would fatten a man rapidly, and in Cardan's experience had been found able to bring back a hectic person from the gates of death. He also advised soup made of snails, and suggested that frogs might be employed in the kitchens of the Britons as they sometimes were in Italy. A soup, made of thick barley water with chicken broth, flavoured with wine and a little cinnamon or ginger, he also strongly recommended as an easily digested and fattening article of diet.

He added a great number of medical prescriptions to be used in various emergencies, some of them taken from the chief authorities in medicine—Greek, Roman and Arabic—and closed the list with the recommendation of an issue under each knee, to be established, however, only as a last resort if other remedies should fail.

It is evident in all this that while Cardan followed the rules established by authority, in his practical treatment of the case he really was guided by an experienced common sense. The check put upon the Archbishop's appetite, the limitation of his hours of business, the rest of ten hours in the night on a suitable bed, the morning shower-bath, a strict fast enjoined during the period of an attack, and an infrequent though nutritious diet at other times, improved the Archbishop's health quickly. Cardan remained in Edinburgh for thirty-five days after his own treatment of the Archbishop had been begun. During that time Scottish nobles flocked to him and paid liberally for his advice. From the grateful Archbishop he had already received 300 gold crowns for travelling expenses, and had been promised 10 crowns a day during his stay in Edinburgh. His Grace now gave him 1400 crowns for himself and 400 for his five attendants, as well as a gold chain worth 125 crowns, and other gifts, including a valuable horse.

In return for all this liberality, Cardan at his departure handed to the Archbishop a document distinct from the long written opinion already mentioned, containing careful and elaborate directions for the patient's private use.[1] This gave directions against all sorts of contingencies and was meant as a substitute for Cardan's own presence in Edinburgh. On his morning walk, the Archbishop was to chew a couple of tears of mastic gum to promote the beneficial flow of water from the mouth.[2] As he got better, he was to breakfast at nine o'clock, eating first the liver of a fowl with two or three grains of ginger, after that some bread soaked in gravy, and about two ounces of white wine, and afterwards he might eat at his discretion some chicken, roasted or stewed, and drink wine four or five times in the forenoon, but in all not more than ten ounces. The four hours after

---

[1] Cardan: "Consilia Medica," included in Opera, Vol. IX, p. 225 et seq.
[2] This accords well with modern American fashion.

noon were to be the hours of business, during which, however, he was not to write letters with his own hand.　　At four o'clock he was to go out for an hour's ride on horseback, and, having returned, he might give audience to persons desiring to see him.　　Towards seven o'clock he was to take the second meal of the day. This should commence with a spoonful of pure honey, and an excellent supper might often be made of bread and goat's milk, as was done by a Cardinal whom Cardan knew in Milan.　　At eight or half-past eight, the Archbishop should retire to bed and should secure ten hours of continued sleep, which would make his hour of rising about 6 a.m.　　For securing punctuality in carrying out the system laid down, Cardan suggested to His Grace to purchase a good clock, for, he said, every Italian prince had many and good clocks.　　When they parted, Archbishop Hamilton promised to follow the régime for two years, and then to send a report of the result to Cardan at Milan.

Cardan also considered it advisable to give his patient the following piece of counsel, which at the present day seems superfluous in the case of an Archbishop :—

De Venere.　　Certe non est bona, neque utilis ; ubi tamen contingat necessitas, debet uti ea inter duos somnos, scilicet post mediam noctem, et melius est exercere eam ter in sex diebus pro exemplo, ita ut singulis duobus diebus semel, quam bis in una die, etiam quod staret per decem dies.[1]

At the end of two years and one month, a Scotsman arrived in Milan, bearing a letter from the Archbishop to Cardan.　　In the course of this, His Grace said : " I thank you not only for your various and very welcome little gifts, but also for my health, that is in great part restored, for the almost complete subjugation of my disease, for strength regained ; in fine, I may say, for life recovered. All those good things, and this body of mine itself, I hold as received from you . . . the accustomed attacks now scarcely occur once a month, and sometimes once in two months ; then, too, they are not urgent and pressing, as they used to be, but are felt very slightly."

The century closed with a tragedy for the medical profession in Edinburgh. Robert Auchmowtie, cherurgeane, a burgess of Edinburgh, was indited for the slaughter in a single combat or duel of James Wauchope, son of George Wauchope of Cleghorn, a merchant burgess of Edinburgh.

The facts of this case appear to be that Auchmowtie and James Wauchope had quarrelled in April, 1600, and had agreed to meet upon St. Leonard's Crags in the King's Park, near Holyrood.　　Here a little dell on the top of an eminence formed a favourite place for such meetings. They fought with swords and Wauchope was killed.　　His relatives lodged a complaint that Auchmowtie had set upon him with two accomplices

---

[1] Cardan : " Consilia Medica," Vol. IX, p. 135.

"and maist schamefullie and crewallie, with swordis, straik him in the face and vpoune the heid, and gaif him foure bludie woundis thairon ; and thairbye maist barborouslie, crewallie and tyrannouslie slew the said vmquhile [*late*] James Vauchope, vpoune set purpois, provisioune and foirthocht fellonye." There appears, however, to have been no justification for saying that this was anything but a regular and fairly-fought duel. At the trial, various objections were lodged, and the Court appears to have been inclined to postpone and dismiss the matter.

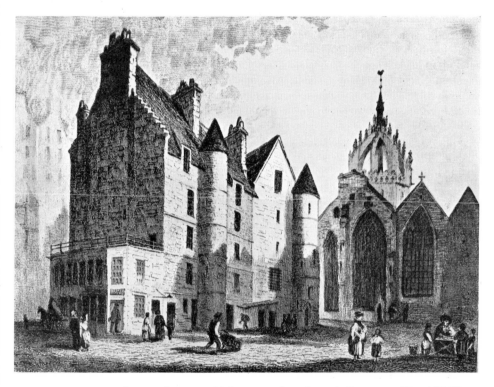

OLD TOLBOOTH (demolished in 1817), WITH ST. GILES' CHURCH, EDINBURGH

Drawn by Sir Daniel Wilson

The pursuers, however, produced three letters from King James, written to the Justice Clerk and Deputies from Stirling, in May, and from Falkland, in June, in which he urged diligence upon the Court, and finally ordered Auchmowtie to be put to an assize. The reason for the King's prejudice against Auchmowtie does not appear, but in view of these royal commands, the issue was clear, and Auchmowtie was convicted of the slaughter and condemned to death.

Still, with the dice of justice loaded against him, Auchmowtie made one more bold bid for freedom.　　Being put in ward in the Tolbooth, he declared that he was sick and could not bear the light.　　He hung one cloak outside the bars of his window and another on the inner side and " he had *aqua fortis* continuallie seithing at the irone window, quhill at lest the irone window wes eittine throw."　　Then one morning he arranged with his prentice to give him a signal by waving his handkerchief at the time when the Town Guard was removed, and hanging out a rope, he prepared to descend.　　The Guard, unfortunately, had seen the signal, and so Auchmowtie was recaptured. He was beheaded at the Market Cross.[1]

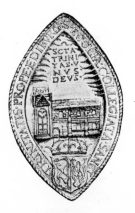

SEAL OF TRINITY HOSPITAL
After the Reformation

---

[1] Pitcairn : " Criminal Trials in Scotland," Vol. II, pp. 112–124.

CHAPTER V

EARLY PUBLIC HEALTH REGULATIONS AND THE PLAGUE

In the year 1498, the plague, which had appeared in the south of Europe about a century and a half previously, attained alarming dimensions in Edinburgh, and a series of regulations was made by the Town Council with the object of stamping it out in the city. The regulations began on 28th March, 1498, and on 17th November, 1498, the Provost, Baillies and Council, referring to the danger of perilous sickness or pestilence now risen in the east part and largely spread, forbade anyone in the burgh to harbour or receive any traveller on foot or horseback, rich or poor, without first obtaining permission from the Baillies, the penalty for contravention being confiscation of all goods and banishment from the town.

Glasgow seems to have been suspected of harbouring the plague, because anyone passing to Glasgow without permission was subject to quarantine of forty days outside the town. In the following year, further regulations were made against bringing in merchandise, such as wool, skins, hides, or cloth or any kind of food, without permission of the Baillies. Some of the parishes close to Edinburgh, as well as Haddington and Kelso, were in this year afflicted by the plague and it was forbidden to receive any persons coming from these places. Contravention of these regulations was to be punished by branding on the cheek and banishing from the town.

In 1499, the plague appears to have broken out in Edinburgh, and more stringent regulations were adopted. Dogs and " swyne " were to be kept " in hous and band," or, if found in the streets and lanes, were to be slaughtered. Children under fifteen years of age were forbidden to wander in the streets under pain of being put in the stocks and beaten. The schools were to be closed, the booths were not to be opened nor markets to be held, and intercourse with Leith was forbidden. The following is the text of the regulations introduced to deal with these matters[1] :—

6 FEBRUARY, 1499

" It is avysit and statute, in augmentatioun of the first statute,[2] that na maner of persoun pas furth of this toune to bye or bring in within this towne ony maner of merchandise, sic as woll, skynnis, hyds, or clayth, bot gif thai haif licence of the baillies and counsale, and with that that thai bring sufficient testimonialls that thai ar cum in furth of clene places, vnder the payne of byrning of the stufe and halding furth of the persouns brekares of this statute furth of the town.

" Item, that na maner of stufe nor victuallis be brocht nor resauit into this towne out of na maner of suspect places, vnder payne of byrning and banesing of the bringares.

---

[1] " Extracts from the Records of the Burgh of Edinburgh, 1403-1528," pp. 72, 74-76.
[2] 17th November 1498.

27 April, 1499

"It is statute and forbidden that ony persouns dwelling within this towne howse harbery or resett ony persouns of Hadingtoun (or) Kelso, considering the seikness is largelie spred thair, vnder the payne of deid, and als that nane of thame cum within this towne vnder payne of byrning on thair cheiks with hett yrne and banesing furth of the same.

"Item, that na maner of persoun indwellare of this towne pas till Peblis for ony maner of airandis without leif askit and obtenit fra the officeris, provest or baillies, vnder the payne of withalding furth of the town and banesing but favouris."

8 June, 1499

"It is statute and ordanit that all maner of persouns within this burgh, haffand dogs or swyne, sall observe and keip thame in hous and band, swa that quhair thai may be fundin in the contrair within this burgh, in hie streits or venellis, thai to be slayne be the persouns limit thairto.

"Item, that na maner of bairnis within xv yeirs of aige be fundin on the gaitt or in streitts or in the kirk, vagand, vnder the payne to the said bairnis of putting of thame in the stoks and scurgeing of thame with wands.

"Item, it is forbidden that ony scholes be halden be ony maner of persouns, men or women, vnder the payne to the haldare of bannesing this towne.

"Item, it is forbidden that ony maner of buithes be oppin to mak merchandice into, or that ony merkett be maid at the ports of this burgh or thairabout, vnder the payne of escheitt of the guidis quhair it may be fundin, bot favouris.

"Item, that all persouns of this towne haiffand ony vittales of corn, wyne and floure in Leyth, that thai bring up the samyn to this towne in all guidlie and possibill haist, for thai heif declairit to the keperis and rewlares of Leyth that thai latt in na persouns thairin to by ony maner of vittales."

In 1499, the Magistrates became much concerned with regard to the dirty state of the city, and in November of that year they appointed several cleansers to clean houses with a view to disinfection, at a cost of ten shillings to men of substance, five shillings to others, and to the poor according to their faculty of paying. The official cleansers were to have for wages twelve pence daily, a large sum in those days for a day labourer, because the work was arduous and dangerous.

In the beginning of the next year (1500), the Provost and Baillies made further regulations with regard to houses and clothing presumed to be infected. The chief means of disinfection was an order to wash furniture and clothing in the running Water of Leith, washing in the various lochs round the town being forbidden. The official cleansers were now five in number, and they were to carry, as a badge of office, a little wand with a hoop of white iron at the end. They were to hear mass in the Hospital of St. Mary's Wynd, and their wages were now reduced to six pence a day, but they were to have fees for burials and the cleansing of houses.[1]

On 27th September, 1509, a more definite arrangement regarding the town cleansing was reached. Thomas Jhonstoun and Jhone Broun were appointed

---

[1] pp. 76–78: " Extracts from the Records of the Burgh of Edinburgh, 1403–1528."

cleansers, with the duty of keeping the High Street clean from the Castlehill to the head of Leith Wynd, and of setting down yearly forty roods of new causeway wherever it should be most required. For this service each inhabitant of the High Street was assessed four pence in the year, while fleshers and fishmongers, because of " thair inhonestie and filth of the same," were to pay sixteen pence in the year, with additional charges for the cleansing of their stands.[1]   Still later, in 1527, a whole-time officer in the person of Alexander Pennecuik was appointed to see that the causeway was " dicht and clengeit sufficiently " every eight days, being provided with twelve servants for this purpose, and receiving the sum of twenty pounds yearly.[2]

Stringent regulations were made in the year 1500 against servants buying clothing without the knowledge of their master or mistress, against the holding of markets until the ensuing St. Giles' Day, and against receiving any goods from the country without leave of the town's officers.   Beggars and vagabonds not provided with tokens from the Magistracy were ordered to leave the town on pain of death.   The penalty to the citizens for disobeying these regulations was branding on the cheek and banishing from the town, in the case of a woman, while a man was to have his hand struck off and similarly to be banished.[3]

These penalties were no idle threat, for on 31st December, 1502, there is a note that a certain Harvy was convicted of breaking the acts of the town, for which he was adjudged to be taken to the Tron, have his hand struck off and be banished from the town.   It does not say what specific act he broke, but it appears from the context that he had broken some of the regulations directed against the plague.[4] Also on 27th May, 1521, a certain Bessye Symourtoun, who was taken by the watch in the act of hiding plague-infected gear under a pile of wood at the end of Fowler's Close, was adjudged to be branded on the cheek and banished from the town.[5]

As time went on and the plague approached nearer to Edinburgh, the regulations of the Town Council became more strict.   In 1502, people other than officerswere for bidden to hold any intercourse with infected persons in the town, under the usual penalties, and everyone appearing after 9 o'clock at night in the High Street had to carry a light.[6]   Any persons or goods which had been taken to the Water of Leith for cleansing had to receive a permit in writing to re-enter the town, and the space of time which had to elapse for cleansing and drying the goods was eight to ten days, after which an isolation period of five or six days had to be passed in the house.   Before re-entry to the house, fumigation with heather was ordained.

The persons employed to bury the dead were forbidden to mix with the other citizens.[7]   It is interesting that three days after the Seal of Cause had

---

[1] pp. 124 and 125, [2] p. 232, [3] p. 78, [4] p. 96, [5] p. 204, [6] p. 96. [7] pp. 100 and 101: " Extracts from the Records of the Burgh of Edinburgh, 1403–1528."

been granted to the Surgeons and Barbers, viz., on 4th July, 1505, a number of further regulations were made in regard to plague. The first example of notification of an infectious disease occurs in the rules that all cases of plague must be revealed to the officers of the town within twenty-four hours of onset.[1] Three months later the duty of notification was imposed upon the " folkis haiffand the rewle and gouernance of that house," and the time for notification was shortened to twelve hours, under pains of branding and banishing.[2]

An officer was provided with a horse and close cart and two servants to cleanse the High Street daily, and it was forbidden to leave any filth on the street longer than twenty-four hours. The sale of second-hand clothes and the shaking or hanging of skins in front of houses was forbidden.[3]

The plague seems to have died out for some time, but on 14th October, 1512, the Magistrates appear to have thought it necessary to recapitulate all the rules in regard to notification of cases of the plague, exclusion of strangers, shutting up of dogs and swine, cleansing of infected goods, etc., and on the 17th January following, a letter, under the Great Seal, was issued by James IV., containing practically the same provisions. In this letter a quarantine period of forty days is imposed upon infected persons.[4] In 1514, the town was divided into four quarters assigned to four baillies for supervision.[5]

It appears that the practice of using the Burgh Muir for disinfection, and also for burying persons dead of the plague, had gradually grown up. All goods to be disinfected, and corpses to be buried, were to be removed between nine in the evening and five in the morning.[6]   Beggars and others who were excluded from the town had apparently taken up their quarters in houses and barns on the Burgh Muir, which, therefore, were ordered by the Town Council to be unroofed on 3rd April, 1520.[7]   As time went on, the regulations against possible infection became stronger and on 27th August, 1519, it was ordained by the Town Council that persons coming from suspected places or entering the burgh with pestilence upon them would do so under pain of death.[8]

After this time the plague again seems to have died out for some years, but in 1529 the regulations against infection were renewed. Dundee, Perth, Cupar and other towns beyond the Forth were now suspected, and no one was to come to the Fair of Hallowmass from these places.[9] Alane Blair having, despite these regulations, come from the town of St. Andrews, the Provost and Baillies were graciously pleased to have " dispensit wit his lyf," but they banished him from the town for all the days of his life under pain of death.[10] Dauid Scot, who had entered the town, despite his having been twice banished before for breaking of the plague statutes, was now scourged and banished anew for all the days of his life under

---

[1] pp. 104 and 105, [2] p. 106, [3] pp. 105–107, [4] pp. 136–141, [5] pp. 149 and 150, [6] pp. 176 and 177, [7] p. 196, [8] p. 190 " Extracts from the Records of the Burgh ol Edinburgh, 1403–1528."
[9], [10] pp. 10 and 11 : "Extracts from the Records of the Burgh of Edinburgh, 1528–1557."

pain of death.[1]   In this year the plague was apparently severe in St. Andrews, for not only were Edinburgh citizens forbidden to cross the Forth, but they were forbidden to receive anyone from St. Andrews under pain of death.[1]

Margaret Cok, being convicted by an assize of coming from St. Andrews with infected gear, was branded on both cheeks, her clothes burned, and herself banished from the town, under pain of death.[2]   A similar regulation was passed with regard to St. Monance on 20th February, 1530, and numerous other banishments are recorded about this time.[3]

Despite all these stringent regulations, the plague appears to have broken out in the city in May, 1530.   The regulations were again promulgated, communication with St. Andrews, wandering of swine about the town, and bringing in of clothing forbidden.   It was found that great filth had accumulated both on the High Street and in the closes as well as in the gutters of the town, and therefore every man and woman was bidden to " dicht and mak clene befor ther durris and closis," under pain of banishment at the Provost's pleasure.

At the same time, Issobell Forsyth, who had mixed with infected folk and taken the sickness herself, was branded on the cheek, banished for life from the town, and meantime ordained to be taken to the Burgh Muir until she should be recovered. Issobell Cattall also, for keeping secret the sickness of her daughter within her house for three days without revealing it to the officers of the town, was branded, and she with all her children was banished from the town to remain meantime on the Burgh Muir until they were cleansed.[4]

The striking off of the hand of male offenders does not seem, however, to have been so rigorously enforced, for on 25th June, 1530, George M'Turk and Male Mudy, his spouse, Marione Suddirland and Alisone Bird, for having a child sick in their house for three days without revealing it to the officers until the child died, were all branded on the cheek, while Marione Suddirland, who was supposed to have been the source of the infection, was banished for life under pain of death, and the other three banished during the town's pleasure.

Patrik Gowanlok, for harbouring an infected woman for ten days in the lodging of the Abbot of Melrose, was banished for ever, while the servant, Jonet Cowane, who was the cause of the trouble, was sentenced to be branded on both cheeks and banished.   A general invitation was issued to those of the townspeople who liked to see justice executed, to come incontinently to the Greyfriars Port where they would see this carried out.[5]   After three months' banishment, the Provost and Baillies relented and allowed Patrik Gowanlok to " cum and duell within this toune as he wes wont till do."   There appears, however, to have been no relenting towards Jonet Cowane.[6]

---

[1] pp. 15 and 16, [2] p. 19, [3] p. 20, [4] pp. 28–30, [5] pp. 35–37, [6] p. 42 : " Extracts from the Records of the Burgh of Edinburgh, 1528–1557."

An aggravated offence was committed by Dauid Duly, tailor, who had kept his wife, being sick of the plague, for two days in his house until she died, without revealing the same to the officers, and in the meantime had gone to mass at St. Giles' Kirk on Sunday " amangis the cleyne pepill, his wife beand *in extremis* in the said seiknes." As, in the opinion of the Town Council, he had done what was in him to infect all the town, he was adjudged to be hanged on a gibbet before his own door. The Council, however, seems to have been somewhat half-hearted in its wrath, because after the gibbet had been erected, it is related that Dauid " at the will of God eschapit," through the rope having broken. As he was " ane pure man with small bairns," the Provost and Baillies took pity on him and commuted his sentence to banishment for life. Willie Myllar, another tailor, for putting out of his house a woman sick of the plague without revealing this to the officers of the town, on the same day received the lesser punishment of being branded on the cheek and banished from the town.[1]

It was evidently regarded as a very serious crime for anyone who was sick or who was in contact with the sick, to appear at Church, and in October of this year Marione Clerk was tried by an assize for appearing at mass in the Chapel of St. Mary's Wynd, and for going to her sister's house and other places while the pestilence was upon her. For this she was adjudged to be taken to " the quarell hollis, and thair to be drounit quhill scho be deid."[2] Issobell Bowy and Kate Boyd, who had been shut up in their houses for suspicion of the plague, were tried for having opened a feather bed and sold half a stone of feathers to Besse Andirsone, thus running the risk of infecting the whole town, for which the three women were banished.[3]

During this epidemic, many people fled from the town, and were forbidden to return without permission from the Council. At various periods, edicts were issued for cleansing the goods of persons who had remained. There are numerous references to infected persons being transferred to the Burgh Muir south of the town (the district now occupied by Bruntsfield Links, the Grange and North Morningside, southwards to the Jordan or Pow Burn and eastwards to Dalkeith Road).

The favourite place for cleansing goods was in the Water of Leith at Drumsheugh.[4] The goods and clothes of infected people in the Muir were apparently stored in St. Roch's Chapel (which stood near the present Grange Loan) and an intimation was made in December, 1530, that people could now claim these, or if they were unclaimed, they were to be burned.[5] In the severe epidemic which again broke out in 1585, St. Roch's Chapel was used as an isolation place for persons suspected of having the plague.[6]

---

[1] pp. 35–37, [2] p. 43, [3] p. 42, [4] pp. 37–39, [5] p. 45 : " Extracts from the Records of the Burgh of Edinburgh, 1528–1557."
[6] p. 416 : " Extracts," 1573–1589."

Persons who had been taken to the Burgh Muir for isolation were forbidden to come back to town, and especially to St. Giles's Church, until they had a licence from the Baillies. In September, 1530, the Provost and Baillies intimated that although, through pity, several persons had not been punished for concealing the plague, they would be visited with still severer pains in the future for any failure to comply with the strict regulations.[1]   As a result of the strict measures which had been taken, the Town Council was able to announce on 8th October, 1530, that all danger was over and that there had been no appearance of any infection for eight days past.   Still they thought it was " verray proffittable " that the rules should be observed for a year to come.[2]

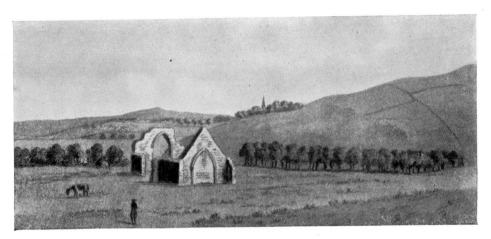

CHAPEL OF ST. ROCH

In the Burgh Muir of Edinburgh early in the 19th Century

In the next few years the regulations are mainly concerned with care to keep out the plague, which was still prevalent in other places.   Intercourse with Leith, where the plague was still active at the end of 1530, was forbidden.[3] Various regulations were passed regarding cleansing.[4]   Ships coming from Bordeaux, Spain and other places from which wine was imported, from Dantzig especially, and from various other towns where plague was rife, were forbidden to come to land, and watches were set at Newhaven and Leith for the purpose of preventing this.   The plan of dealing with these ships appears to have been to allow them to land their goods for a time upon one of the islands in the Forth, and after an interval to allow the goods to be brought into one of the ports.[5]

---

[1] p. 41, [2] p. 43, [3] pp. 44 and 45, [4] p. 120, [5] pp. 227 and 228 : " Extracts from the Records of the Burgh of Edinburgh, 1528–1557."

There seems to have been a small outbreak of plague also about 1568, when the sick were again isolated on the Burgh Muir. Cleansers for clothes and houses were appointed at a salary of eight pounds monthly, and buriers of the dead at five pounds each. These were provided with a gown of grey, bearing a white St. Andrew's Cross on front and back, and with a staff having a white cloth on the end. Two biers were furnished, covered with black and carrying a bell so that people might be given warning of the approach of a plague-stricken corpse. Bodies buried in the Greyfriars Churchyard were to be interred at a depth of seven feet. Persons wishing to visit their friends on the Muir were allowed to do so at eleven in the forenoon in company with the officer appointed for the day, but at no other time.[1] It is interesting to note that eight days were apparently regarded as the necessary isolation period, for there is a notice that, in 1564, George Younger, furrier, after being cleansed, was ordained to pass to some quiet house outside the town for the space of eight days and thereafter, if in good health, was to be allowed to resort to the town.[2]

In 1568, one of the regulations was that any person falling sick within the burgh, no matter what the sickness was, must, along with all those in the house, remain there until the Baillie of the quarter had been notified and his instructions received. When it was discovered that the house was infected with plague, the whole household with their goods were forthwith dispatched to the Muir, the dead buried, and the houses cleansed.[3] Wooden huts had been built for the reception of the sick on the Muir, to which they, as well as suspects at a later date, were immediately conveyed from the town. Various references are made to a Baillie being in charge of the sick folk on the Muir, and an official cleanser was also established here. In November, 1568, Jhonn Forrest was put in charge of the cleansing on the Muir, and the post was so responsible that his appointment was made on terms of the pain of death for any fault.[4] This outbreak died out in the winter of 1569, when Jhonn Legait, master of the deserted Muir, was cleansed, brought home and paid.[5] On 30th December, 1569, an announcement was made that the pest was over, and that all who had been sick in the hospital of the Senys Convent were to be taken to the Muir and cleansed.[6]

Another outbreak of the plague took place in 1574, beginning in October of that year at Leith, and being present also at Kirkcaldy. The Town Council of Edinburgh ordained anew that any sick should go to the hospital at Senys, and ordered vagabonds to leave the town within forty-eight hours. On 15th November, 1574, Jhonn Forrest, cordinar (shoemaker), was again elected to be master cleanser of the " folkis mendit of the pest, and to haue the charge of thair guddis and of the tovne mure." He was to have a servant, to receive six

---

[1] pp. 253-255, [2] p. 184, [3] p. 255, [4] p. 256, [5] p. 265, [6] p. 267 : " Extracts from the Records of the Burgh of Edinburgh, 1557-1571."

pounds monthly, to keep the people under his charge isolated, clean their goods in sufficient manner, and to work under the ominous regulation that if any infection should happen afterwards through insufficient cleansing of the said goods, he was " to suffer the deith thairfor." At the same time, a more efficient method of disinfection was introduced by the Town Council, who authorised their treasurer to buy a cauldron for cleansing of the foul goods. This method of disinfection by boiling was adopted in all subsequent outbreaks of the plague.[1] In the following January, a house called " lytill Loundoun " on the links at Leith was prepared for the cleansed people on the said links, and the house was to be watched night and day that no one should enter except the officers deputed by the town for the purpose.[2] This outbreak was over by 18th February, 1575, when the sick were brought back to town.[3]

Still another outbreak was threatened in the autumn of 1580, by ships coming from Dantzig, and from Bruges and Maine, in the Low Countries. Elaborate rules were made as to the isolation of their crews and disinfection of their goods on the islands in the Firth of Forth.[4] By the end of the year this threatened attack was over, and those who had been isolated on Inchkeith and Inchcolm were allowed to return.[5]

In the middle of 1584, plague again threatened at Wemyss and other places on the north shore of the Forth. Androw Sclater and James Henrysoun, chirurgeane, on 22nd July, 1584, were sent to see the conditions in Wester Wemyss so that the Council might take the steps necessary to avoid the pest. Regulations were instituted against bringing goods from Flanders, for the examination of persons coming ashore at Leith, and forbidding any intercourse with Dysart, Kirkcaldy or Wemyss.[6]

The people of Edinburgh appear to have been very charitable with regard to the plague-stricken poor in other places, for in August, 1584, a collection was made for the sick at Wemyss; in December, for the sick at Perth; and in May, 1585, the large sum of £201 was collected from the advocates and their servants, and £43 from the writers, on behalf of the sick in the latter place.[7] In October, 1584, two burgesses were sent to inspect the town of Dysart with regard to the occurrence of plague, and, following upon their report that Dysart was in need of help, the Town Council of Edinburgh sent them a present of food and almost one ton of soap.[8] At last, in April, 1585, a woman died at Edinburgh in the Fish Market Close. Despite the fact that all those who had been in contact with her were isolated in their house, and that the usual regulations for cleansing streets, preventing swine from wandering, etc., were enforced, two of the contacts died. The house was cleansed with

---

[1] pp. 28–30, [2] p. 35, [3] p. 36, [4] pp. 178–181, [5] pp. 189, 556 and 557, [6] pp. 344, 345, 346, 347 and 351, [7] pp. 346, 381, 418 and 419, [8] pp. 358 and 360 : " Extracts from the Records of the Burgh of Edinburgh, 1573–1589."

diligence, the contacts were now transferred to a house near St. Roch's Chapel, but, notwithstanding, the plague broke out.   A gibbet was set up on the Muir, apparently to form a visible reminder of the public health regulations. A temporary hospital consisting of wooden huts was set up near the Kirk of the Seynis, and five or six other shelters were built on the Muir.   The anxiety of the Baillies was now thoroughly roused.   Alexander Fraynche, the "clenger," was exhorted to be true and diligent in his office on the Muir, and he was promised, as a reward for diligent execution of his duties, a house, rent-free, and a pension for life.   The Council also ordered Dustefute (the hangman) to slay all swine, dogs and cats wherever he might apprehend them.   The Council further decided to meet every day for urgent business connected with the plague.

The Muir appears to have been divided into two parts, the clean or west Muir (St. Roch's Hospital), where contacts were isolated, and the foul or east Muir (Sienna or Sciennes Hospital) where the sick were treated.

The Chapel of St. Roque, or Roch (in Gaelic "Maroch"), at the bridge-end of had been founded by James IV. in 1499, and dedicated to the "Patron of Stirling Pestilences."   The Chapel of St. Roque on the Burgh Muir at Edinburgh was established by the same monarch some years later, and around it an isolation station, for "contacts" with the plague, was formed at various times during the 16th century.[1]

In 1532, the Hospital of St. Laurence, situated on the west side of the Royal Burgh of Haddington was formally annexed to the Nunnery of the Sciennes. This Hospital had been founded by Richard Guthrie, Abbot of the Monastery of St. Thomas at Arbroath, and out of the revenues a contribution had been made annually to the burgh leper-house at Haddington.   The Haddington Hospital was apparently closed shortly afterwards.   This must have been a small hospital, as the annual value of its revenues did not exceed £9 sterling.[2]   The Hospital of the Sciennes was some years later used for the treatment of cases of plague.

Although it is probable that in previous outbreaks, the town had always consulted some of the surgeons with regard to treatment and isolation regulations for the sick, the Baillies now, on 26th May, 1585, definitely appointed James Henrysoun, chirurgeane, to take care of the sick, to visit all the hospitals of the burgh and the poor who were sick or hurt, whatever their sickness might be. He was to be at the disposal of the Council day and night, and the town was to furnish him with whatever "vngnents, drogs, implasteris and vther mendicaments" he might require.   He was to have a yearly stipend of twenty pounds for life. Jhonn Forrest was again appointed cleanser on the clean Muir at ten pounds per month, with various assistants and watchmen.   Leave of absence was granted

---

[1] Moir Bryce : "The Burgh Muir of Edinburgh," Old Edinburgh Club, Edinburgh, 1918, p. 172.
[2] Moir Bryce : "The Burgh Muir of Edinburgh," Old Edinburgh Club, Edinburgh, 1918, p. 122.

to Robert Rollok and Duncane Nairne, the masters of the College, to leave the town, because all the students had fled through fear of the pestilence. Other measures taken were the erection of a gibbet on the western Muir, the purchase of a small kettle for disinfecting the clothes of the poor, the erection of a wooden shed at the Greyfriars port to keep infected goods, the housing of homeless children in the Chapel of St. Mary's Wynd, the raising by tax of one thousand pounds for the support of the sick poor, and distribution of food to the latter. A curious regulation was that the sale of " any sybois, leiks or vngyeouns " (sives, leeks or onions) was prohibited during the plague. There were instances of private charity, as, for example, that the tenants of the Laird of Inverleith in the West Port and Potterrow, who took sick, were placed on a separate part of the Muir at his expense.[1] Robert Fairlie of Braid also offered his house of " Littill Egipt," near the Muir for any suitable use.[2] The Council ordered a heavy bier to be employed for burying the dead on the Muir, and forbade that bodies should be carried upon the backs of men or on sledges through the laziness of the buriers. Apparently some of the officials on the Muir had not behaved themselves, for in July, 1585, Smythtie, " the fowle hangman," was ordained to be laid in irons and bound to the gibbet till further order, while the rest of the servants on the Muir who had not obeyed the orders of the Baillies were to be discharged.

The isolation period was increased in August, 1585, to fifteen days, and anyone returning from the Muir was to remain in his house for this period before he mixed with the townspeople generally. All gatherings at this time, except at Kirk and market, were forbidden, and there appears to have been a great scarcity of town officers and of ministers, even the Provost having absented himself from the town.[3] On 17th December, 1585, the plague had so far abated that the Council was able to place the infected persons in a single house (the White House) which they leased for a certain time. For further purification of suspected goods, it was ordered, in December, 1585, that all such suspected of infection, even if they had been cleansed, should be laid out in yards or other suitable places during the time of the frost.[4] The timber used in the lodges on the Muir was brought in next spring and stored in a vault of the Town's College against the outbreak of some further epidemic.[5] James Henrysoun, chirurgeane, was thanked for his good services, especially as he had contracted the plague himself and had lost his wife from the same cause. He was exempted from all burgh taxes for the rest of his life.[6]

Once again, in November, 1587, the pest appeared at Leith, and the usual regulations were adopted. The gibbets were set up in the town, a watch was kept on the gates to prevent the entrance of undesirable persons, and the sick were taken to the hospital of the Seynis. This outbreak, however, does not appear to have been of any great severity.[7] There were various other smaller outbreaks, as,

---

[1] pp. 413–426, [2] p. 436, [3] pp. 430–434, [4] pp. 444 and 445, [5] p. 452, [6] pp. 436 and 437, [7] pp. 504–506 : " Extracts from the Records of the Burgh of Edinburgh, 1573–1589."

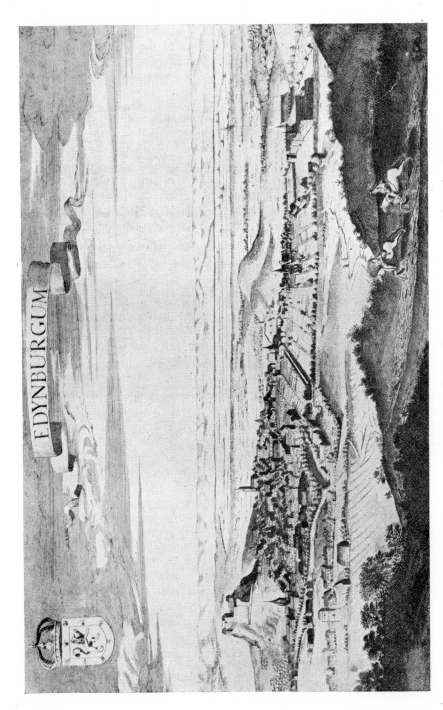

VIEW OF EDINBURGH FROM THE SOUTH-EAST, EARLY IN THE 17TH CENTURY
Showing the beginning of the Burgh Muir in the left foreground
(From an engraving by Rombout van den Hoyen)

for example, when in 1593 a ship from an English port, with persons suspected of the plague, was quarantined at Inchcolm.   Again in 1597, the pest began in Leith, and many persons fled from Edinburgh, but the epidemic was over by the end of the harvest.[1]

During the latter half of the 16th century, Aberdeen had remained curiously immune from the plague.   This may have been in large part due to the severe regulations which had been early introduced.   In May, 1585, the Magistrates had erected three gibbets, "ane at the mercat cross, ane other at the brig of Dee, and the third at the haven mouth, that in case ony infectit person arrive or repair by sea or land to this burgh, or in case ony indweller of this burgh receive, house, or harbour, or give meat or drink to the infectit person or persons, the man be hangit and the woman drownit."[2]

From 1603 to 1609, plague was present in one place or another throughout Scotland, but there was no serious epidemic.   In 1644, it again appeared in Edinburgh, Kelso, Bo'ness, Perth and other places.   At Edinburgh the plague-stricken were housed in huts in the King's Park below Salisbury Crags, and at Perth the epidemic is said to have given rise to the story of Bessie Bell and Mary Gray, who fled from the plague-stricken city and "biggit a bower on yon burn brae, and theekit it ower wi' rashes."[3]   At Glasgow, the infection was severe from 1646 to 1648, but this year is the last in which plague is heard of in Scotland.[2]

It is surprising that in their regulations against dogs and swine and dirt in the streets, and the chance of infection by persons coming to the town, the Baillies of Edinburgh did not suspect the rats as a possible cause of plague.   The black rat which brought plague into Europe from the East in the 14th century had reached Scotland before the 16th century, and was plentiful in many places throughout the country.

A curious fact which may explain the comparative immunity of the northern city from the plague is that rats were unable to subsist in Aberdeen. Bishop Leslie, in 1578, records in regard to Aberdeenshire: "In this cuntrey na Rattoune is bred, or, brocht in frome ony vthir place, thair may lyue [live]."   A similar fact is recorded in the 17th century with regard to Sutherlandshire, and in Liddesdale the same tradition was long preserved.[4]

---

[1] Creighton : "History of Epidemics in Britain," I, p. 369.
[2] Creighton : "History of Epidemics in Britain," I, pp. 371 and 563.
[3] Chambers : "Domestic Annals of Scotland," Vol. II, pp. 166 and 167
[4] Ritchie : "Animal Life in Scotland," p. 426.

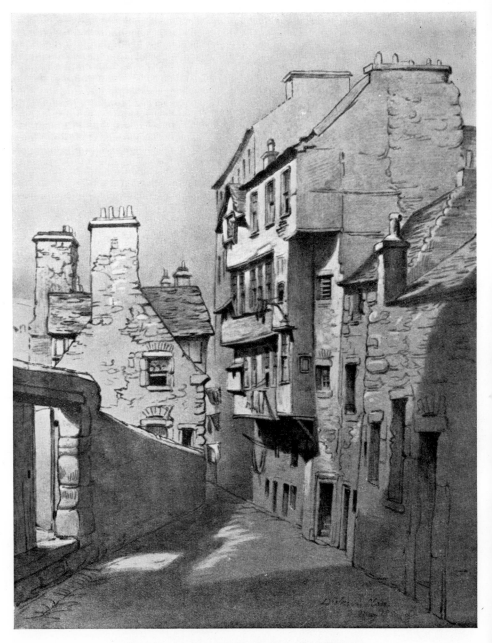

HOUSE IN DICKSON'S CLOSE, EDINBURGH
(From a sketch by James Drummond, R.S.A., in 1850)

Where in 1647 "three rowmes of ane tenement" were taken as a Convening House for the surgeons and barbers
The stair and walls are still standing (1927), though the timber front has been removed

CHAPTER VI

THE SURGEONS OF EDINBURGH IN THE SEVENTEENTH CENTURY

AFTER the recognition of the combined surgeons and barbers as one of the guilds of craftsmen in Edinburgh, a definite history commences, which has extended up to the present day. The united guild originally stood ninth or tenth in order of seniority, but, partly by virtue of its important nature and partly owing to the high social position of the surgeons included in it, the guild of surgeons and barbers gradually attained the first position. Under Gilbert Primrose as Deacon, in 1582, this craft took precedence as the first of fourteen then in existence. Many of the surgeons were men of wealth and owned lands near Edinburgh, such as James Borthwick of Stow, Alexander Pennycuik of Newhall, and Christopher Irving of Bonschaw. During the 17th century, three Deacons of the surgeons, viz., James Borthwick, in 1661, Arthur Temple, in 1669, and George Stirling, in 1689, held the position of one of the two members returned by Edinburgh to the Scottish Parliament.[1]

The place of meeting of the crafts at this time was the Magdalen Chapel in the Cowgate, which belonged to the Guild of Hammermen. From the year 1581, also, the barber-surgeons appear to have held regular meetings, of which they kept minutes, and in this year the craft included sixteen masters, together with their apprentices.

It should be mentioned in passing that the surgeons signed the National Covenant on 25th August, 1638, and ordained all their apprentices and servants to subscribe it as well, declaring that no apprentice or servant should be admitted in future except such as should subscribe the Covenant.

Shortly after this time, a change took place in the nature of the craft. Pharmacy was now taught along with the art of surgery, whereas previously a surgeon had sometimes been an apothecary as well, but, as a rule, had not. The apothecary's calling appears to have been regarded as of higher standing than that of the surgeon, if we may judge from the fact that James Borthwick, who had been a very prominent member of the surgeons' incorporation, was described on his tombstone as "pharmacopœus" only.[2] Troubles also arose in connection with the extension of the city, for the rights of monopoly possessed by the surgeons and barbers in Edinburgh did not extend to the Canongate and other suburbs. It must be remembered that, at this time, anyone who desired to practise medicine and surgery in Scotland might do so without let or hindrance,

---

[1] John Gairdner, M.D. : "Historical Sketch of the Royal College of Surgeons of Edinburgh," Edinburgh, 1860, p. 10.
[2] Maitland: "History of Edinburgh," p. 193.

so long as he did not invade the district in and around Glasgow supervised by the Faculty of Physicians and Surgeons, or practise as a barber-surgeon in one of the burghs where a guild existed. The necessary qualification elsewhere consisted simply in the ability to obtain patients.

From 1657 onwards, when Borthwick and Kincaid set up as surgeon-apothecaries, pharmacy had a greater attraction to the apprentices than the barber craft. Barber-surgeons who practised shaving, hair-cutting and minor surgery thus fell off in numbers, so much so that in 1682 the Town Council made a complaint to the incorporation that there were only six barbers following the trade within the city walls.[1] The change in medical practice in Edinburgh at this time was a very complicated one. Simple barbers, as they were called, who had no desire to practise minor surgery, set up shops ; simple apothecaries also, who did not practise surgery, possessed shops for the sale of spices, drugs and similar commodities. A careful watch was kept by the incorporation of surgeons upon these to see that the privileges of the incorporation were not invaded, and numerous prosecutions took place and fines were levied. The simple barbers, whose trade in wig-making at the end of the 17th century had, owing to the prevailing fashion, become very profitable, wished to be free of surgery and the surgeons; and

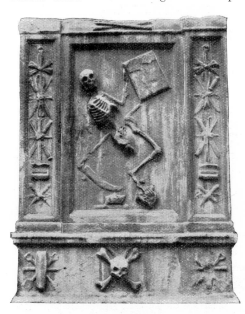

JAMES BORTHWICK'S TOMBSTONE IN GREYFRIARS CHURCHYARD, EDINBURGH

Note the 17th century representations of surgical instruments in the panels

accordingly, as the result of an action brought in 1718, a final cleavage between these two crafts took place. In 1682, the apothecaries had come under the protection of the College of Physicians, founded in 1681, and could to a large extent bid defiance to the surgeons, so long as they did not grossly offend by performing any serious operation.

In other parts of Scotland, the surgeon-apothecary, during the course of the 17th century, became the type of practitioner who looked after the health of the community, and lost all connection with the calling of the barber. His training consisted solely in an apprenticeship, usually of five years, to an

[1] C. H. Creswell: "The Royal College of Surgeons of Edinburgh," Edinburgh, 1926, p. 103.

established practitioner, although, in the case of a man who wished to attain reputation and success in practice, he had usually taken occasion in his youth to hear lectures at one of the Universities or in some Continental Medical School.

On 22nd May, 1778, a charter was granted to the incorporation, embodying it anew under the name and title of the Royal College of Surgeons of the City of Edinburgh, and thus the final separation from barbers on the one hand and apothecaries on the other was legally ratified. In 1798, the College petitioned the East India Company to recognise a diploma issued by the College as sufficient evidence of qualification for appointment to their service without further examination, and this request was granted. About 1808, the diploma was similarly recognised by the Army Medical Board after a revisal of the laws relative to examination in 1806. More stringent regulations regarding the diploma were made in 1816 ; and after the passing of the Medical Act of 1858, the College of Surgeons and the College of Physicians instituted a double qualification. In 1884, these two Colleges joined with the Faculty of Physicians and Surgeons

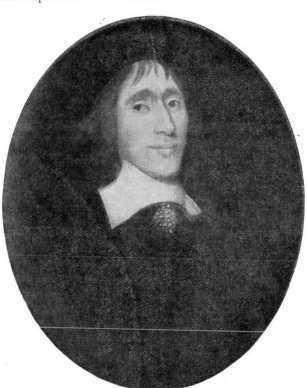

JAMES BORTHWICK (1615–1675)
(Original in the Royal College of Surgeons, Edinburgh)

of Glasgow to establish the Triple Qualification by which the licentiates of all three bodies might have the qualification necessary for practice, viz., of holding a diploma in both medicine and surgery.

From an early period of its existence, the craft of surgeons and barbers had taken an interest in the study of anatomy, and had been granted, in 1505, the privilege in this respect conveyed by the Seal of Cause. In terms of the Seal of Cause, instruction in anatomy was given by the members in rotation for more than a century, but when we come to the year 1645 we find for the first time a

definite teacher of Anatomy mentioned.   In this year James Borthwick, a burgess
of Edinburgh, having duly passed his examination, was admitted as a Master
Surgeon for the special purpose of " desceting of anatomie for the farder instruction of prentissis and servandis."   Borthwick's admission was a special one :
he paid 200 pounds of entry fee instead of the statutory five pounds.[1]   Instead
of the usual apprenticeship, he had served abroad as a surgeon along with Alexander
Pennycuik.   Pennycuik was Deacon of the Craft in 1645, and had been surgeon
to General Banner (Commander of the Swedish Forces in the Thirty Years' War),
and later Chirurgeon-General to the Auxiliary Scots Army in England during the
Civil War, and to the Scots troops with Prince Charles in 1650.[2]   A petition of
1663, which indicates the important military services of Alexander Pennycuik,
was recommended by Commissioners after the Civil War for payment by His
Majesty Charles II.   Pennycuik had accompanied the Scottish Army, fighting
for Charles II., and had been present at the battles of Preston and Worcester.   He
petitioned for a sum of £3668 6s. 8d. as balance of pay and disbursements made
by him during six years' service.   He also claimed £166 13s 4d. for damage done
to his lands and plundering of his house in Edinburgh by the " Inglish usurpers."[3]

It had been the custom till now to hold the meetings of the Craft in the house
of the Deacon for the time being, and one can imagine that the anatomical
instruction must have caused some awkwardness in his domestic arrangements.
In 1647, however, David Kennedy and James Borthwick reported that they had
taken as a place of meeting, " three rowmes of ane tenement of land in Diksone
Close, for payment of fourtie poundis zeirlie."[4]

By 1669, it was found that even this was unsuitable, and the Craft decided
to build a " convening house " on a piece of ground, in the south-east angle of the
city wall, presented to them by the Town Council in 1656, each member subscribing
£100 for that purpose.[5]   On 24th October, 1694, a member of the Incorporation,
Alexander Monteath, apparently on the instigation of Dr. Pitcairne, obtained from
the Town Council a gift for thirteen years " of those bodies that dye in the
correction-house," and of " the bodies of fundlings that dye upon the breast,"
together with a room for dissections.   Immediately the other members of the
Incorporation presented a petition (2nd November, 1694) for similar privileges.
The ingenuity of the Town Council was somewhat taxed to discover other sources
of anatomical material, but they succeeded by granting " the bodies of fundlings
who dye betwixt the tyme that they are weaned and their being put to schools
or trades ; also the dead bodies of such as are stiflet in the birth, which are exposed,
and have none to owne them ; as also the dead bodies of such as are felo de se,
and have none to owne them ; likewayes the bodies of such as are put to death

---

[1] " Records of the College of Surgeons," 20th March, 1645.
[2] " Works of Alexander Pennecuik," Leith, 1815, p. 2.
[3] " Acts of the Scottish Parliament," Vol. VII, Appendix, p. 101.
[4] " Records of the College of Surgeons," 26th September, 1591, and 15th July, 1647.
[5] Ibid. 18th May, and 26th May, 1669.

by sentence of the magistrat, and have none to owne them."   The grant was to take effect in the winter time, and there was an important condition attached, that the petitioners should, by Michaelmas, 1697, build, repair and have in readiness an anatomical theatre for public dissections, the hall of 1669 being apparently not large enough, or otherwise unsuitable.[1]

The new Surgeons' Hall was ready on the site of the old one, and the gift confirmed by December, 1697, and from this time the teaching of anatomy in Edinburgh became systematic.   The surgeons also laid out round the Hall a garden in which medicinal herbs were grown, and, at a later date, established a bath in connection with their premises.

Pitcairne and Monteath joined other members of the Incorporation in giving combined anatomical demonstrations, and we find Pitcairne writing, in 1694, to a friend in London that he proposed " to make better improvements in anatomy than have been made in Leyden these thirty years.[2]

There is a minute of the Incorporation for January, 1703, showing how the anatomical demonstrations were then (November, 1702) carried out by the various members appointed for the purpose : *First day*, a general discourse on anatomy, and the common teguments and muscles of the abdomen, by James Hamilton, the Deacon.   *Second day*, the peritoneum, omentum, stomach, intestines, mesentery and pancreas, by John Baillie.   *Third day*, the liver, spleen, kidneys, ureters, bladder and parts of generation, by Alexander Monteath. *Fourth day*, the brain and its membranes, with a discourse of the animal spirits, by David Fyfe.   *Fifth day*, the muscles of the extremities, by Hugh Paterson. *Sixth day*, the skeleton in general, with the head, by Robert Clerk.   *Seventh* day, the articulations and the rest of the skeleton, by James Auchinleck. *Eighth day*, the epilogue, by Dr. Pitcairne.[3]

Another and longer course of ten demonstrations is minuted in the records of the surgeons (18th May, 1704) as having taken place in the preceding April.

About the year 1705, there appears to have been a general desire that one man should take over the management of these lectures, and there was considerable competition for the privilege of being appointed to do this.   Robert Eliot was chosen by the Incorporation as " public dissector," and later in the same year (29th August, 1705) he also received from the Town Council a salary of £15 per annum.   Eliot was thus the first " Professor of Anatomy " in the Town's College, and the earliest professor of this subject in Britain.   The appointment was a double one, the town providing the salary and the surgeons supplying the theatre. In 1708, at his request, Adam Drummond was conjoined with him in this post, receiving half of the salary.[4]

---

[1] John Gairdner : " Historical Sketch of the Royal College of Surgeons of Edinburgh," Edinburgh, 1860, pp. 16 and 17.
[2] A. Bower : " History of the University of Edinburgh," 1817, Vol. II, p. 149.
[3] C. H. Creswell : " The Royal College of Surgeons of Edinburgh," Edinburgh, 1926, pp. 123-194.
[4] J. Struthers : " The Edinburgh Anatomical School," Edinburgh, 1867, p. 14.

G

Anatomy now became a very popular study, and the supply of bodies from the sources already mentioned proving inadequate, recourse was had to body-snatching. As early as 1711, there were great complaints of graves in Edinburgh being rifled. The Incorporation of Surgeons felt themselves called upon to forward to the Magistrates a memorial which, in the first place, denounced this as "a scandalous report, most maliciously spread about the town," and entreated the Magistrates to exert their utmost power for the "discovery of such an atrocious and wicked crime." Expulsion from the Incorporation was also threatened against any of its members or apprentices who should be found concerned in the foresaid crimes. The whole memorial, however, sounds rather exculpatory than sincere, and the practice probably continued, though with greater precaution.[1]

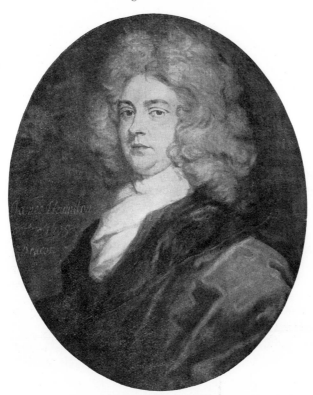

JAMES HAMILTON
Deacon of Surgeons, 1702
(Original in the Royal College of Surgeons, Edinburgh)

On the death of Robert Eliot, in 1714, John M'Gill was associated with Adam Drummond as Joint Professor of Anatomy in the Town's College. Two years later they resigned their posts—"as the state of their health and business were such that they could not duly attend the said professorships"—in favour of Alexander Monro (primus). Monro (1697–1767), a young man of twenty-two, had been particularly educated by his father John Monro, an old army surgeon, to fill this post. John Monro had been a pupil of Pitcairne[2] at Leyden in 1692, so that he readily fell in with the schemes of the latter for the establishment of a medical school at Edinburgh, and continued to work for the foundation of a

[1] A. Bower : "History of the University of Edinburgh," 1817, Vol. II, p. 163.
[2] Album Studiosorum Acad., Lugduno-Batav., 1575–1875.

hospital there after Pitcairne's death.   Alexander Monro had a special knowledge of anatomy, had studied under Cheselden in London, and had been admitted
a Master of the Calling three months previously.   He was now (29th January,
1720) elected " Professor of Anatomy in this city (Edinburgh) and college," the
yearly salary of £15 being continued.   On 14th March, 1722, Monro's appointment
was confirmed *aut vitam aut culpam*,
instead of the previous tenure of office
" during the Council's pleasure." [1]

In 1718, Alexander Monro had presented to the surgeons "some anatomical
pieces done by himself," including an
articulated skeleton in a glass case, and
dissections preserved in spirit ; of which
the skeleton and case are still extant.
Monro lectured in the Hall of the Surgeons from 1719 till 1725, when, following
upon a public riot directed against body-
snatching, he removed his preparations
for greater security within the walls of
the University, as the Town's College had
come by this time to be called.[2]   Once
more on this occasion (17th April,
1725) the Incorporation of Chirurgeons
published a notice, which was
printed and distributed through the
town, deprecating and denying body-
snatching.   It contains the following
curious passage :—

" As also, the Incorporation understanding that country people and servants
in town are frightened by a villainous
report that they are in danger of being
attacked and seized by Chirurgeons'
apprentices in order to be dissected ; and

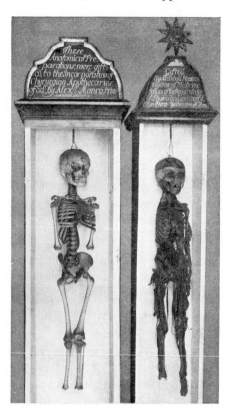

DISSECTIONS BY ALEXANDER MONRO
(primus) AND ARCHIBALD PITCAIRNE
*(Preserved in the Royal College of Surgeons at
Edinburgh)*

although this report will appear ridiculous and incredible to any thinking person,
yet the Incorporation, for finding out the foundation and rise thereof, do promise
a reward of five pounds stg. for discovering such as have given just ground for
this report, whether they be Chirurgeons' apprentices or others personating them
in their rambles or using this cover for executing their other villainous designs."

[1] Bower : Vol. II, p. 182.
[2] Bower : Vol. II, p. 184.

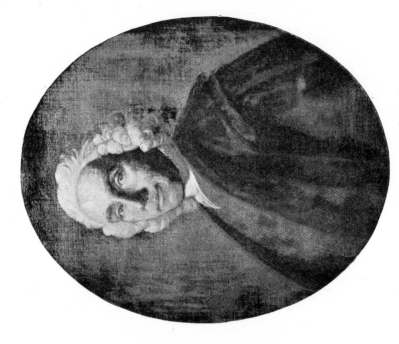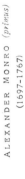

ALEXANDER MONRO (*primus*)
(1697-1767)

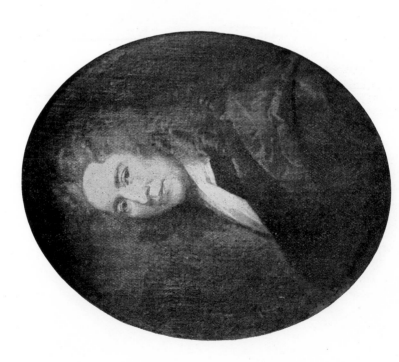

JOHN MONRO
Deacon of Surgeons 1712 ; died about 1737

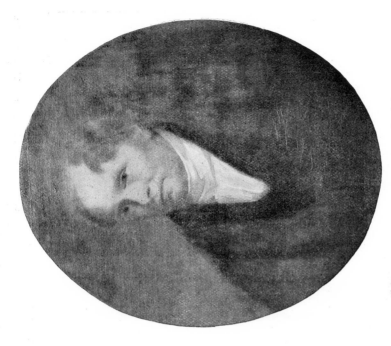

ALEXANDER MONRO (*tertius*)
(1773–1859)

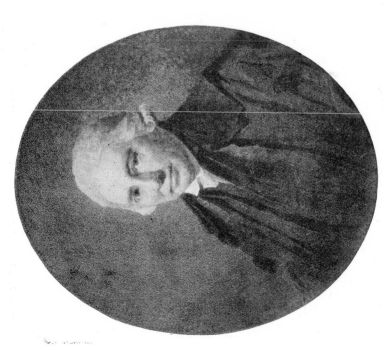

ALEXANDER MONRO (*secundus*)
(1733–1817)

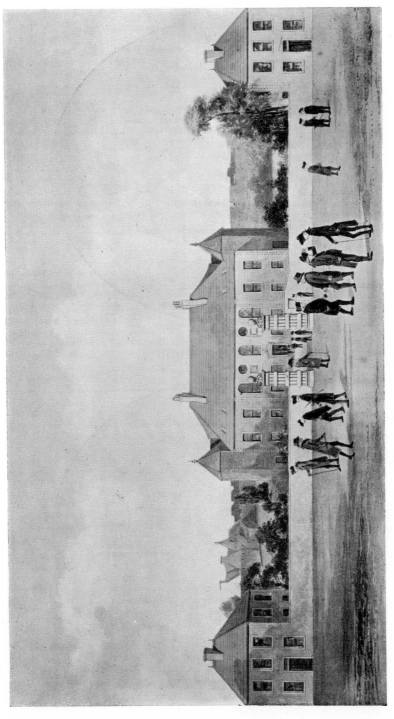

SURGEONS' HALL OF 1697

The figures in front include Benjamin Bell, A. Monro (*secundus*), and Alexander Wood: the city wall and Curriehill House appear in the background. The ground flat, with the door and date, still remains: a third flat has been added

(*Original in the Royal College of Surgeons, Edinburgh*)

There are, however, records which give some colour to this report; for example, in 1724, after a woman had been executed, there ensued a fight between her friends and some surgeon-apprentices for possession of the body. In the middle of the fracas the supposed corpse came to life, and lived for many years with the popular appellation of "half hangit Maggie Dickson." It was not till a century later that the report received dreadful confirmation in the revelations at the trial of Burke and Hare.[1]

Monro (*primus*), being appointed Professor of Anatomy, immediately introduced an extended course of instruction lasting from October to May, and embracing the following subjects: He began with a history of anatomy, which he apparently treated very fully. Next he took up osteology, dealing not only with the form and structure of the bones, but also with their uses and the diseases and accidents to which each is liable. Next he demonstrated on adult subjects— the muscles, viscera and brain, and on the bodies of children, the nerves and blood-vessels, again dealing not only with anatomy as we regard it, but with disease in the various organs. He further illustrated the anatomy of the human body by the dissection of various quadrupeds, fowls and fishes, comparing the structure and uses of their organs with those of the human body. He proceeded then to consider the diseases for which chirurgical operations were commonly undertaken, and to demonstrate the operations on the cadaver, as well as the bandages and various instruments and appliances used in surgery. Finally, he concluded his winter course with some general lectures on physiology.[2]

From 1726 onwards, the anatomical lectures were conducted in the Town's College, and the progress of anatomy became part of the history of the Medical Faculty in the University for three-quarters of a century.

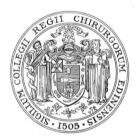

SEAL
ROYAL COLLEGE OF SURGEONS
EDINBURGH

---

[1] C. H. Creswell: "The Royal College of Surgeons: Anatomy in the Early Days," *Edin. Med. Journ.*, 1914, p. 150.
[2] "Works of Alexander Monro," published by his son, Edinburgh, 1781.

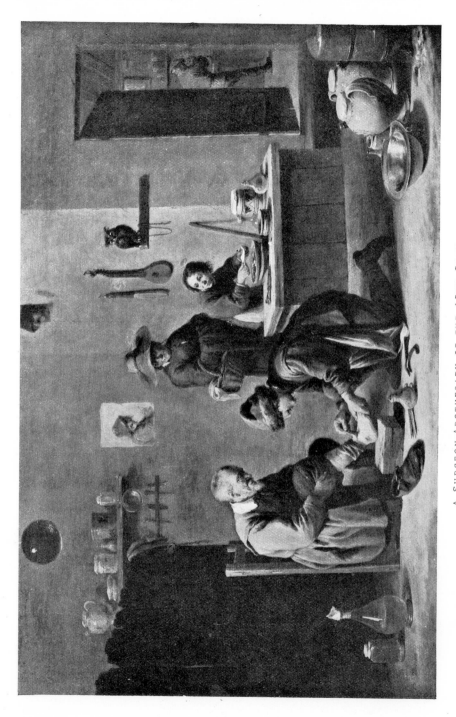

A SURGEON-APOTHECARY OF THE 17TH CENTURY

The picture, painted by David Teniers, the Younger (1610-1690), at Brussels, gives an impression, applicable to Scotland, of the conditions of general practice in the latter half of this century

CHAPTER VII

GENERAL PRACTICE IN THE SEVENTEENTH AND EIGHTEENTH CENTURIES

DURING the 17th century, Scotland was an extremely poor country. The southern and more wealthy part had been wasted by the English Wars in the middle of the 16th century, by the plague, and by the internal political troubles associated with the period of the Reformation. About the middle of the 17th century, the country was still further impoverished by the Civil Wars, the efforts made in 1650 on behalf of Prince Charles, and the great fines subsequently imposed by Cromwell. The 17th century accordingly was one which showed only a very gradual development in medicine. Opportunities for medical education were few, and means of transport were extremely bad and slow, so that it was difficult for medical practitioners to travel any great distance to see patients, except in the case of the wealthy, or, indeed, to subsist at all in country places. With the exception of a few roads between the principal towns, there were no routes over which wheeled vehicles could pass, and such roads as existed were of very poor quality. Communication in country districts was carried out entirely on foot or horseback. Even carts were not introduced till late in the 17th century, and merchandise was transported on rough sledges or by horse panniers. Horse litters also had been used from early times by wealthy and sickly people.

So late as 1658, a stage-coach passed between London and Edinburgh only once in three weeks.[1] Two places so near as Edinburgh and Haddington were connected by stage-coach only twice weekly in the year 1678, while the first stage-coaches between Edinburgh and Glasgow were set up in this year, subsidised by the municipalities, and even so, were unsuccessful. A traveller in Scotland, in 1688, says that there were then no stage-coaches, although the great men of the country often travelled by a coach and six, exercising great caution, with a footman running on each side. Letters were carried by foot-post and carriers, and so late as 1749, communication between Edinburgh and Glasgow (now occupying sixty-five minutes) was effected by a covered spring-cart twice in the week, which took a day and a half on the journey.[2] In 1716 a traveller proceeding from Edinburgh to Ross-shire got as far as Queensferry in a coach and then had to proceed on horseback, taking six days to cover 170 miles.[3] Even in 1740, Lord Lovat, having occasion to travel from Inverness to Edinburgh with his two daughters, had to carry a wheelwright with him in order to repair his coach on the journey,

---

[1] Chambers : " Domestic Annals of Scotland," 1859, Vol. II, p. 247.
[2] Chambers : " Domestic Annals of Scotland," Vol. II, p. 393.
[3] Op. cit., Vol. III, p. 407.

which occupied twelve days, and was attended by numerous accidents.[1] The famous roads through the Highlands, begun by General Wade in 1726 (the year in which the Medical Faculty at Edinburgh was founded), did much to accelerate communication between certain places, but only 260 miles of road were affected, and these were not finished until late in the century.

Inns, too, were of late development in Scotland. Fynes Moryson, a gentleman who made a tour in Scotland about the year 1598, and published his " Itinerary " in 1617, stated that there were no inns as in England, but in all places some houses were known where passengers might have meat and lodging. He, however, records the great hospitality with which he met.[2] This isolation had a paralysing effect upon all attempts to improve medical practice or better the practitioner's knowledge.

As an example of the sparseness of medical practitioners in country districts, it is said that there was only one medical man on the main road for fifty miles north of Aberdeen at the beginning of the 18th century, Dr. Beattie, in the Garioch. " In his later days he used to be seen visiting patients mounted on a shaggy pony. His professional dress was a greatcoat, so frayed by time and weather that its original colour was undiscernible, and he wore a yellow wig." [3]

In the absence of local medical practitioners, it was necessary that the clergyman and the Laird should know something about medicine, and they had often picked up some rudiments of this during their College course. In the case of the wealthy, physicians and surgeons were frequently brought from a long distance to attend during an illness, while the great nobles and the Highland chiefs had their private medical attendants, who could give assistance to the poor retainers of their patrons.

An interesting proprietary remedy, introduced early in the 17th century, was Anderson's Scots Pills. Dr. Patrick Anderson, who practised at Edinburgh, London and Paris, speaks in a little book, which he wrote on their virtues, of having got the receipt in Venice about 1603. Their main constituent was aloes, and they were widely used for headache, stomach troubles, constipation, rheumatism, etc. Indeed, several men who were early principals and regents in the Town's College, wrote elegant Latin verses on their usefulness. These pills were widely used for 300 years, and were still on sale in the year 1910.[4]

An indication of professional fees charged at the end of the 17th century may be gained from two examples. In 1689, Dr. David Mitchell, of Edinburgh, under sanction of the Privy Council, undertook the charge of Alexander Irvine, of

[1] Spalding's " Miscellany," Vol. II, p. 5.

[2] Chambers : " Domestic Annals of Scotland," Vol. I, p. 299.

[3] E. H. B. Rodger : " Aberdeen Doctors," 1893, p. 25.

[4] Anderson : " Grana Angelica," Edinburgh, 1635 ; and Wootton : " Chronicles of Pharmacy," London, 1910 Vol. II, p. 168.

Drum, in Aberdeenshire, a mentally defective person.   He hired some additional rooms and made the necessary furnishings, thus establishing one of the first nursing-homes on record.   After one month, however, with Dr. Mitchell, the Laird of Drum was persuaded by Marjory Forbes to marry her, and left his medical protector.   Dr. Mitchell was allowed by the Lords of the Privy Council a sum of £500 Scots, or £41 13s. 4d., in addition to twenty pieces, for a professional visit to the Laird in Aberdeenshire.[1]

The Earl of Home, in 1695, was placed under arrest and ordered to repair to Edinburgh Castle.   As he represented his indisposition of body to be such that this was impossible, the Privy Council ordered Sir Thomas Burnet, the King's physician, and Gideon Elliot, chirurgeon, to proceed to the Hirsel in Berwickshire and report upon the Earl's state of health.   The doctor and surgeon reported in such terms that the Earl was allowed to remain at his house, the Hirsel, and for their pains in travelling fifty miles and back and giving this medical report, Dr. Burnet was allowed 200 merks (£11 2s. 2d.), and Mr. Gideon Elliot 100 merks (£5 11s. 1d.).[2]   The relative importance of the physician and surgeon towards the end of the 17th century may thus be estimated.

Scottish military surgeons, during the 17th century, appear to have occupied a position of good standing and to have been well paid.   In 1644, four surgeons were appointed to the Army, each to have charge of two regiments forming a brigade in the Army sent into England.   Each of these was provided with two surgeon's mates.   The names of the surgeons were David Kennedie, James Ker, Thomas Kincaid and Nehemiah Touche.   Each of the surgeons received an allowance of £15 for furnishing his " kist."   The pay was at the rate of 5s. daily for a surgeon, and 4s. for his two mates, with an additional allowance of 3s. daily for their three riding horses, and 2s. 6d. for two baggage horses to carry their equipment.[3]   In 1646, the pay was raised so that the surgeons, of whom one was now allowed to each regiment, received 20s. daily, this being the same rate as that for a Lieutenant of Foot and an Ensign of Dragoons.[4]

In 1649, when the Scottish Army was being re-formed in Perth and the neighbourhood, a generous scale of allowances was sanctioned, and the Army appears to have been well equipped, although it met with disaster at Worcester two years later.   Among its general officers were two surgeons-general, each of whom was promised £40 per month.   It may be mentioned in passing that each of eight ministers, similarly classed as generals, received £66 13s. 4d. monthly, while the Army, which set out with high hopes for a premature Restoration, included a " writer of the History of the Times," at a salary of £200 per month.[5]

---

[1] Chambers : " Domestic Annals of Scotland," Vol. III, p. 22.
[2] Chambers : Op. cit., Vol. III, p. 117.
[3] " Acts of the Scottish Parliament," Vol. VI, i, p. 74.
[4] " Acts of the Scottish Parliament," Vol. VI, i, p. 620.
[5] " Acts of the Scottish Parliament," Vol. VI, ii, p. 448.

During the 17th century, surgery appears to have been of a rough and ready type, although no doubt gradual progress was made.   Most of the foundation hospitals which had existed before the Reformation had fallen into neglect, or their buildings and revenues had been appropriated by the proprietors of neighbouring lands, or by persons possessing sufficient influence with the Reforming powers ;   and the voluntary hospital movement of the 18th century had not yet begun. There were thus few facilities available for surgeons who wished to improve their methods. As an illustration of surgical practice at its best, a few quotations may be given from Richard Wiseman, " the father of English surgery." Wiseman accompanied Prince Charles (later Charles II.) from Holland to Scotland in 1650, as his medical attendant and surgeon to his troops, and took part in the operations against Cromwell, which ended with the battle of Worcester. He practised

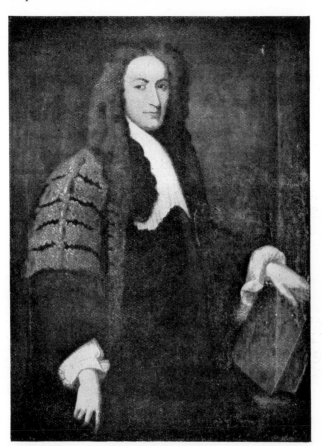

RICHARD WISEMAN (1620-1676)
(From the original in the Wellcome Historical Medical Museum)

for about a year in Stirling and Perth, for after the disaster at Dunbar, Charles was still left with a Royalist Army in the neighbourhood of Perth.

Speaking of the type of wounds with which surgeons then had to deal, and which were found in the Covenanters who had managed to escape from Cromwell's horsemen at Dunbar, Wiseman says :—

" I shall now consider of Wounds with losse of Substance made by Bill, Pole-axe, Sword, etc., some cutting twice or thrice in one or near one place, whereby the Wound is large, transverse, yea and oblique, at the same time, and the Lips contracted various ways, and so the Cure is rendred much more difficult.   These kind of Wounds are not so often seen in times of Peace, but in the Wars they are frequent, especially when the Horse-men fall in amongst the Infantry, and cruelly hack them ; the poor Souldiers the while sheltring their Heads with their Arms, sometime with the one, then the other, untill they be both most cruelly mangled : and yet the Head fareth little the better the while for their Defence, many of them not escaping with lesse then two or three Wounds through the Scull to the Membranes, and often into the Brain.   And if the man fly, and the Enemy pursue, his Hinder parts meet with great Wounds, as over the Thighs, Back, Shoulders and Neck. . . . At Sterling in Scotland Mr. John Chace, Apothecary to his Majesty, helped me in the like work.   One of the Souldiers had such a gash thwart the Nape of his Neck, that it was a wonder to us he lived.   His Wound was full of Maggots ; and so were those of all the rest that were inflicted on the Hinder parts, they having been some days undrest." [1]

In discussing wounds of the brain, Wiseman gives, among others, the following instance of success following trephining.   The servant maid must have been a hardy lass, to be able to attend him daily as an out-patient after a trephine opening had been made in her skull.   The Mr. Penycuke, whom Wiseman mentions, was Alexander Pennycuik, who entered the Edinburgh Incorporation of Surgeons and Barbers in the year 1640.   His father was the Laird of Pennycuik, and Alexander sold this estate and bought Newhall in Midlothian. He had been surgeon to General Banner in the Thirty Years' War, and was, at the time of his connection with Wiseman, surgeon-general to the Scottish troops.

" At Sterling Mr. John Chace was present when a poor Servant-maid came to me to be drest of a Wound she had received on her Head by a Musket-shot, in the taking of Calendar-House by the Enemy.   There was a Fracture with a Depression of the Scull. I set on a Trepan for the elevation of the deprest Bone, and for discharge of the Sanies. She had laboured under this Fracture at least a week before she came to me, yet had none of those Symptoms aforementioned.   But after Perforation, and raising up this deprest Bone, and dressing her Wound, she went her way, and came daily thither to be drest, as if it had been onely a simple Wound of the Hairy scalp.   Mr. Penycuke, an eminent Chirurgeon of that Nation, did assist me in this work.   I think the Brain it self was wounded.   I left her in his hands, who I suppose finished the Cure." [2]

The following quotation illustrates a point upon which Wiseman and his contemporaries often insisted, that gun-shot wounds were not poisonous because of anything connected with the powder, but that their tendency to inflammation was due to failure on the surgeon's part to purify the wound properly :—

" Nay, while any of the Rags remain in the Wound, it will never cure : but the extraneous bodies drawn out, there is little difficulty in the healing these Simple Wounds, if drest rationally.

" An Instance whereof I shall give you in a poor Souldier, who was shot at the Castle of Dunbar with a Musket-bullet a little above the left Clavicle, in amongst the Muscles of that Scapula.   The Bullet was drawn out by one of my Servants, and the Wound drest up with Digestives.   But some days after, he being brought to Saint-Johnston's (Perth), I found it inflamed and very much swelled.   We dressed it up according to the method set down in this Treatise ; but it apostemated, and mattered very much.

---

[1] Richard Wiseman : " Severall Chirurgicall Treatises," London, 1676, p. 348.
[2] Richard Wiseman : " Severall Chirurgicall Treatises," London, 1676, p. 401.

After several unsuccessful Applications, I made an Incision by the side of the Scapula into the Cavity, and pulled out the Rags that had been carried in by the Shot: and from that time all Accidents ceased, and the Wound cured soon after. But if such be handled as some have lately taught, they are so many poisoned Gun-shot Wounds."[1]

Gun-shot wounds of the chest were apparently treated with success in Wiseman's time, as the following quotation shows. He seems somewhat sarcastic as to the great cures performed by the Scottish leeches in such cases by virtue of balsams given internally:—

" From the Defeat of the Scotish Army near Dunbar there came many of the wounded to Saint-Johnston's (*Perth*), and amongst them there were severall wounded into the Breast. They who were so shot as to have the Ribs broken, were in extreme Pain from the Shivers: whereas the rest whose Bones were not hurt had scarce any Pain at all, but what proceeded from Difficulty of breathing; they all coughing up a stinking Sanies both before and after the separation of the Sloughs. One of them cought a very great proportion daily of thin Matter, of a brown colour and ranck smell. None but this died under my hands; the rest after some while retiring to their homes, where (as I have often heard them say) their Leeches performed great Cures, by virtue of some Plants which they gave internally, and which with Fats they made Balsams of. Yet I believe this man died tabid."[2]

About the middle of the 17th century, Sydenham, in London, introduced a new method of treating fevers. Hitherto, it had been the custom to treat the patient in a fever by heaping clothes upon him in bed, closing up the room in which he lay, lighting a large fire, and supplying the patient with cordials and stimulants. Sydenham, however, insisted on opening windows, banishing fires and providing only the ordinary bed-clothes. The sick man was to be well supplied with bland fluids, of which Sydenham specially commended small beer, and in the case of smallpox he recommended the use of syrup of white poppies, and of a vomit of antimonial wine, as well as blood-letting in moderate degree, according to circumstances.

In 1687, Sydenham was visited by Dr. Andrew Broun, of Edinburgh, who, in 1691, published a small book called " A Vindicatory Schedule concerning the New Cure of Fevers." Broun, who is commonly called " Dolphinton," from his estate in Lanarkshire, was an Edinburgh physician, and spent several months as a pupil of Sydenham, whom he eulogises in his book. The book provoked a spirited controversy in Edinburgh medical circles of the time, and in the Royal College of Physicians at Edinburgh there are preserved some fourteen pamphlets published between 1691 and 1709, of refutations, defences, letters, etc., in regard to the new method of Sydenham's treatment, which Broun strove to introduce. The most interesting of these is one of 1692, entitled " In Speculo teipsum Contemplare," an imaginary and very abusive dialogue between Dr. Brown and a hypothetical Dr. Black.

---

[1] Richard Wiseman : " Severall Chirurgicall Treatises," London, 1676, pp. 410 and 411.
[2] Richard Wiseman : " Severall Chirurgicall Treatises," London, 1676, p. 436.

The general contention on the part of Andrew Broun and his supporters, following Sydenham, was that in fevers cathartics gave relief, and might be combined with blood-letting and restrained by paregoric.   Help might also be had from fixed and volatile salts as well as alkaline concretions, and by cupping, leeches and frictions.   Vomiting, too, was supposed to aid the elimination of the poisonous material.   For those persons who were able to go about, horseback exercise was recommended on account of its influence in " jogging the humours."   Towards the end of this discussion, Dr. Archibald Pitcairne and Sir Robert Sibbald were brought in on a side issue, and the whole question seems to have caused great heart-burning for nearly twenty years in Edinburgh medical circles.   It appears from incidental references in these controversies that the chief medical authorities used in Scotland at that date were the " Practice of Medicine," of Riverius, and " The Practice of Medicine " of Sylvius.

The Pharmacopœia issued by the Royal College of Physicians of Edinburgh in 1699, did much to standardise medical prescriptions and the substances used in treatment.   Hitherto a knowledge of remedies had been gained from ancient writers, such as Dioscorides, commentaries like that of Matthiolus, and herbals, either preserved in manuscript form, or printed like those of Gerard and Culpepper.   The Pharmacopœia is a small duodecimo volume containing a long list of simple medicaments, mostly of vegetable origin, with instructions for the preparation from them of various waters, syrups, powders, lozenges, pills, ointments and tinctures.

Among the more striking preparations contained in it is a compound powder of crabs' claws, which contains various substances such as powdered red coral, crabs' claws, etc., but whose impressiveness is enormously enhanced by the inclusion of bezoar stone and prepared pearls.   It must have been a most expensive form of prescription for carbonate of lime.   Another noteworthy preparation is the " Mithridatium Damocratis," which contains no fewer than forty-eight ingredients, chiefly flowers, seeds, gums and oils, of which opium seems to be the most active.   It was given in cases of poisoning.   There is nothing in this first Pharmacopœia that could be called disgusting, and this official list of medicines stands in marked contrast to the popular medicine of the day, represented, for example, by the receipts of John Moncrief of Tippermalloch, which will be mentioned later.   It contrasts very favourably also with the Pharmacopœia of corresponding date issued by the College of Physicians in London.

A second edition of the Pharmacopœia was issued in 1722, and a third in 1735.   By this time various animal substances had been introduced, possibly as a concession to popular medicine.   Thus, a method of preparing dried goats' blood is given.   Urine mixed with salt is used to prepare sal ammoniac.   Prepared millipedes (slaters) are to be dried at a gentle heat and used as an

ingredient of various medicines, probably for the stimulating properties of the
formic acid they contained.   Dried bees are used in a similar manner.   Crabs'
claws and pearls are employed as before.   One of the most striking additions
to the materia medica is " Bufo præparatus," for which the recipe is that " living
toads are to be set in an earthen pot, desiccated at a moderate heat and reduced
to powder."   It seems hard on the toads that they should have been alive at
the beginning of the preparation, but it has been found in recent years that the
skin of the toad contains a valuable glucoside, having an action similar to that of
digitalis.[1]   This was half a century before William Withering, an Edinburgh
graduate, who had settled near Birmingham, investigated, in 1776, the medicinal
properties of the foxglove.

There was a great deal of irregular practice in the early part of the
18th century.   The country was invaded by mountebanks, who came especially
from Germany and the Low Countries, set up stages in the towns and treated
people wholesale.   Partly owing to the scarcity of doctors and partly perhaps
from want of faith in some of those who were provided with University degrees, a
great number of books on simple forms of medical treatment were also in vogue.

This general attitude is illustrated by the case of Sir John Clerk, of Penicuick,
who, in 1710, fell ill of a great cold, tried several doctors and medicines, and finally
rode to Bath " contrary to the advice of Physitians at Edin., for they all agreed
that the Bath Water wou'd prove hurtful."   He, however, found that the change
of air contributed to his recovery, and that he was cured by taking the " Elixir
Proprietatis cum spiritu sulphuris."   This was a nostrum composed by
Dr. George Thomson, who wrote " The Direct Method of Curing Chymically,"
London, 1675.[2]   This book was typical of many others.

A book of simple, harmless and generally useful remedies, which had an
enormous vogue in England, and which was occasionally found in Scotland, was
" Primitive Physic, or an Easy and Natural Method of Curing Most Diseases,"
composed by the Rev. John Wesley (1703–1791), and sold at the Methodist
preaching-houses throughout England.   It had reached its 21st edition by 1785.

In Scotland several books were in use, designed for those who knew a little
medicine, such as the clergymen, lairds or great ladies who took an interest in
their retainers.   Of these books, one of the best known was " The Poor Man's
Physician, or the Receits of the Famous John Moncrief of Tippermalloch."
This, as its title-page records, is " a choice collection of simple and easy
remedies for most distempers, very useful for all persons, especially those
of a poorer condition."   The first edition was published in 1712, and the
third edition in 1731.

---

[1] See Abel & Macht : " J. Pharm. Exp. Therap.," Vol. III, 1912, p. 319 ; and Shimizu : " J. Pharm. Exp. Therap.,"
Vol. VIII, 1916, p. 347.
[2] " Sir John Clerk's Memoirs, 1676–1755," Scottish Hist. Soc., Edinburgh, 1892, p. 77.

Tippermalloch's little book consists of a long list of remedies divided under diseases of the head, diseases of the nostrils, diseases of the liver, and so on through other parts of the body, taking up the various diseases affecting each part.   There is no attempt at explanation, but after each heading is given a selection of remedies.   Some of these appear to be quite natural and salutary, and some can only be described as extremely disgusting.   No doubt his intention was to mention remedies likely to be favoured by different types of person, so that people who liked heroic or disgusting things could get what they liked.   For the scurvey, which was a troublesome disease at the time, he sensibly recommends to " take of clear Juice of Water-cresses and Brook-lime, of each one Ounce, the Juice of Fumitory two Ounces, white Sugar two Drams.   Make a Potion." [1]   For the itch, another very troublesome disease of the time, he recommends the standard remedy of brimstone, with nitre, rubbed on.

The following is a fair average sample of the book :—

" 38. *For the Colick.*

1. The Hoofs of living Creatures are singularly good, being drunk. *Rhasis.*   Or dry Oxdung drunk in Broth, or the Juice pressed from the Ox-dung drunk, is better. *Gesnerus.*   2. The Heart of a Lark bound to the Thigh, is excellent against the Colick, and some have eaten it raw with very good Success. *A Spaniard.*   3. This is certain, that a Wolf's Dung, Guts, or Skin eaten, will cure the Colick, or if you do but carry them about you ; for they strengthen the Choler. *Cardanus.*" [2]

Some of his remedies have apparently come down by tradition as old folk-medicine.   Others, such as the following, suggest a derivation from some of the ancient classic writers like Scribonius Largus, possibly through old monastic sources.   As a cure for the falling sickness in children, he gives the following prescription :—

" 8. *Of the Falling-sickness in Children.*

3. Take a little black sucking Puppy (but for a Girl take a Bitch-whelp), choke it, open it, and take out the Gall, which hath not above three or four Drops of pure Choler : Give it all to the Child in the Time of the Fit, with a little Tiletree-flower Water, and you shall see him cured, as it were by a Miracle, presently." [3]

Towards the end of the 18th century, as regular medicine became more easily available, these ancient recipes passed out of use, and excited a great deal of ridicule, as in the sarcastic poem of Robert Burns on " Death and Dr. Hornbook " :

" Calces o' fossils, earth, and trees ;
True sal-marinum o' the seas ;
The farina of beans an' pease,
    He has't in plenty ;
Aqua-fontis, what you please,
    He can content ye.

---

[1], [2], [3], Moncrief : " The Poor Man's Physician," Edinburgh, 1731, pp. 40, 182 and 4.

> Forbye some new, uncommon weapons,
> Urinus spiritus of capons;
> Or mite-horn shavings, filings, scrapings,
>   Distill'd *per se*;
> Sal-alkali o' midge-tail-clippings,
>   And monie mae."

Among the diseases of the 17th and 18th centuries, which those medical practitioners who happened to be available found themselves frequently called upon to treat, were smallpox and ague.

Smallpox appeared at recurring intervals in epidemics, which were sufficiently noteworthy to be recorded by the historians of the time, although in Scotland this disease does not seem to have attained the universality with which it afflicted England, if we may judge by Macaulay's words. Referring to the death of Queen Mary in 1694, Macaulay says:—

> "That disease, over which science has since achieved a succession of glorious and beneficent victories, was then the most terrible of all the ministers of death. The havoc of the plague had been far more rapid: but plague had visited our shores only once or twice within living memory; and the smallpox was always present, filling the churchyards with corpses, tormenting with constant fears all whom it had not yet stricken, leaving on those whose lives it spared the hideous traces of its power, turning the babe into a changeling at which the mother shuddered, and making the eyes and cheeks of the betrothed maiden objects of horror to the lover."[1]

In Scotland, however, the epidemics of smallpox were sufficiently severe. In 1610, there was a great visitation of the young children of Aberdeen with the plague of the pocks, which was attributed to "the sins of the land." In 1635, the smallpox raged for six or seven months with great severity among the young in Scotland, and, what was remarked as unusual, some persons took the disease for the second time.[2] Again, in August, 1641, Aberdeen was greatly afflicted for:

> "In this month, ane great death, both in burgh and land, of young bairns in the pox; so that nine or ten children would be buried in New Aberdeen in one day, and continued a long time. . . . There was reckoned buried in Aberdeen about twelve score bairns in this disease."[3]

In April, 1672, it is recorded that smallpox was present in Glasgow, and had raged for six months previously, so that hardly a family escaped the infection, and eight hundred deaths and upwards occurred.[4] This was extremely serious for a small town of about 12,000 inhabitants, which Glasgow then contained. Still another record of December, 1713, mentions that in Eglesham parish the smallpox was severe and eighty children died.[5]

Dr. Archibald Pitcairne's method of curing the smallpox, written in the year 1704 (that is before the introduction of inoculation), for the use of the noble and

---

[1] Macaulay: "History of England," Vol. IV, p. 532.
[2] p. 85, [3] p. 140, [4] p. 347, Chambers: "Domestic Annals," Vol. II.
[5] Chambers: Op. cit., Vol. III, p. 387.

honourable family of March, may be given here as an example of 17th century medical treatment :—

" If a Child, or any Person grow sick, feverish, or has a Pain in the Back, or Slot of the Breast, Loss of Appetite, Drowsiness, short Cough, Sneezing, watery Eyes or some of these ; but always accompanied with some Heat, and frequent Pulse, or Drought. In this case Blood is to be taken at the Arm, or with Loch-Leeches ; and if the Fever ceases not, tho' the Pox appear, let Blood a second or third time.   Meantime give the Child a Spoonful of Syrup of White Poppies at Night, and in the Night-time, also till Sleep or Ease comes.

" After the Pox appears, and Fever is gone, then steep a Handful of Sheeps' Purles in a large Mutchkin[1] of Carduus-water, or Hysop-water, or Fountain-water, for 5 or 6 Hours ; then pour it off without straining, and sweeten it with Syrup of red Poppies.   Give of this a Spoonful or two, every 4th or 5th Hour, to make the Pox fill, and preserve the Throat.   Always at Night-time, and in the Night, give a Spoonful or two of the Syrup of white Poppies for a Cordial, that keeps down the Fever, and keeps up the Pox.

" If the Pox run together in the Face (which is the only thing that brings Hazard) use the Infusion of the Purles, and the Syrup of white Poppies oftner than in other Cases ; also about the eighth Day from the appearing of the Pox, or a little before that, give the Child to drink of Barley-water, sweetned with Syrup of white Poppies ; this will make the Child spit, which saves the Child.

" The Child's Drink may be Milk and Water at other times, or Emulsion, but use the first rather.

" Apply nothing to the Face.   Use no Wine, or Winish Possets.

" If any Loosness comes before the 4th Day of the Eruption, stop it with Syrup of Poppies, and five or seven Drops of liquid Laudanum given now and then till it be stopt.

" Let the Child's Diet be all along a thin *Bread-Berry* in the Morning, a weak Broth, and soft Bread for Dinner, and Milk and Bread at night, or Sugar-Bisket and Milk, and about the fifth Day from the Eruption, give the Child Water-gruel sometimes.

" *Note.*—If at any time the *Small-Pox* disappear, with a Raving before the 5th, 6th, or 8th Day from the Eruption, then let Blood again, and apply a large Blistering Plaister between the Shoulders, and give an Emulsion.

" If the Small-Pox fall down, without Raving, then apply a Blistering Plaister large between the Shoulders, and give an Emulsion, and boyl in a Gill of Water, and as much White or Red Wine, half a Dram or a Dram of Zedoary-Root sliced, 2 Figgs, and 2 Scruples of Theriac or Diascordium ; sweeten it with Syrup of Kermes and white Poppies, each half an Ounce.

" In the End of the Disease, that is, about the 10th, 11th, 14th, &c., Day, after the Eruption ; if the Child's Defluxion is gross, either apply a new Vesicatory, or give often the Spirit of Hart-horn, in Syrup of Violets, or a Vomitor.

" *Lastly*, When the Pox is blackened sufficiently, or about the 14th Day from the Eruption, let the Child drink Whey, eat Pottage, &c.   Broth with Prunes, unless the Child's Belly is open enough of it self.

" But if the Child is so young or unlucky, as not to cough heartily, and force up the Defluxions ; or if the Frost thickens it, apply to the *Slot* of his Breast a Pultess of Theriac,

---

[1] A Pint Measure.

Diascordium, Alkermes, Oyl of Rosemary, and Cinammon with warm Claret, in a double Linnen Cloath often.

" And to the Throat apply, in a double Linnen Cloath, a Pultess of Cow's Dung boil'd with Milk, and soft white Bread : Put a little Brandy to as much as you apply at a time.

" For the Defluxion also give inwardly some of this, which has a Dram of *Sperma Cœti*, well mix'd in a Glass-Mortar (not a Brass one) with fine Sugar ; to which add at leisure Syrup of Violets, or Balsamick, or Poppy Syrup, with some Spirit of Harthorn.

" If the Pox was confluent or run together on the Face, then, after the Person is recovered, give a Purgative, to bring away the Remainder of the Pox within the Guts."[1]

The practice of inoculation was introduced into London on the recommendation of Lady Mary Wortley Montagu in the year 1721. Dr. Peter Kennedy, a Scotsman practising ophthalmic surgery in London, had already, in 1715, written of the good effects that he had seen from inoculation in Constantinople.[2] Maitland, a Scottish surgeon, who had attended the Embassy in Constantinople, was employed, in 1721, to carry out the experimental inoculations upon condemned criminals, conducted by Sir Hans Sloane at the instance of King George I.[3]

The practice of inoculation against the natural smallpox, having proved effective in England, was adopted in Scotland some five years later, and appears to have been very successful in diminishing or preventing the epidemics which had occurred in previous centuries. In a statistical account of Scotland, published in 1791, the former ravages of smallpox are declared to be much abated owing to the parish ministers performing inoculation in children. The epidemical disease most dreaded was still said to be the natural smallpox, which occurred about once in every seven years and swept away a number of children. This was attributed to the neglect of inoculation, and there are numerous complaints at this time of the absence of doctors or surgeons in country districts. A plan was proposed that the students of divinity at the University of Edinburgh should be instructed in the art of performing inoculation, "which the physicians of that city generously and humanely proposed to do, without putting them to any expense." As an example of the success of inoculation, it is mentioned that among one thousand patients inoculated by Dr. Lindsay, in Jedburgh, only two died, and these were believed to have been infected in the natural way.[4]

The method of performing inoculation about fifty years after its introduction is given in a letter by Professor William Cullen to a young practitioner in the south of Scotland, as follows :—

To Mr. Michael Gardiner, on Inoculation,

DEAR SIR,—Lord Stonefield proposes to have his son Mr. Willie inoculated this harvest, and as he is to be under your care his Lop. desires me to give you my opinion concerning

---

[1] Pitcairne : " The Method of Curing the Small-Pox ; Written in the Year 1704. For the Use of the Noble and Honourable Family of March," Printed 1715.

[2] Kennedy : " An Essay on External Remedies," London, 1715, Chap. 37, p. 153.

[3] Creighton : " History of Epidemics in Britain," Vol. II, p. 467.

[4] Sinclair : " Statistical Account of Scotland," Edinburgh, 1791, Vol. I, pp. 3 and 263, Vol. II, p. 126, and Vol. IV, pp. 527 and 548.

the best manner of managing this matter. With regard to the ordinary practice I know that I need not instruct you, and shall therefor say only what relates to the particular patient, or to new and late improvements in the general practice which you may not have had experience of.

I think he should not be inoculated for ten or twelve days after he goes to the country that you may be certain he has catched no cold in changing quarters, and farther that the hot season may be over.

During this time there is to be no change of the diet he has been on for some time past, which is milk, grain and vegetables, and entirely without animal food, and this diet is to be continued during the whole course of the disease.

In the time which is to pass before inoculation you may purge him twice, giving one grain of Calomel overnight and a Senna infusion in the morning. The same purging is to be repeated twice between the Inoculation and Sickening, and in both cases the doses are to be given at the interval of three or four days.

The inoculation is better performed by a Lancet whose point has been dipt in a pustule than by a thread as formerly; but if you cannot have the opportunity of preparing a lancet within a few days before your intended inoculation, you must employ a thread as usual. In employing the lancet if the matter upon it happens to be dry, you must hold it a little over the steam of warm water before you employ it. In employing it you have only to insinuate it under the cuticle without going deeper, and when you have withdrawn the Lancet you have only to press down again the cuticle, and tie a bit of rag upon it which rather does harm. (*sic.*)

Every day both before and after inoculation and every day during the course of the disease, your patient must walk out or be carried out into the fresh air and be very much in it. When rains or high wind render it inconvenient for him to be abroad the windows of his chamber must be kept open for the most part. In short, he can hardly have too much fresh air; but it is by no means necessary to expose him either to a stream of air or to any moisture, so that these ordinary causes of cold may still be avoided. I say farther that before Inoculation, and from thence to the Sickening, there is no occasion to seek for much cold, and therefor to push him constantly out of the house, but it may be enough to avoid heat, to keep his chamber cool, and to have him often abroad. When the weather is warm he may be cooler within doors than abroad, and this minds to say that when he is abroad he must keep out of the sun and avoid any exercise that may heat him. The less exercise he takes the better. This is the management till he sickens, and when that happens there must be more pains taken to cool him. If any fever appears if it is in the day-time let him be carried abroad to sit in the Shade, and if there is a little Stream of air to fan him it is the better. If it rains or he is so sick as to be averse to sit up, let the windows and even opposite windows be open, and while he lies upon his bed if this does not cool him let him be carried near to the window and held in the stream of air. This is to be done also in the night-time, and if it is fair without high wind I think even in the night-time carrying the patient abroad into the open air is safer than keeping him at a window. When by any of these means the heat delirium, or other symptoms of fever are much abated, he is to be laid abed but he must not be immediately covered with blankets but should be for some time with only a single sheet upon him. Let this be observed that the fever is most liable to come on in the Evening and forepart of the night, and therefor at this time the cooling measures are most necessary; but that after two or three o'Clock the fever usually declines, and both from this consideration and from the measures employed before, the patient may be covered towards morning and especially during sleep at this time. Upon the whole I think it is found from much experience that external cold is the surest and generally a safe means of moderating the eruptive fever, and in proportion of rendering the small pox few and of a good kind. I have given you hints of the particular execution, but some part of it must be left to your own discretion upon understanding the general plan.   I have only to add that these cooling practices are especially necessary during the eruptive fever, and are to be continued if the small pox should after all prove numerous or be attended with any other unfavourable circumstance. But if upon eruption they are very few and of a good kind, hardly any measures at all are necessary, and the patient may go abroad or stay at home as in ordinary health, or as directed above for the time before sickening.   In case of any sharp fever at eruption, besides the cooling I have spoken of it is also proper the day after sickening to give such a dose of Calomel and Physic as above mentioned, and this may be repeated during the course of the disease, and once or twice after it.   I have thus given you my plan I hope fully enough ; but if any doubt or difficulties remain, you have still enough to have them solved, and I shall be glad to hear from you being very much.—Dear Michael your &cc.

W. C.

EDINR., 8th Augt., 1771. [1]

The procedure of vaccination, which completely superseded inoculation, was introduced by Edward Jenner in 1796, and within a few years came into general use in Scotland.   One of the earliest persons to publish an extended inquiry into its good effects was Dr. William Pulteney Alison, at Edinburgh, in 1817.

Ague or malaria was a disease which occasioned much trouble in the 17th and 18th centuries.   It prevailed particularly among the labouring classes, to such a serious extent that frequently the cultivation of the ground in spring could not be performed.   By the end of the 18th century ague had almost disappeared from Scotland.   The records of Kelso Dispensary show that the number of cases treated there in 1781 was 161, after which a gradual fall took place, so that by 1797 they did not exceed ten in any one year, and after 1840, disappeared altogether.   This was probably due to the disappearance of bog land by drainage and cultivation.[2]

Two peculiarly Scottish diseases of the 18th century were sibbens and croup. Sibbens was a troublesome infectious disease prevailing in the south-west of Scotland.   It appeared first as a sore throat with glandular enlargement, and later produced on the skin pustules, which ulcerated deeply, together with small hard knots of a reddish colour, later developing into excrescences resembling raspberries.   It is supposed to have been introduced by Cromwell's soldiers, and to have been identical with yaws, a disease prevalent in West Africa, and carried by negro slaves to the West Indies.[3]   It gradually died out.

Croup was an old Scottish name for an acute disease of the throat accompanied by harsh breathing and hoarse coughing.   It had been prevalent in the south-east of Scotland, but had not been described until 1765, when Professor Francis Home, of Edinburgh, published an account of the disease.   A little later we find the parish ministers deploring the uncommon mortality due to epidemical sore throat, the fatal issue of which they believed might be prevented by proper

---

[1] From MS. Letter-books of William Cullen, preserved in the Royal College of Physicians, Edinburgh.
[2] Ritchie : " Animal Life in Scotland," Cambridge, 1920, p. 510.
[3] G. Matheson Cullen : " Concerning Sibbens and the Scottish Yaws," *Caledonian Medical Journal*, April, 1911.

care.[1]   Dr. Francis Home says that his description is the first account of the disease, which seldom occurred in Edinburgh, but was frequent in Fife, Ayrshire, Galloway, and other parts near the sea.   He described the " white, soft, thick preternatural coat or membrane " covering the air passages of the children who died, " like the blankets of a bed that has been laid in," and he suggested tracheotomy for its relief.[2]   This account was issued more than half a century before the celebrated treatise of Pierre Bretonneau, who gave to the disease the name " La Diphthérite," and who is generally regarded as its discoverer.

Various family accounts for medical expenses have been preserved by the descendants of families living in country districts.   For example, in the middle of the 18th century, the family of Lumsden of Cushnie, in Aberdeenshire, had occasion to call Dr. Gregory, mediciner of King's College, and Dr. James Gordon, professor in Marischal College, for attendance in the fatal illness of Mistress Bettie Lumsden.   The account

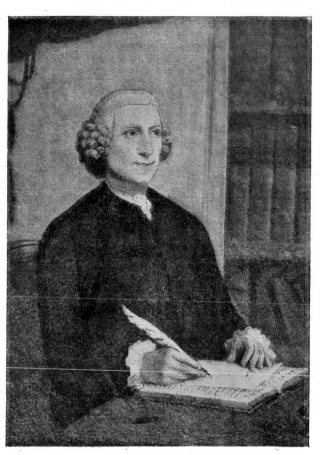

FRANCIS HOME (1719-1813)

of the former amounted to £33 18s. Scots, and of the latter to £37 16s.   The lady's illness also incurred a long bill from Francis Legatt, chirurgeon-apothecary, in which such items are mentioned as 8 oz. of cordial mixture at 4s. ; 3 vomits at 2s. 6d. each ; 2 drachms of cephalick spirit, 4d. ; 2 bloodings, 2s. 6d. each ; eyewater, 1s. ; anodyne purgative 1s. ; " blistering plaster for your back," 1s.[3]

[1] Sinclair : " Statistical Account of Scotland," 1791, Vol. XXI, p. 75.
[2] Francis Home : " An Enquiry into the Nature, Cause and Cure of the Croup," Edinburgh, 1765.
[3] E. H. B. Rodger : " Aberdeen Doctors," p. 18.

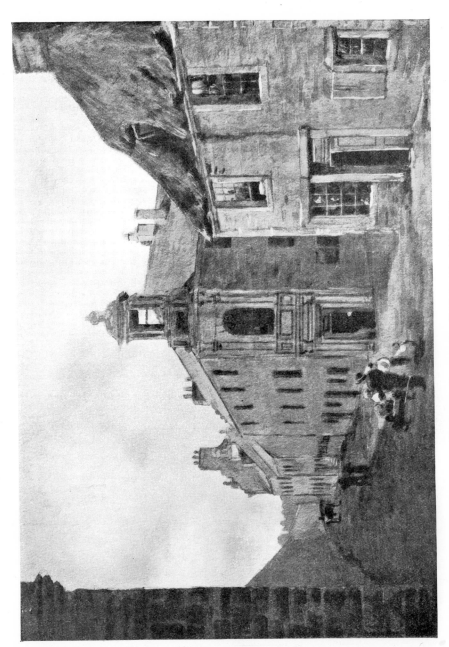

WILLIAM CULLEN'S HOUSE IN HAMILTON

The house is on the right of the picture

(Original picture in the Hall of the Royal Faculty of Physicians and Surgeons of Glasgow)

A good idea of practice in the country from the middle of the 18th century onwards, can be gained from the account-book containing the record of medicines furnished by Dr. William Cullen, at Hamilton, from September, 1737, to October, 1741, which is preserved in the Library of the Royal College of Physicians at Edinburgh.   The doctor appears to have obtained some of his drugs wholesale from the "Chymicall Laberatory at Edinburgh," and these included such substances as tinctura antimonialis, sweet spirit of nitre, oil of absinth, oil of cinnamon, oil of lavender, oil of rue, oil of savin, extract of chamomile, extract of Peruvian bark, extract of gentian, flowers of benzoin, white precipitate of mercury, red precipitate, green precipitate, sal ammoniac crystallised, and rectified sal volatile.

Hamilton was a large enough place to possess a druggist, and from Mrs. Johnston, who managed the druggist's shop, Cullen obtained oil of turpentine, spirit of wine, oil of origanon, oil of vitriol, English crocus, white arsenic, borax, hellebore root, white wax, lard, gum benzoin, gum elemi, coral, cubebs, sandalwood, oil of anise, levigating marble, Florence flasks, castor, cinnabar, Venetian treacle, mithridaticum, pepper, gentian root, valerian root, laurel berries, Venice turpentine, etc., etc.

He made up these substances into ointments, elixirs, cordials, draughts, enemata, stomachic drops, apozemata, electuaries, etc., at charges from 3d. to a few shillings each.   His account to Her Grace the Duchess of Hamilton, from November 5, 1741, to April 15, 1742, included such items as 2 ownces of senna, 1s. ; a glass of specific balsam ; a Blistering plaister for ye Ear, 6d ; a glass of hysteric drops, 6d. ; a glass of cordiall mixture, 3s. ; ane anodyne Draught, 1s., etc.   It is noteworthy that "drugs for the horses" came to much more than those for the family.   Chocolate was a dear commodity, as two pounds are set down at 10s.

A method of treatment which was much recommended by practitioners in Scotland during the 18th century was the whey cure.   This, which involved early rising, spare diet, and was carried out in a country district, was of great value at a time when people were apt to exceed both in eating and drinking.   The method is concisely expressed in a letter from William Cullen to a patient. The letter is dated from Edinburgh in May, 1768, the year before that in which Cullen first gave a course of lectures in practice of medicine, and runs as follows :—

"For Governor Glen

Goat Whey.

When the stomach is well suited to digest Goat whey, the drinking of this for some weeks at a proper Season is of great Service to many constitutions & the best management for a Goat whey course I take to be the following.

Let the milk be taken from Goats that feed in a mountainous pasture & the higher the better.

Let the Goats be milked early in the morning & if possible let the rennet be put to the milk while it is yet warm from the Goat.

Let that part of whey only be taken that parts readily and entirely from the Curd.

In drinking the whey it is always proper to begin with a small quantity about a gill[1] to continue this for two days & afterwards by slow degrees to increase the dose till it arises to a muchkin[2] and half or a chopin[3] in a morning & above this it is hardly ever proper to go.

Whenever the quantity taken in a morning goes above a Gill it is always proper to divide it into different draughts & to take these at an interval of half an hour or more between them.

It is always best to take the whey betimes in the morning but sooner or later according to the habits that people are in of getting up in the morning. The first draught may be taken a bed but a person should be up to take the second ; if the weather allows of it, it is usefull to walk about in the open air between the draughts & for a little after the whole is taken.

When the whey happens to sit heavy or prove windy on the stomach, it may be somewhat corrected by taking a teaspoonfull of Aniseed Sugar in the first draught of the whey or by eating a little Sugared Carraway Seed between the draughts.

The whey operates most properly when it keeps the belly regular without purging & when the most part of whey goes of by Urine.

When the whey does not even keep the belly regular, it is proper to take along with it every day or every second day a Dose of the Soluble Tartar ordered below. The Dose should be such as to keep the body open & no more for I think purging might be hurtfull to the Governor.

Breakfast should not be taken till an hour after the whole of the whey is taken.

The Diet along with Goat whey may be the same as at other times only the stomach should be kept always light. Fish should be taken seldom & very sparingly & much of greens or Roots especially of the Colder or more windy kinds should be avoided.

In drink all kinds of fermented liquors whether wines or Ales are improper & if any Strong drink is necessary the best is water with a little Spirits without any Sowring and with very little or no Sugar. However if this is disagreeable & wine has been usually taken a little Madeira or sherry may be taken at dinner & Supper.

Nothing secures the good effects of Goat whey more than being much in the Open Air & taking a great deal of gentle Exercise on horseback or in a Carriage.

I should have said above that is enough to take the Goat whey once a day for the Evening hardly affords a Convenient time for it unless a person can take it alone for supper.

WILLIAM CULLEN.

EDINR., 30th. May, 1768.
For Governor Glen.
Tartar. Solubil ℥ ii
Sacchar. alb. duriss. ℥ i

Terito simul in pulverem & mitte in Phiala patuli oris bene obturata.

Signa. Aperient salts two, three or four teaspoonfulls for a dose to be taken in a draught of Goat whey.

W. C.

30th May, 1768.[4]

---

[1] One quarter pint.
[2] One pint.
[3] One English quart.
[4] From William Cullen's letter-books.

The following description of an 18th century Scottish country practitioner is given by Lonsdale in regard to the grandfather of John Goodsir, the anatomist :—

"Nearly a century ago (1768), Dr. John Goodsir was among the best-known men in the East Neuk of Fife.   Born in the parish of Wemyss in 1746, he became a graduate of the University of Edinburgh, and settled at Largo.   Known at home for his skill, affability and other good parts, his essays in ' Duncan's Annals of Medicine ' gained for him reputation in the Edinburgh circle.   This big-nosed, long-headed, large-hearted disciple of Galen and Lucina, was a fine specimen of the eighteenth century country medical practitioner—hatted, coated, booted and spurred, *à la mode.*   Wiry in build, thoughtful and successful in practice, aye ready with his ' mull ' (*Scotticé* for snuff-box), and aye ready to help a neighbour as well as to uphold the interests and character of ' canny Fife,' he was among the most popular of men.   The customs of the period were primitive and curious, and the practice of the healing art in rural districts was carried on in pack-saddle fashion and regularity.   Dr. Goodsir would start from Largo on Monday, caparisoned

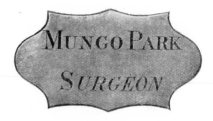

EIGHTEENTH CENTURY DOORPLATE FROM THE HOUSE OF DR. MUNGO PARK AT PEEBLES
(*Preserved in the Royal Scottish Museum of Antiquities*)

for the week with drugs and surgical appliances, and not return home till Friday—as itinerant with his physic as the ancient Peripatetic with his philosophy. . . . To obviate the dangers of travelling by night, he carried a lantern, fastened by a strap above his knee.   The bull's-eye of the doctor's lantern was often signalled, in moonless nights, heralding the comforting assurance of an obstetric deliverance.   His regularity in his rounds vied with the carrier of His Majesty's mails, and the saddle-bags of the one and surgical accoutrements of the other were similarly horsed, so that the Laird of Largo, scanning the roads, used to say :   ' It's either the doctor or the post that's coming.' "[1]

Another well-known Scottish practitioner at the end of the 18th century was Mungo Park, who studied medicine at Edinburgh from 1789 to 1791. After some years' travel in Africa, recorded in his celebrated " Travels in the Interior of Africa," he settled in practice at Peebles in 1799.   He afterwards undertook another journey of exploration to the Dark Continent, from which he did not return.

---

[1] " The Anatomical Memoirs of John Goodsir." Edited by William Turner, M.B., Edinburgh, 1868, Vol. I, pp. 7 and 8.

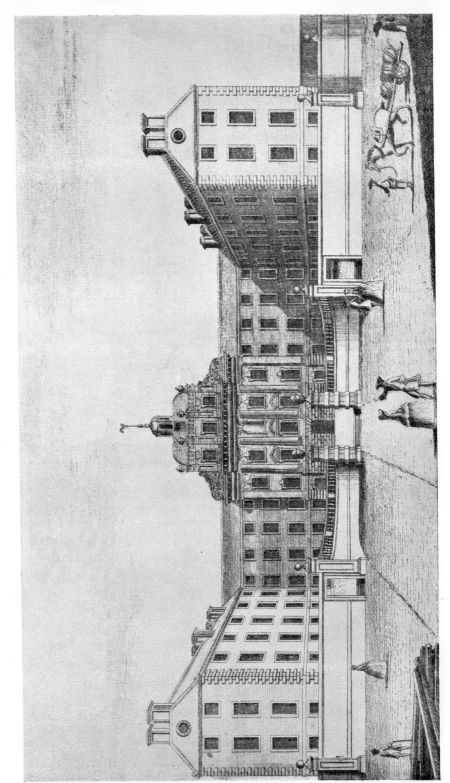

ROYAL INFIRMARY, EDINBURGH

Foundation Stone laid 1738: opened 1741: demolished about 1879

Chapter VIII

The Eighteenth Century Voluntary Hospital Movement

THE early part of the 18th century in Scottish medicine was specially characterised by the movement for the erection of hospitals. Up to the Reformation, the country had been well provided with hospitals for the treatment of chronic, aged and infirm cases, but most of these foundations had disappeared with the decay and suppression of the religious orders. The 17th century, in consequence, had been very deficient as regards progress in medicine and surgery, apart from attempts to regulate and organise the practice of medicine. It is true that the Faculty of Physicians and Surgeons in Glasgow, and the Royal College of Physicians in Edinburgh, had given advice and medicines gratuitously to sick persons in their halls and had visited the poor at their own homes, but so far as the study of disease was concerned, these efforts had produced little result.

In the end of the 17th century some of the Fellows of the Royal College of Physicians at Edinburgh had taken tentative steps for the establishment of a complete medical school in that city, and this involved the idea of building a hospital. The first definite steps were taken by the College of Physicians in 1725, when the foundation of a building, into which the sick could be received for treatment, was proposed. In 1726, the minutes of the College mention that subscriptions had already been set on foot with " pretty good success," and the Fellows of the College were now joined in their scheme by the members of the Incorporation of Surgeons, as well as receiving substantial encouragement from charitable people in many quarters. It was considered that the sum of £2000 was the smallest which would suffice for the purpose, and, this sum having been speedily collected, the Committee charged with the object decided to hire a small house, for receiving sick poor, out of the annual proceeds of the capital sum, and at the same time appointed twenty managers to control it. This " small hired house " stood at the head of Robertson's Close and provided accommodation for six patients. It was formally opened on 6th August, 1729.[1]

On the following page is a list of the thirty-five patients who were treated in the first year of the little hospital's existence. It is interesting both as showing the wide area from which patients were received and the diseases from which they suffered. It is noticeable that most of the patients suffered from chronic conditions, and formed the same type of invalid who would have been a bedesman in one of the 15th or 16th century hospitals :—

---

[1] " The History and Statutes of the Royal Infirmary of Edinburgh," 1778, pp. 7 et seq.

Patients' Names	Parish	Admitted and Discharged 1729-1730	Diseases
Elizabeth Sinclair	Caithness	6. 8.29—19.11.29 recovered	Chlorosis
Barbara Hastie	Edinburgh	7. 8.29—19. 8.29 dismissed	Pain in the Thigh, and Looseness
Hew Richmond	Ochiltry	11. 8.29—19. 8.29 dismissed	Cancer in the Face
Isabel Brown	Dunbar	22. 8.29—10. 9.29 cured	Inflammation of the Eyes
Farquhar Mackinnan, Soldier	....	25. 8.29— 6. 9.29 cured	Pain of the Liver with hectick Fever
John Simson	West-Kirk	25. 8.29—28. 9.29 cured	Scorbutick painful Tumor of the Knee
Helen Allan	Edinburgh	12. 9.29—23. 9.29 dismissed	Hysterick Disorders
Mary Dickson	Canongate	23. 9.29—31.10.29 cured	Bloody Flux
Hector Morison	Isle of Mull	23. 9.29—30. 9.29 dismissed	Consumption
James Short	Edinburgh	1.10.29— 9.10.29 cured	Beginning Consumption
Katharine Macfarline	Edinburgh	4.10.29— 4.11.29 cured	Obstructions
Jean Cunningham	West-Kirk	13.10.29—30.11.29 cured	Cancer of the Breast
Mary Walker	Congalton	31.10.29—17.11.29 cured	Tertian Ague and Sore Eyes
Robert Brown, Dragoon	....	18.11.29— 8. 1.30 cured	Quartan Ague
Alexander Lamb	....	18.11.29—25.11.29 cured	Flux
William Lindsay	Edinburgh	28.11.29—22.12.29 dismissed	Pain and Swelling of the Belly
Mary Sheriff	West-Kirk	1.12.29—17.12.29 cured	Bloody Flux
Ebenezer Tweedie	Edinburgh	5.12.29—23.12.29 cured	Melancholy
Elizabeth Hog	Ormistoun	17.12.29— 9. 3.30 recovered	Dropsy of the Belly
James Ladlie	Arnistoun	23.12.29—27. 3.30 dead	Consumption
James M'Naughton	Canongate	8. 1.30—29. 1.30 cured	Palsy of the Hand
David Lighton	Edinburgh	22. 1.30—10. 4.30 cured	Universal Palsy
Sarah M'Laughlan	....	25. 1.30—16. 3.30 recovered	Pthisick and Tumor of the Belly after a Quartan Ague
Mary Bowman	Haddingtoun	16. 3.30— 7. 5.30 cured	Hysterick Disorders
Margaret Doig	Dundee	24. 3.30— 2. 7.30 cured	Tympany after a most irregular Ague
George Somervile	Gingle-Kirk	4. 4.30— 1. 5.30 recovered	Pthisick with Fistulous Ulcer of the Leg
Margaret Johnston	Canongate	13. 4.30—14. 7.30 cured	Cancerous Tumor of the Side
Jean Robertson	Peterhead	7. 5.30—In the Infirmary	Inveterate Scorbutick Ulcer of the Leg
Mary Hood	Canongate	7. 5.30— 1. 7.30 cured	Fistula lachrymalis and Ulcer of the Toe
Thomas Middleton	Edinburgh	1. 7.30—In the Infirmary	Old Scorbutick Ulcer of the Leg
Thomas Smart	South Leith	2. 7.30—28. 7.30 cured	Bloody Flux
Margaret Young	Edinburgh	2. 7.30—28. 7.30 recovered	Vertigo, Deafness, and other Affections of the Nerves
Helen Waddel	Elie	28. 7.30—In the Infirmary	Steatom of the Cheek
William Panton	Queensferry	29. 7.30—In the Infirmary	Deep Ulcers of Middle Finger and Palm of the Hand
James Mills	West-Kirk	4. 8.30—In the Infirmary	Cancer of the Lip

Cured	...	...	...	...	...	...	...	19

Recovered so as to go about their ordinary Affairs and requiring only some
    Time to confirm their Health, and to restore their Strength fully   ... 05

Dismissed either as incurable or for Irregularities			...		...		...	05
Dead	...	...	...	...	...	...	...	01
In the Infirmary ...	...	...	...	...	...	...	05

Total this first year   ...   . 35 [1]

In 1736, the Surgeons also opened a small hospital, which they continued successfully for two years; but they then joined the Royal Infirmary, handing over to the latter Institution the funds they had collected.

The Managers obtained a Royal Charter from His Majesty George II., dated 25th August, 1736, in which the hospital is designated the Royal Infirmary of Edinburgh, and, by 2nd August, 1738, the foundation stone of a permanent hospital was ceremoniously laid. This building consisted of a "body with two wings, each of three full stories and an attic one, with garrets above." The body was 210 feet long and each wing extended 70 feet, with a large theatre where more than 200 students could see operations, and which was also a convenient chapel. The house was designed for 228 sick people "each in a distinct bed," and on the ground floor there were twelve cells for mad people. Round the hospital was an area of two acres, with grass walks for the patients to walk in. The patients previously had the privilege of walking in the neighbouring Physic Garden of the Town's College, which had been leased in 1724 to Dr. Rutherford and some of his colleagues for the purpose of rearing medicinal plants.

The building of this hospital appears to have commended itself to all classes. The Assembly of the Church of Scotland ordered collections to be made at all church-doors, benefit nights were given at the theatre, most of the societies in and about Edinburgh sent money, merchants sent presents of timber, stone and other materials, farmers and carters supplied carriages, and mechanics and labourers gave so many days' work gratis. In addition, the Managers dispersed copies of their prospectus to England, Ireland and the British Plantations, from all of which countries considerable subscriptions were received. In the credit assigned to the founders of the hospital, one of the most active deserving recognition was George Drummond, Commissioner of Excise, who held the office of Lord Provost of Edinburgh six times. Finally, the Infirmary was fitted up and the sick were received into it in December, 1741.

In 1745 and 1746, the affairs of the Infirmary, as well as of the whole country, were thrown into confusion by the Rebellion, and the Infirmary was converted into a general hospital for sick and wounded soldiers, of whom several hundreds were attended and dressed by the surgeons. From the commencement of the hospital in 1729, the surgeon-apothecaries had not only attended without fee, but each had furnished the medicines necessary out of his own shop. In 1748,

---

[1] "An Account of the Rise and Establishment of the Infirmary," Edinburgh, 1730.

however, the Managers decided to fit up an apothecary's shop in the institution, from which both in-patients and out-patients could be served.

By 1778, when a new appeal was issued, it had been found that the original twelve cells for mad people were unnecessary, and some of them had, therefore, been converted to other uses.   On the upper floor, a ward had also been established " for lying-in women, sufficiently separated from the rest of the house, and under the direction of the professor of midwifery," Professor Thomas Young.   On the attic storey, and in a remote part of the house, a salivating ward for female patients containing twelve beds, had also been established.   " This ward was fitted up in consequence of a few female patients, who, being sufferers, not by any fault of their own, but by that of their husbands, or from suckling infected children, had applied to be taken under cure in the hospital."   By this time, too, it is recorded that " in the west wing are one cold, and two hot baths, with their respective dressing-rooms," while in the east wing " is a bath for the patients of the house, so constructed, that it may be occasionally used either as a cold or a hot bath."   The report continues: " Those in the west wing are intended for people of the city ; no patient in the Hospital having, at any time, admittance to them." These three baths seem to have been the only provision, in the middle of the 18th century, by which the inhabitants of Edinburgh could carry out complete ablution otherwise than in a stream or in the sea, and the baths were a source or revenue to the charitable institution.   At an earlier date, the College of Physicians had established a cold bath in the garden of the Hall near the Cowgate ; and, later, the Incorporation of Surgeons also instituted a bath.

Another considerable source of revenue was tapped in 1746, when the Managers of the Infirmary and of the town's workhouse took a joint lease of the hall where the weekly assemblies at Edinburgh for dancing were held. Several ladies of quality and rank undertook to act in turn as directresses of the weekly assemblies, and the profits arising from these brought to the Infirmary a revenue of about £100 per annum.

It is interesting to note that the Royal Infirmary of Edinburgh in the 18th century affords an example of the modern movement for the payment of hospital staffs.   In January, 1751, the Managers elected Dr. David Clerk and Dr. Colin Drummond physicians in ordinary to the Infirmary, each with a salary of £30. This was to supersede the old arrangement by which each of the Fellows of the College of Physicians had in turn attended the Infirmary for a month, but this arrangement seems again to have lapsed at a later period.   Similarly, all the members of the Incorporation of Surgeons up to 1766 attended the surgical cases in rotation, but in July of that year, the Managers appointed James Rae, Peter Addis, John Balfour and Andrew Wood as surgeons to the hospital. For a time, also, the practice of having paying patients was introduced, and the charge for these was at the rate of 6d. per day.

After the Peace of 1763, a great number of sick and lamed soldiers presented themselves at the Infirmary, and in the same year Dr. Adam Austin was appointed by the Commander-in-Chief to visit the military wards regularly and to report thereon. Every assistance was given by the Managers and staff of the house to Dr. Austin in the execution of these duties.   Excluding the military ward and the wards reserved for special types of case, some sixty beds appear to have been available for ordinary free patients.   With these, the Infirmary continued for about half a century, but in 1828 the old High School, vacated by the transference of that institution to a site on the Calton Hill, was acquired, and this, along with an intermediate building connecting it with the original Infirmary structure, became the surgical hospital.   This part of the old Infirmary is still standing, though the original building of 1741 has long since disappeared.   Lister's Wards were subse-

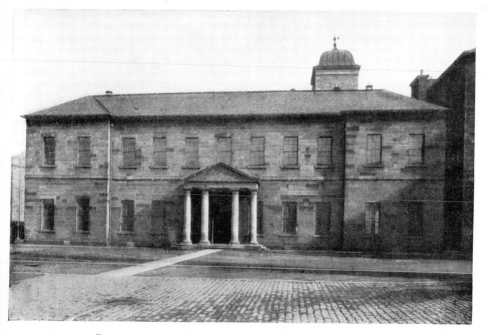

PART OF THE OLD ROYAL INFIRMARY, EDINBURGH

This building was originally the High School, later was occupied by surgical wards (under the charge of Professor Joseph Lister), later was part of the Hospital for Infectious Diseases, and is now (1927) the Engineering Department of Edinburgh University

quently situated in the part which had been the High School, and is now (1927) the Engineering Department of the University.   Between 1860 and 1870, much discussion took place as to whether the Infirmary should be rebuilt or whether a new Infirmary should be erected on a different site.   The latter alternative was adopted, in great part owing to the advocacy of Professor Syme.   The site selected was that of George Watson's Hospital, between Heriot's Hospital and the Meadows.   Here, the foundation stone of the present Infirmary buildings was laid on 13th October, 1870. The present Royal Infirmary was opened on 29th October, 1879.

One of the most important developments in the relationship of the Royal Infirmary to the Edinburgh Medical School commenced when John Rutherford, Professor of Practice of Physic in the University, obtained permission from the Managers, on 1st February, 1748, to give a course of clinical lectures in the Royal Infirmary.   He had already, however, according to Bower, given these lectures for two years.[1]   These were perhaps the first courses of clinical lectures delivered in this country, and were organised by Rutherford on the model of lectures which he had attended in the hospital at Leyden.   Very soon other professors of the Medical Faculty began to co-operate with Rutherford, and the fame of the clinical teaching at Edinburgh increased, especially in the hands of William Cullen, who commenced to give clinical lectures in 1757, and became Professor of Practice of Physic in 1773.

An interesting account is given by Dr. Graves of Dublin, of clinical teaching at Edinburgh when he was a student there in 1819.   Two clinical clerks, he said, were appointed for the male and female wards, selected by the physician from among the senior pupils.   Their business was to write an accurate history of the cases, to report the effects of medicines and to record the symptoms which might have occurred since the physician's last visit.   At his daily visit, the physician stood at the bed of each patient, and, having received the necessary information from his clerk, he examined the patient, interrogating him in a loud voice, while the clerk repeated the patient's answers in a tone of voice equally loud.   This was done to enable the whole audience to understand what was going on, and required an exertion almost stentorian to render this conversation between the physician and his patient audible by the more distant members of the class.   Every word was attentively listened to and forthwith registered most faithfully in each student's case-book, and afterwards all the observations of the professors, made in their clinical lectures, were taken down with equal care and fidelity.[2]   According to Graves, this method of instruction was indeed very useful and nothing better could be devised for a beginner.

The Royal Hospital for Sick Children at Edinburgh was the first hospital in Scotland devoted to this special type of sickness, and was opened in 1860 at Lauriston Lane with twenty-four cots.   In 1864, it was transferred to Meadowside House in the immediate neighbourhood, where there was accommodation for forty patients, including fever cases.   The present building was erected after 1890.

The Royal Maternity and Simpson Memorial Hospital at Edinburgh developed out of the attic storey of the old Royal Infirmary, which, under Professor Thomas Young, had been devoted by the Managers of that institution to the treatment of lying-in women.   Here practical instruction in obstetrics was given by Professor Young and continued by his successor in the Chair, Dr. Alexander

---

[1] Bower : " History of the University of Edinburgh," Vol. II, p. 213.
[2] " Edinburgh Hospital Reports," Vol. I, Pentland, Edinburgh and London, 1893, pp. 10 and 11.

Hamilton, under whom, in 1793, a building situated in Park Place was erected as a lying-in hospital.   Attendance on this institution and instruction of students there was carried on by his son, Professor James Hamilton, for forty years. After various transfers, the hospital settled in its present building, which had been erected as a memorial to Sir James Y. Simpson in 1879.

The latter part of the 18th century was notable for the development in many cities in England and Scotland of dispensaries or institutions for the treatment of the sick poor who did not require admission to hospital.   The first of these

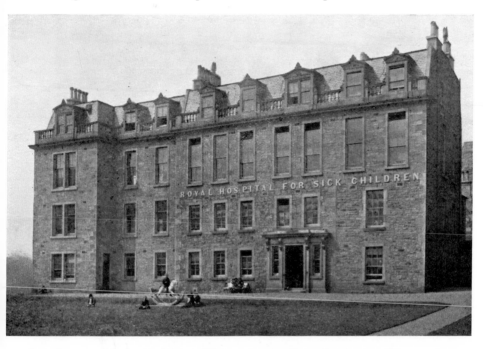

OLD BUILDING OF THE ROYAL HOSPITAL FOR SICK CHILDREN, EDINBURGH
The site is now occupied by the gynæcological block of the Royal Infirmary

in Edinburgh, the Royal Public Dispensary, was founded in the year 1776, mainly through the instrumentality of Dr. Andrew Duncan.   This institution served the double purpose of affording attendance to the sick poor and of giving instruction and an opportunity for practice to senior medical students.   As the town grew, the necessity for another Dispensary was felt, and the New Town Dispensary was instituted in 1815 in Thistle Street.   Other Dispensaries followed at later dates in other parts of the town.

In Glasgow, the Faculty of Physicians and Surgeons, from the time of its inauguration under Maister Peter Lowe, had given gratuitous advice to the poor at its ordinary monthly meetings, and the Town Council had from time to time

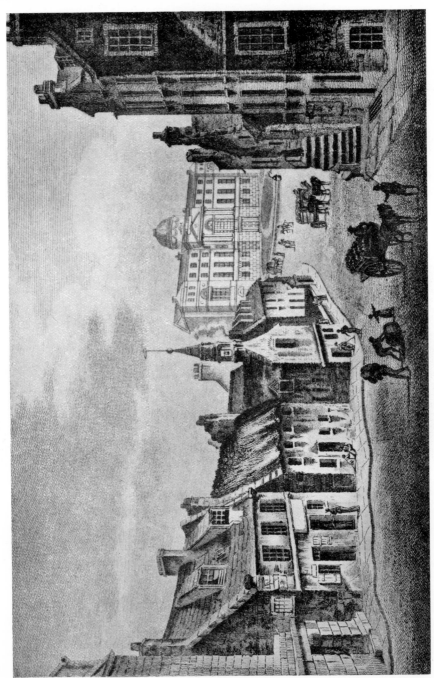

GLASGOW INFIRMARY

(From an engraving published November, 1801, by W. Miller, London).

The plate was engraved by J. C. Fittler after a drawing by J. C. Nattes. The view shows the Royal Infirmary of Glasgow, which opened its doors at the end of 1794. The view shows the Royal Infirmary of Glasgow, which opened its doors at the end of 1794. The main little building with the bell-tower and weather-cock on the left-hand side of the street, is the old Hospital of St. Nicholas, founded by Bishop Muirhead in

subsidised various physicians and surgeons to attend those of poorer means. By 1733, the hospital movement in this city had attained so much force that a Town's Hospital was erected by public subscription on the Old Green near the College, a little west from the Stockwell.   This hospital was maintained by the Town Council, the Merchants' House, the Trades' House and the general Kirk Session, which contributed to it in definite proportions.   The members of Faculty gave their services gratuitously in rotation.   No provision, however, was made here for clinical teaching, nor indeed was there a sufficiently large medical school in

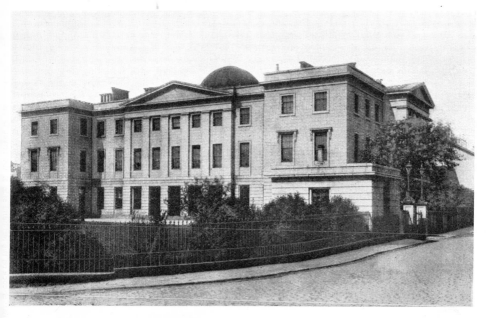

ABERDEEN ROYAL INFIRMARY
Erected in 1840

Glasgow at this time to require it.[1]   Towards the end of the century, this Town's Hospital was felt to be insufficient, and in December, 1794, the Royal Infirmary was opened for the reception of patients.   This building was erected on the site of the old palace of the Bishop of Glasgow and was in immediate proximity to the College or University of Glasgow, which stood in the High Street. With regard to the staff, the arrangement was made that the physicians and surgeons of the Faculty should act in rotation, each physician for six months and each surgeon for two months.[2]   Gradually, however, the numbers of the staff were reduced and the tenure of office extended.   The numbers of students attending the Glasgow Medical School almost immediately increased, despite the fact that the Medical

---

[1] " Memorials of the Faculty of Physicians and Surgeons of Glasgow," Maclehose, Glasgow, 1896, pp. 136 and 137.
[2] Op., cit., pp. 137 and 138.

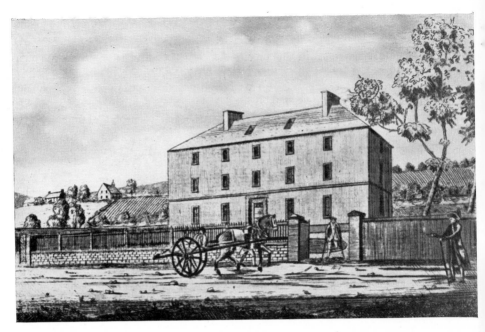

DUMFRIES INFIRMARY, 1776

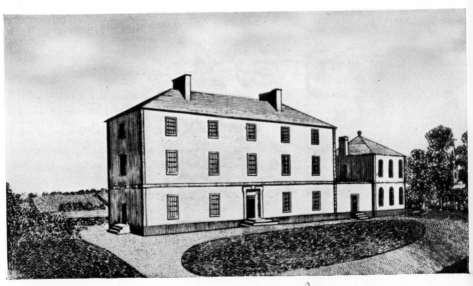

DUMFRIES INFIRMARY, 1781
With Lunatic Asylum, which served for mental patients in the south-west of Scotland till 1839

Faculty of the University was still very incomplete. After the opening of the new University buildings at Gilmorehill, in 1870, a transference of teaching took place from the Royal Infirmary to the newly-erected Western Infirmary beside the University.[1]

The Town Council of Aberdeen, in 1739, convened a public meeting of citizens with the proposal to erect an Infirmary and a workhouse within the burgh. The project was approved by the citizens and, in November, 1739, William Christall, Convener of the Trades, was directed to go to Edinburgh and Glasgow in order to see the hospitals there and to prepare the necessary plans and estimates. These having been passed, the foundation stone of the Aberdeen Infirmary was laid on 1st January, 1740, on a piece of ground at Woolmanhill, gifted by the Town Council. As the building neared completion, it was resolved to make it as extensive and universally useful as possible instead of confining its benefits to the sick poor of Aberdeen. The infirmary was ready for occupation with six beds in the summer of 1742, and Dr. James Gordon was elected physician and surgeon at a salary of ten guineas per annum, he agreeing to supply all the drugs.

The Rebellion of 1745 seriously interfered with the activities of the Hospital, which was first seized by the rebels for the treatment of their wounded, and afterwards was occupied till 1746 by the wounded Government troops. After the Rebellion, Dr. Burnet of Old Aberdeen was appointed physician and surgeon to the institution at the same salary as Dr. Gordon. In 1748 the Town Council decided to lay out a Physic Garden in the immediate neighbourhood of the Infirmary, but this does not appear to have proved a success and was abandoned in 1800. By 1749 the Infirmary had increased to a capacity of nineteen beds, and a few years later two wings were added, bringing the number of beds up to eighty. The important step was taken in 1773 of obtaining a Royal Charter for the Infirmary, which henceforth enjoyed the title of the "Royal Infirmary of Aberdeen." Early in the 19th century it was decided to rebuild the institution, and the new building was completed in 1840, with accommodation for 230 patients. Separate wards for medical and surgical cases were now provided, and two wards were set aside for ophthalmic cases, under the charge of Dr. Cadenhead. Four years later a fever-house was established, and finally, in 1892, a new surgical block, and in 1897 a new medical block were opened in commemoration of Queen Victoria's Jubilees.[2] At the present time (1927) an extensive scheme of reconstruction is under consideration, by which various hospital and public health activities of the city will be concentrated at Forresterhill.

As in Edinburgh, Aberdeen and Glasgow, the other important towns of Scotland undertook the work of building Infirmaries. The Dumfries and Galloway Infirmary was founded in 1776, when a house was opened for

---

[1] Coutts: "History of the University of Glasgow," Glasgow, 1909, p. 586.
[2] "History of the Aberdeen Royal Infirmary," Leng, Dundee, 1904.

eight patients, pending the erection of a special building which was completed in 1778. For this the Town Council granted as a site an acre of the High Dock. The institution of the Infirmary was largely due to the activity of Dr. John Gilchrist, a physician of the town, who had graduated M.D. at Edinburgh, in 1774, with a thesis upon an epidemic fever which had occurred in Dumfries in 1767. The original Infirmary was a building of three storeys, the upper flat being reserved as a military hospital for the sick of troops stationed in Dumfries. One room in the hospital was set aside and divided up into cells for the treatment of lunatics, for whom, however, a separate building was erected in 1781, and continued in use until 1839, when the Crichton Royal Institution was established. In 1807, the institution received a Charter from King George III, and became the "Dumfries and Galloway Royal Infirmary." After considerable additions, the hospital was removed to its present site in 1873.

The Montrose Royal Infirmary and Dispensary was founded in 1782. It had a curiously inverted origin for a hospital, having first of all formed part of the Royal Asylum for the Insane housed in a building on Montrose Links, and occupying a portion of the building not required for the asylum patients. In 1810, the conjoint institution received a Royal Charter as the "Montrose Royal Lunatic Asylum, Infirmary and Dispensary." A considerable amount of inconvenience resulted from this arrangement, and the present Royal Montrose Infirmary was established separately in Bridge Street, Montrose, and opened in 1839.

Dundee Dispensary was founded in 1782, the foundation stone of the Infirmary laid in 1793, and the Royal Infirmary was finally opened for the reception of patients in 1798.

At Paisley, a Dispensary was instituted in 1786, to which a house of recovery was added and in-patients admitted in 1805. After several enlargements, the name of Paisley Infirmary was adopted, and finally the style of the Royal Alexandra Infirmary was used from 1901, when the new building at Barbour Park superseded the old Infirmary.

The Northern Infirmary at Inverness was founded in 1799, and opened for patients in 1804. It undertook the care of both physical and mental disease, the number of beds available for the former being about twenty-five, and for the latter about twelve. This Infirmary, which, with additions, served the needs of the northern part of Scotland for over a century, is at present (1927) being greatly extended.[1]

At Greenock, a house of recovery was added to a previously existing Dispensary in 1807, and opened for the reception of patients in 1809 ; this hospital was largely extended, and the new house was opened in 1868.

---

[1] *Inverness Courier*, January 1, 1926.

At Perth, the County and City of Perth Royal Infirmary was founded in 1834, and opened for patients in 1838.

The Royal Infirmary at Stirling was acquired and opened in 1874.

Like the hospitals for physical disease, asylums for the humane treatment of the insane were established at an early date in Scotland. The Royal Asylum of Montrose was founded in 1779, the buildings completed in 1781, and the first patients admitted early in 1782.

The Royal Edinburgh Asylum for the Insane received a charter in 1807, its foundation stone was laid in 1809, and it was opened for patients a few years later. The founding of this institution was largely the outcome of a suggestion by Dr. Andrew Duncan, who had been greatly impressed by the miserable death of Robert Fergusson, the poet, while confined in the common madhouse in 1774. Professor Duncan obtained a Royal Charter and a Government grant for £2000 towards the erection of this lunatic asylum on modern humane lines at Morningside, Edinburgh. Here instruction by lectures on mental disease was given from a very early date, and has continued ever since.

The Faculty of Physicians and Surgeons of Glasgow in 1810 took a great interest in the promotion of an asylum for the insane, which was opened in 1814 in Parliamentary Road, Glasgow, near the Royal Infirmary. In 1842 this institution was transferred to Gartnavel.

The idea of founding an asylum for the insane at Aberdeen originated in the 18th century, and the property of the old leper hospital was diverted to this purpose. The Asylum was founded in the year 1798, and opened for patients in 1800, a Royal Charter being obtained in 1852.

Dundee Royal Asylum was founded in 1812, and opened for patients in 1820.

James Murray's Royal Asylum, Perth, was endowed in 1814, received a Royal Charter in 1827, and in the same year was opened for patients.

The Crichton Royal Institution at Dumfries was erected between 1835 and 1839 out of a bequest by Dr. James Crichton of Friars' Carse. It had at first been proposed to use this money for founding a fifth Scottish University at Dumfries, but owing to opposition this project fell through, and the money was used for the amelioration of the condition of the insane, for whom at that time insufficient provision could be made by the Dumfries Royal Infirmary. The Institution was opened for patients in 1839.

An important new development in the provision of an institution for the feeble-minded, as distinct from the insane, took place in 1859, with the founding of the Royal Scottish National Institution at Larbert ; this building was opened for patients in 1862, and at the present time (1927) is in process of undergoing great extension in the establishment of a colony for mental defectives.

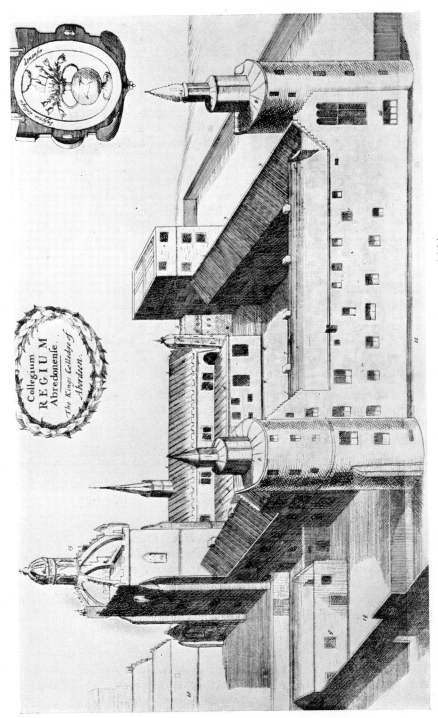

Collegium
REGIUM
Abredonenſe.

The Kings Colledge of
Aberdein.

Joannis
Kingis colleg

KING'S COLLEGE. ABERDEEN, ABOUT 1661

(From Gordon of Rothemay's plan of Aberdeen)

CHAPTER IX

THE MEDICAL SCHOOL OF ABERDEEN

ALTHOUGH the University of Edinburgh was later in its inception than any of the other three, medicine developed earlier at Edinburgh and was more particularly cultivated than in any of the other towns. The University of St. Andrews was founded in the beginning of the 15th century, Glasgow was founded in the middle, and Aberdeen at its close, while Edinburgh University was not founded until a century later, in 1582. As we have seen, however, the Guild of Surgeons and Barbers at Edinburgh was a well-established teaching body by 1505.

The craft of the "Barbours" is mentioned casually several times in the early minutes of the Aberdeen Town Council. Aberdeen received from William the Lion, in the 12th century, a Charter authorising the burgesses to trade, and several important monasteries were founded within its bounds, to one of which, the Trinity Friars, King William gave up his own palace in the Green. The gradual acquisition of medical knowledge by the barbers and their formation into a semi-religious craft would therefore be easy. A Council minute of 10th October, 1494, refers to payment of twenty shillings for the "barbours obeytis,"[1] and on 30th January, 1505, the craft is mentioned as taking part in a pageant.[2] The place of the barbers among the other crafts was a humble one, as appears from their position in the great procession of Corpus Christi Day in 1531, when the barbers walked next to the fleshers, who came lowest in precedence, the hammermen taking the chief position among the seventeen crafts mentioned. In the pageant the barbers represented "Saint Lowrance and his Tormentouris."[3] The Guild of Barbers was incorporated by the Town Council in 1537.[4] Military surgery must have been an important part of the craft, for Aberdeen was an active centre, both during the War of Independence against the English and during the raids by caterans from the north-west, which culminated in the repulse of the Highland hosts at Harlaw in 1411.

There had been a Rector of the Schools at Aberdeen as early as 1262, and numerous subsequent references are found to the Grammar School of Aberdeen. In 1494, Bishop Elphinstone of Aberdeen, obtained permission for the establishment of a "studium generale," or University, in his episcopal See. The Pope thus bestowed the usual privileges of a University, which were to teach, study and confer degrees in theology, canon and civil law, medicine and arts.

---

[1] p. 55, [2] p. 432 : " Extracts from the Council Register of the Burgh of Aberdeen, 1398–1570," Aberdeen, 1844.
[3] " Extracts from the Council Register of the Burgh of Aberdeen," p. 451.
[4] Parker : " Early History of Surgery in Great Britain," London, 1920, p. 93.

Bishop Elphinstone collected a collegiate body and obtained its endowment by his own means and influence, while the young King James IV made a small donation and consented to the annexation of the hospital of St. Germains to assist the revenues. The Bishop's first efforts were to restore the Cathedral and to collect an establishment of forty-two clerics and scholars. The erection of the College of St. Mary of the Nativity, later named King's College, after King James IV, followed in 1500.[1] The first principal was Hector Boece, a native of Forfarshire, who had been a teacher of philosophy in the College Montaigu at Paris. King's College appears to have been completed in the year 1505. With regard to the size of the University, some information is got from a letter written by Randolph, the English Ambassador, who, in 1562, accompanied Queen Mary on a northern progress. He wrote to Cecil from Aberdeen, " The Quene, in her progresse, is now come as far as Olde Aberdine, the Bishop's seat, and where also the Universitie is, or at the least, one college with fiftene or sixteen scollers."[2]

From the beginning, one of the teachers at King's College was a " Mediciner." Thus it was secured that medicine should form an intrinsic part in the teaching of the University, and this was the first University recognition of the subject in Great Britain. Cambridge followed in 1540, Oxford in 1546, and Glasgow in 1637, but Edinburgh did not follow this example until 1685, when three Professors of Medicine were appointed in the Town's College.

The creation of a Chair in medicine must not be misinterpreted, and the whole relations subsisting between a University and medicine in the 16th and 17th centuries will be better understood if the duties of the mediciner are grasped. The study of medicine was, as has been mentioned in connection with the monasteries, regarded as an important branch of scholarship. At this time it was usual for well-educated men to include a knowledge of physic among their literary and philosophical studies, even when there was no intention of adopting medicine as a profession. In outlying districts of the country where the common people were poor and where roads were bad or non-existent, it was difficult for one who practised medicine as his only means of sustenance to exist at all, or, in any case, to visit his patients.

The persons, therefore, who rendered help in time of sickness in country districts, both before and after the Reformation, were the local clergymen or land-owners, who had attended the course at a University and knew something about the medical writings. The students who attended the three or four years required to complete the " studium generale," like the ancient philosophers, took all knowledge for their province. At Edinburgh, as appears from a report by the Commissioners of 1648 to the General Assembly, the anatomy of the human body was described in the third year's course of Arts, while at St. Andrews, in the

---

[1] " Fasti Aberdonenses, 1494–1854," Spalding Club Pub., Aberdeen, 1854, p. v et seq.
[2] Letter to Cecil, 31st August, 1562, quoted in Chalmers' " Life of Ruddiman," p. 7 (note).

last year, the students learned some compend of anatomy, and at Aberdeen some instruction in anatomy and physic was given, apparently at the discretion of the mediciner. The successive mediciners varied in the extent of medicine which they taught to their students, some of them regarding the post as purely titular.[1]

This attitude on the part of the Universities towards the teaching of medicine was reflected in the matter of degrees, when these came to be conferred. The aim was to produce not a practitioner but a scholar, not craftsmanship but erudition. Instruction in medicine, while it might be slight, was associated with a course in arts and philosophy. The person who received a degree was *doctus in medicina*—learned in medicine—but not necessarily a skilled practitioner of the craft. At the University, the same professor often taught medicine with Oriental languages or with mathematics. In the early days, Greek, Latin and Arabic were the languages in which medical knowledge was stored, and from the 17th century onwards the systems of medicine which men strove to establish had a distinct physical or mathematical trend. When a degree in medicine was conferred, it was not given because

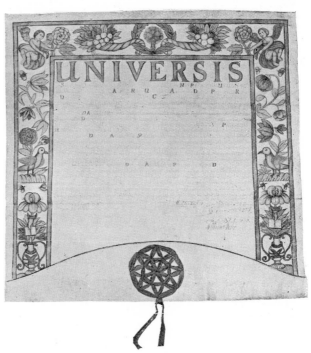

DIPLOMA OF M.D. DEGREE
Conferred on Dr. Archibald Pitcairne by King's College, Aberdeen, signed by Patrick Urquhart, M.D., and dated 7th August, 1699
(Preserved in the Royal Scottish Museum of Antiquities)

of examinations which the student had successfully passed, but as a recognition by the University of general and professional attainments, however acquired. It did not convey the idea of a licence to practise, and it was frequently conferred as an honorary distinction. Thus, the first name mentioned as having received the degree of M.D. from King's College is that of Dr. Joannes Glover, Londonensis, who graduated on 15th May, 1654, and who was already a B.A. of Harvard (1650).[1]

---

[1] "Studies in Hist. and Development of the University of Aberdeen," Ed. P. J. Anderson, p. 308.

Examples of the manner in which the M.D. degree was given for purely honorary reasons and *in absentia* are afforded by two minutes of the Principall and Maisters. " 31st May, 1712 :—Mr. Patrick Blair, apothecary in Cupar, who had been recommended by the bishop of Aberdeen and severall eminent physicians in Angus, was graduated Doctor of Medicine."

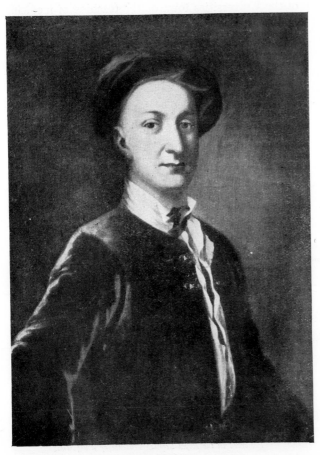

JOHN ARBUTHNOT (1667-1735)
(Original in the Royal Scottish National Portrait Gallery)

" 10th November, 1719, this day, the masters signed a diploma, *gratis*, in favours of Mr. Alexander Anderson, minister at Duffus, as Doctor of Medicine, he being a gentleman of approven skill of physic, as also his father having been once regent, and his grandfather Mr. John Rou, once Principall in this University."[1]

In Marischal College, the first recorded doctor is Richard Stoughton, in 1713 ; two others, Joseph Cam and John Spink, graduated in 1714, and were already licentiates of the Archbishoprick of Canterbury, while for many years those who graduated appear to have been men who had already been for a considerable time in practice or who had published works on medicine and were, in any case, men of recognised distinction.[2]   The same principle applies to the other Universities. At Edinburgh the first M.D. was David Cockburn, A.M., who graduated on 14th May, 1705, and there were twenty-one graduates in medicine prior to 1726, the year in which a Medical Faculty was established in this University.[3]   In Glasgow

---

1 " Fasti Aberdonenses of King's College, 1494-1854," Spalding Club, 1854, pp. 442-444.
2 " Records of Marischal College," Vol. II, p. 111.
3 " Edinburgh Medical Graduates," Edinburgh, 1867.

University the first M.D. degree appears to have been conferred in 1703, and degrees were even conferred on applicants *in absentia*. At St. Andrews University, Dr. John Arbuthnot was the first recorded M.D. He graduated in 1696 and underwent examination. He had studied at Marischal College, Aberdeen, where he graduated in Arts in 1681.[1] In later life he practised in London, being physician to Queen Anne, and the familiar friend of Pope and Swift. St. Andrews University for long continued the custom of conferring degrees only after examination, but without any residence or instruction at the University.

It was not until after the foundation of a Medical Faculty at Edinburgh, in 1726, that the idea came into being in Scotland of conferring the M.D. degree on young men as the consummation of three years' medical study, and to which they were entitled after successful examination.

The following is the list of mediciners at King's College, with their dates of appointment :—

Before	1522	James Cumyne
	1522	Robert Gray
	1556	Gilbert Skeen
	1619	Dr. Patrick Dun
	1632	Dr. William Gordon
	1640	Chair vacant
	1649	Dr. Andrew Moore
	1672	Dr. Patrick Urquhart
	1725	Dr. James Gregory (elder)
	1732	Dr. James Gregory (younger)
	1755	Dr. John Gregory
	1766	Sir Alexander Gordon of Lesmore
	1782	Dr. William Chalmers
	1793	Sir Alexander Burnett Bannerman
	1813	Dr. James Bannerman
	1839	Dr. William Gregory
	1844	Dr. Andrew Fyfe

Master James Cumyne had been brought to Aberdeen about the year 1503 to act as medical officer of the burgh. The Magistrates, on 20th October, 1503, agreed to pay him a retaining fee of ten merks yearly, and later one half of the net fishings at the fords of Dee, on condition that he should " mak personale residence within the said burghe, and cum and vesy tham that beis seik, and schow them his medicin, one thar expensis." It was also stipulated that his " wyf, houshalde, and bairnis " should be brought to reside in the burgh. He was evidently, from his title of " Master," a University graduate.[2]

---

[1] " Records of Marischal College," Vol. II, p. 253.
[2] " Extracts from the Council Register of the Burgh of Aberdeen," p. 431.

Cumyne seems also to have received from the Royal Exchequer a grant mentioned in the year 1502, and continued in subsequent years. It was paid through the Bishop of Aberdeen and charged against the Burgh of Cullen, though the name of the recipient is never stated. "To a doctor graduated in the Faculty of Medicine, reading in the University at Aberdeen, newly founded in the city of Old Aberdeen, receiving annually twelve pounds six shillings from the concession of the King" (James IV.).[1]

Gilbert Skeen, or Skeyne, was born about the year 1522, and after the usual education at the Grammar School and King's College, he took a Master of Arts

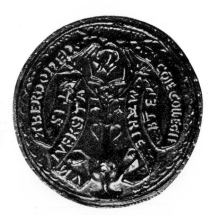

degree and applied himself to the study of medicine, being appointed mediciner to King's College in 1556. While occupying this position, he published "Ane Breve Descriptioun of the Pest," printed at Edinburgh in 1568. Having married, in 1569, Agnes Lawson, the widow of a burgess of Edinburgh, he transferred to this city in 1575 and commenced the practice of medicine in a house at Niddrie Wynd, Edinburgh. Here he rose to considerable celebrity, and on 16th June, 1581, he was appointed physician to His Majesty James VI., receiving a "gift of pension" of "twa hundreth pundis money of our realme."[2] Another small treatise, entitled "Ane Brief Descriptioun

SEAL OF KING'S COLLEGE
ABERDEEN

of the Qualiteis and Effectis of the Well of the Woman Hill besyde Abirdene, Anno Do. 1580," is also attributed to him.[3] He died in 1599.

Gilbert Skeen lived through the worst outbreak of the plague in Edinburgh, but his brief description of the pest, though printed in 1568 at Edinburgh, was written before he left Aberdeen. It is interesting, also, as one of the few examples of books published by Scottish doctors or surgeons in the 16th century, and, like the "Chyrurgerie" of Maister Peter Lowe, it is written in the vernacular. Their vernacular language was also employed about this time by Ambrose Paré, the great Elizabethan surgeons, and Richard Wiseman. This practice gave to such works, unlike those written in Latin, a greater usefulness though a narrower circulation at their time, but conferred on them a more enduring fame. The little treatise on the plague runs to about 10,000 words. The following are Skeen's views as to the cause of plague:—

---

[1] "Exchequer Rolls of Scotland," Vol. XII, p. 106.
[2] "Tracts by Dr. Gilbert Skeyne, Medicinar to His Majesty," Bannatyne Club Reprint, Edinburgh, 1860 ,pp. vii-ix.
[3] See reprint in facsimile, Edmond & Spark, Aberdeen, 1884.

" The cause of pest in ane privat Citie is stinkand corruptioun and filth, quhilkis occupeis the commune streittis and gaittis, greit reik of colis *(smoke of coals)* without vinde to dispache the sam, corruptioun of Herbis, sic as Caill and growand Treis, Moist heuie sauer *(smell)* of Lynt, Hemp, & Ledder steipit in Vater.   Ane priuat house infectis ather of stinkand closettis, or corrupte Carioun thairin, or neir by, or gif the inhabitantis hes inuiseit vther infectit Rowmis, or drinking corrupte Vatter, eating of Fruttis, or vder meitctis quhilkis ar corrupte, as we see dalie the pure mair subiecte to sic calamitie, nor the potent, quha ar constrynit be pouertie to eit ewill and corrupte meittis, and diseisis contractit heirof ar callit Pandemiall."[1]

The diagnostic signs of plague are given by him as follows, and he also has a long section upon the signs of death : —

" Thair is mony notis quhilkis schauis ane man infectit be pest.   First gif the exteriour partis of the bodie be caulde, and the interiour partis of the bodie vehement hait.   As gif the hoill bodie be heauie with oft scharpe punctiounis, stinkand sueiting tyritnes of bodie, ganting of mowthe, detestable brathe with greit difficultie, at sumtyme vehement feuer rather on nycht nor day.   Greit doloure of heid with heauynes, sollicitude & sadnes of mynd : greit displesour with sowning *(swooning)*, quhairefter followis haistelie deth.   As greit appetit and propensnes to sleip albeit on day, rauing and walking occupeis the last.   Cruell inspectioun of the ene, quhilkis apperis of sindre colouris, maist variant dolour of the stomak inlak of appetite, vehement doloure of heart, with greit attractioun of Air : intolerable thirst, frequent vomitting of diuers colouris or greit appetit by daylie accustum to Vomit, without effecte : Bitternes of mowth, and toung with blaiknit colour thairof & greit drouth : frequent puls small & profund quhais vrine for the maist part is turbide thik & stinkand or first vaterie colourit thairefter of bilious colour, last confusit and turbide, or at the beginning is zallow inclyning to greine (callit citrine collour) and confusit, thairefter becummis reid without contentis.   Albeit sum of thir properteis may be sene in haill mennis vater, quhairby mony ar deceauit abydand Helth of the patient, quhan sic vater is maist manifest sing of deth, because the haill venome & cause coniunit thairwith, leauand the naturall partis occupeis the hart and nobillest interioure partis of the body.   Last of all and maiste certane, gif with constant feuer, by the earis, vnder the oxtaris, or by the secrete membres maist frequentlie apperis apostumis *(abscesses)* callit Bubones, without ony other manifest cause, or gif the charbunkil apperis hastelie in ony other part, quhilk gif it dois, in the begining, testifeis strenthe of nature helth, and the laitter sic thingis appeir, and apperand, it is the mair deidlie.   At sumtym in ane criticall day mony accidentis apperis principalie vomiteing, spitting of blude, with sweit, flux of womb, bylis, scabe with dyuers other symptomis, maist heauie and detestable."[2]

The chief part of the little book is devoted to the means by which those exposed to plague may avoid infection, and to the treatment which Skeen has found useful in cases of the plague :—

" Euacuatioun is perfitit be blude drawing, befoir or efter that ony persone hes bene in suspect place, in speciall of the Vaine callit Mediana of the richt arme takand in quantitie as strenth, temperament, consuetude, aige, and tyme may suffir.   Euerilk ane remouand

---

[1] pp. 6 and 7, [2] pp. 12-14, " Tracts by Dr. Gilbert Skeyne," reprinted by The Bannatyne Club, Edinburgh, 1860.
                                                                                            K

thame self fra cuntrey, town, and Air, infectit or suspect and quha may not do the samyn, or mowit be Christiane Cheritie will not, man be studious to liue in fre Air. . . ." [1]

" Fyre made of fir or akin tymmer ar maist lowable, makand suffumigatioun thairwith of the tre of Aloes, Calamus callit Aromaticall. . . ."

" Perfumand also al claithis in priuat lugeingis with the reik of sandal, rose vater or sic lyke other materialis.   And as ony of the simplis befoir written seruis, siclyk compositionis may be maide of the sam, in forme of trociseis, thik pulderis, candillis or pomis odoratiue in this maneir.   Rec. storac, calamint. vnc. duas, rasuræ ligni Iuniperj vnc. sex. masticis vnc. vnam, benio. vnc. duas, paretur, puluis. . . ." [2]

" Four scrupulis of the pil. of Ruffus ar maist profitable, quhilkis beand tane oft befoir (sayis Ruffus) preseruis maist surlie fra the pest, & ar callit be some, pilulæ communes, be vtheris pilulæ Arabicæ, vel pilulæ contra pestem, quhilkis are dyuerse vayis dispensit, as followis. Rec. aloes Hepatici partes duas, ammoniaci electissimi partes duas, myrrhæ electæ partem vnam, cum vino odorato formentur. . . ." [3]

" Twichand meittis, flesche is maist proper quhilk generis louable humoris, & is of facill digestioun, Sic as Pertrik, Phasiane, Lauerok (lark), Hen, Turture, Kid, Mottoun, Cunning (rabbit), Veill, & siclyk otheris, vsand thairwith Garyophillis (cloves), and Cannell pulderit. . . ." [4]

The part devoted to the cure contains a great many prescriptions for ointments, mixtures, plasters, etc., which are almost all derived from vegetable sources and are mainly of the nature of volatile oils.

" Of fructis, feggis, bytter almondis, dry rasingis, sowr apill or peir, orange, citroun, or limown, caperis, soure prunis, or cheryis, with daylie use of vinagir or vergeus with all sortis of meittis : drinkand cleir quhyt odoratiue Vyne, temperat with vater, veschand face, mouthe, & handis, at morning with vyne temperat with rois vater, drawand at neis the decoctioun, of the leauis of laure, onytand the eiris with oile de spica, hauand in mouthe the seid of citroun, abstenand fra sleip on day lycht, Ire, crying, Venus playis, as fra maist dangerous enemeis." [5]

With regard to the treatment of the bubos, he recommends early opening by a " chirurgical hand," after which various maturative materials or suppuratives may be applied, for which he gives several prescriptions, again consisting of aromatic substances.   Gangrene, which he says is wont to appear, also demands the hand of the surgeon, and is to be treated by maturatives and washed with turpentine spirit and other substances which we should call antiseptics. A curative plaster is finally to be applied.

Patrick Dun, a native of Aberdeen, was M.D. of Basel, and held office both in King's and Marischal Colleges.   He was a benefactor both of the Grammar School and of Marischal College, to which he gave 2000 merks for repair of damage

---

[1] p. 18, [2] p. 19, [3] p. 23, [4] p. 25, [5] p. 26 : " Tracts by Dr. Gilbert Skeyne."

caused by a fire in 1639. In the latter College he held successively the posts of Regent, Professor of Logic (1610), Rector (1619) and Principal (1621). He was the author of " Themata medica de dolore colico," Basel (1607), and edited Liddell's " Ars conservandi sanitatem " (1651).[1]

William Gordon, mediciner at King's College in the year 1636, appears to have taken a serious view of his duties, and in this year petitioned the Lords of the Privy Council, that seeing he was appointed to teach medicine and anatomy, and had exercised his students sufficiently for two years past in the dissection of beasts, he desired the Lords to give him opportunities for the practical teaching of human anatomy. He mentions in his petition that it was usual for the Magistrates of cities in which Universities were situated to deliver two bodies of men and two of women in each year to be publicly anatomised. The Privy Council met his request by

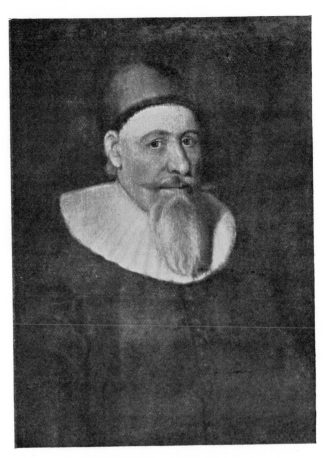

PATRICK DUN (Died 1649)
(Original picture, by Jamesone, in the Grammar School, Aberdeen)

directing the Sheriffs, Provost and Baillies of Aberdeen and Banff to deliver to the suppliant two bodies of executed malefactors, especially of rebels or outlaws, or failing that, bodies of the poorer sort, who had few friends or acquaintances to take exception.[2] Some of his successors in the post, however, were less thorough in their desire to teach, and some of them gave up lecturing on medicine altogether.

---

[1] " Records of Marischal College," New Spalding Club, 1898, Vol. II, p. 28, and Vol. I, p. 231.
[2] " Miscellany of the Spalding Club," Aberdeen, 1842, Vol. II, p. 71.

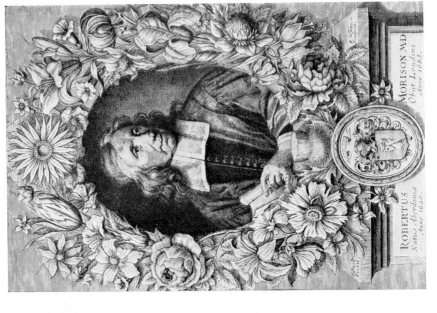

ROBERT MORISON, M.D. (1620–1683)

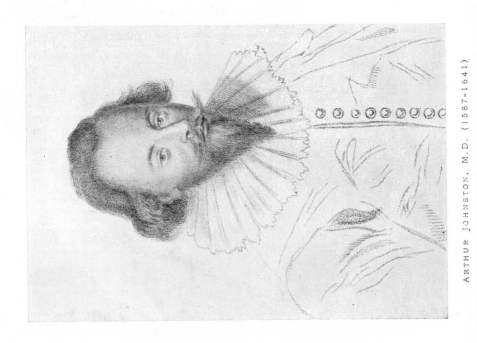

ARTHUR JOHNSTON, M.D. (1587–1641)

A distinguished Rector of King's College, in 1637 (though not a mediciner), was Arthur Johnston (1587–1641), of Caskieben (now called Keith Hall, near Inverurie), who had taken the M.D. of Padua in 1610. He became physician-in-ordinary to Charles I., and his talent as a writer of Latin verse was pronounced by some authorities to be superior to that of George Buchanan. He had practised medicine in France, and his famous translation of the Psalms was published at Aberdeen in 1637, although his duties as Court Physician kept him mainly in England. Numerous other Aberdonians of this period were celebrated as medical practitioners outside Aberdeen, such as Robert Straloch, who taught medicine at Paris; Gilbert Jack (1578–1628), who taught at Leyden and published the " Institutiones Medicæ "; Alexander Reid, physician to Charles I., who published treatises on anatomy and surgery (1634); and Robert Morison (1620–1683), physician to Charles II., and professor of botany in Oxford.[1]

Among the mediciners of King's College are four of the family of Gregory. This family produced no fewer than sixteen professors in Aberdeen, Edinburgh and other Universities. The earliest to attain professorial rank was James Gregory, professor of mathematics in St. Andrews and Edinburgh, who married a daughter of George Jamesone, the Scottish Vandyke. His son, Professor James Gregory, the elder, became mediciner at King's College in 1725, and was succeeded by his son James Gregory, the younger, who in turn was followed as mediciner by his younger brother, Dr. John Gregory, who for a time had been professor of natural philosophy in King's College. This Dr. John Gregory was also one of the early physicians of the Aberdeen Infirmary. He had begun life by working in the shop of his brother, a chemist of Aberdeen, and thus obtained a thorough knowledge of drugs. He also studied at Leyden before finally settling down in Aberdeen. Thinking Aberdeen too small for the exercise of his abilities, he tried medical practice in London for twelve months, and eventually settled in Edinburgh, where he was elected to the Chair of Medicine in 1766, in succession to Robert Whytt. He in turn was succeeded in the Edinburgh Chair by the illustrious William Cullen. The part of his career spent in Aberdeen is better known than that in Edinburgh, because, in the latter place, he was overshadowed by his more distinguished son, James Gregory, who succeeded Cullen as Professor of Medicine in 1790.

The Gregorys were of the same family as the MacGregors, and at the time of the Jacobite Rebellion in 1745, Rob Roy, who was hiding in Aberdeenshire, paid an uninvited visit to his cousin, the mediciner of King's College. Seeing young James Gregory, then a sturdy child, he declared he would take James with him to the Highlands and " make a man of him." The respectable mediciner of King's College was horrified at the idea, and was much relieved when, as he was walking

---

[1] " Studies in the History of the University of Aberdeen," Edited by P. J. Anderson, M.A.; Article on " Four Centuries of Medicine in Aberdeen," Stephenson, Aberdeen, 1906, pp. 305 and 306.

FAMILY OF GREGORY

Showing the number of Professors, with their Universities, Chairs and dates of tenure.

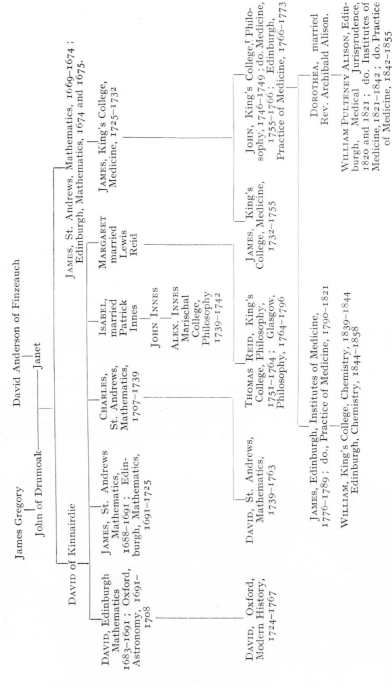

As compiled by Anderson for " Fasti Academiae Mariscallanae Aberdonensis," Vol. I., p. 203.

one day with Rob Roy in the Castlegate, a troop of soldiers appeared from the barracks. "If those lads are stirring, I had better be off," said the cateran, and disappeared up a neighbouring Close and so from Aberdeen, leaving James Gregory to become ultimately a celebrated Edinburgh professor.[1] Dr. John Gregory, in his early days, had studied at Leyden with a little group of Scottish students, which also included the Rev. Alexander Carlyle, later of Inveresk, who, in his autobiography, gives an account of this University, the favourite resort for Scottish students of the time.[2] Carlyle describes John Gregory, when tried by the ardent spirits of Edinburgh, as being adjudged "cold, selfish and cunning," and pretending to "professional arts to get into business." This, however, he denies, and having had him as family physician at a later period, he found Gregory "friendly, affectionate and generous."[3]

John Gregory published "The Elements of the Practice of Physic," but is better known as the author of "Lectures on the Duties and Qualifications of a Physician," published

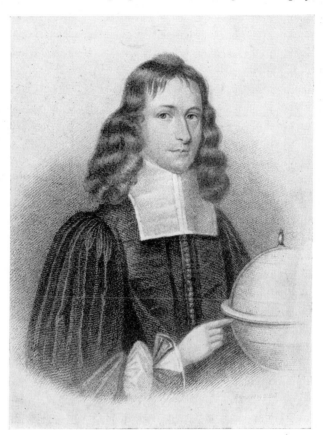

JAMES GREGORY, M.A. (ABERDEEN) (1638-1675)
Professor of Mathematics in St. Andrews and Edinburgh, and the first Professor of this family

in 1772. This was a series of six lectures delivered to his students and intended as a guide to recently qualified practitioners for their conduct in practice. Although somewhat diffuse, after the manner of writings of the

[1] E. H. B. Rodger: "Aberdeen Doctors," 1893, p. 75. This story is also told by Sir Walter Scott in his introduction to "Rob Roy."
[2] "Autobiography of the Rev. Alexander Carlyle," Edinburgh, 1860.
[3] Carlyle: Op. cit., pp. 178 and 179.

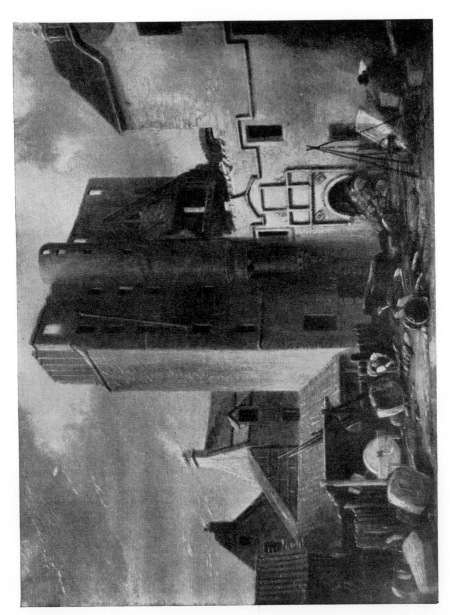

OLD MARISCHAL COLLEGE
In process of demolition in 1840
(Original painting by Auld, in the University of Aberdeen)

18th century generally, it is still well worth reading.[1]   The following quotation, which is the last paragraph of the book, gives a general idea of the whole :—

" I hope I have advanced no opinions in these lectures that tend to lessen the dignity of a profession which has always been considered as most honourable and important.   But, I apprehend, this dignity is not to be supported by a narrow, selfish, corporation-spirit ; by self-importance ; a formality in dress and manners ; or by an affectation of mystery.   The true dignity of physic is to be maintained by the superior learning and abilities of those who profess it, by the liberal manners of gentlemen, and by that openness and candour, which disdain all artifice, which invite to a free enquiry, and thus boldly bid defiance to all that illiberal ridicule and abuse to which medicine has been so much and so long exposed."

Gregory's works in four volumes were published after his death at Edinburgh in 1778.

After John Gregory left Aberdeen in 1766, the duties of the mediciner at King's College appear to have been carried out with little energy.   It is said that the two Bannermans, who held the post from 1793 to 1838, never lectured.[2]

On the death of the younger Bannerman, William Gregory, grandson of Dr. John Gregory, was appointed to the post of mediciner.   William Gregory took a special interest in chemistry, and five years later, in 1844, was appointed professor of chemistry in Edinburgh University, when he was succeeded at King's College by Andrew Fyfe, who had been assistant to Professor Hope in Edinburgh. Fyfe became Professor of Chemistry at the University of Aberdeen in 1860.

Marischal College and University was founded on the site of the Greyfriars Monastery by George Keith, 5th Earl Marischal of Scotland, in 1593, out of the former possessions of the Grey Friars, Black Friars and White Friars of Aberdeen, because of his knowledge of the lack of means in the north of Scotland for obtaining a liberal and Christian education.   The Earls Marischal continued as hereditary Chancellors of this College until their forfeiture following the Rebellion of 1715. William, 9th Earl Marischal, erected a professorship of medicine in Marischal College on 8th August, 1700, and nominated for the post Mr. Patrick Chalmers of Fedrett, M.D., "to be Professor of Medicine in our Colledge and University."[3]   No remuneration apparently was attached to the post, but on 31st May, 1712, Queen Anne granted £210 from the Civil List to the Principal and Professors of Marischal and King's Colleges for the augmentation of their salaries.   The share of the professor of medicine at Marischal College appears to have been £10 10s. yearly.[4]

[1] John Gregory : " Lectures on the Duties and Qualifications of a Physician," London, 1772.
[2] " Studies in the History of the University," Edited by P. J. Anderson, Aberdeen, 1906, p. 312.
[3] " Fasti Academiae Mariscallanae Aberdonensis," New Spalding Club, Aberdeen, 1889.   Edited by P. J. Anderson, M.A., LL.B., Vol. I, p. 381.
[4] Op. cit., p. 395.

In 1717, the Crown nominated Dr. Matthew Mackaile to succeed Chalmers, who had been ejected by the Commission of Visitation, probably in consequence of Jacobite sympathies.   The following is a list of the professors of medicine in Marischal College, with their dates of appointment :—

1700	Patrick Chalmers
1717	Matthew Mackaile
1734	James Gordon
1755	Alexander Donaldson
1793	William Livingston
1823	Charles Skene
1839	John Macrobin

Their duties were probably very similar to those of the mediciners in the neighbouring King's College, although they appear to have carried these out with greater energy.

The ledger of Patrick Chalmers has been preserved, and some of its details afford an interesting picture of the work and especially of the remuneration of a physician in Aberdeen at the close of the 17th and beginning of the 18th centuries.

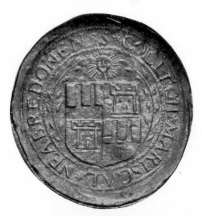

SEAL OF MARISCHAL COLLEGE
ABERDEEN

Chalmers settled in Aberdeen in medical practice in the year 1682, having already studied medicine according to the practice of the time at the Universities of Leyden, Paris and Padua, in each of which Universities he took the M.D. degree. His professional income appears to have increased from £384 16s. Scots in 1684, to £1084 2s. 2d. in 1694. This was, however, a particularly good year, and his average income seems to have been about £600 Scots. His patients included many of the county families of Aberdeenshire. Among the diseases most frequently mentioned in the ledger are fever and ague, rheumatism, scrofula, pleurisy, cholera, flux, smallpox and hydropsie. There are frequent entries of payments by the Earle of Aberdeine, including one of £67 in 1686, and the fees vary from sums of about this amount to £8 for delivery and medical attendance on a baillie's wife, and £6 paid by Captain David Garioch for " drunkenness."   There are frequent entries of accounts to ladies for cure of " the vapours," and ague seems to have been a very common complaint.   The Sheriff of Murray paid £6 9s. for treatment of the itch, and Mrs. Helen Leslie for vapours and itch, £6 6s.; while Mrs. Duncan " in gratitude for her salvation " paid £12 18s.   Presents in kind seem often to have been tendered by way of payment, from meal and malt down to a hat in 1692.

These presents are duly valued and entered, and their amount varied from £40 down to £9 in the year.[1]

Matthew Mackaile was also regent in 1729. He was the son of the better known Matthew Mackaile, an apothecary and burgess of Edinburgh, who later practised in Aberdeen and who was the author of several books, especially one on "The Diversite of Salts and Spirits" (1683), and another dealing with the waters of Moffat and of St. Catherine's Well near Liberton (1664).[2] The father's portrait hangs in the Great Hall at Marischal College.

James Gordon was the son of Dr. John Gordon, a physician of Aberdeen.[3]

Alexander Donaldson succeeded his father as professor of Oriental languages in 1754, and continued to hold this post along with that of mediciner till his death in 1793.[4]

William Livingston was the son of Dr. Thomas Livingston, a physician of Aberdeen.[5] He was an early President of the Medical Society, and its library and museum were kept in his house.

Charles Skene was a son of George Skene, professor of natural history.[6]

John Macrobin was an M.D. of Edinburgh. When the two Colleges were united in 1860, Macrobin became Professor of Practice of Medicine in the University of Aberdeen. He was the author of an "Introduction to the Study of Practical Medicine."[7]

King's and Marischal Colleges co-existed for a long period as independent and rival institutions, but an attempt was made during the reign of Charles I, in 1641, to combine them into one academic body. This attempt, however, appears to have been abortive, and they again fell apart. Various attempts at rapprochement were made from time to time. Thus, in a scheme of union in 1707, a joint school of medicine was a prominent feature. Again, in 1818, an attempt which lasted for some years was made to combine the two medical schools. In 1826, a Commission was appointed by Sir Robert Peel to investigate the state of affairs in the Scottish Universities, and their report in 1830 suggested that in Aberdeen the fusion of the two Colleges would create an efficient Medical School. A Bill was proposed in 1836, under the title "The United University of Aberdeen," but, owing to opposition, was withdrawn, and local jealousies kept the two schools apart until their final fusion in 1860.[8]

At Marischal College, professors of chemistry had existed in the persons of George French, appointed in 1793, and Thomas Clark, appointed in 1833. Dr. George French, the son of an Aberdeen advocate, was one of the surgeons

[1] John I. Chalmers : "Proceedings of the Society of Antiquaries of Scotland," Vol. IV, pp. 181–185.
[2] "Aberdeen Public Library Catalogue of Local Collection," p. 226.
[3], [4], [5], [6], [7] "Records of Marischal College," New Spalding Club, Aberdeen, 1898, Vol. II, pp. 55 and 56.
[8] J. Scott Riddell : "Records of the Aberdeen Medico-Chirurgical Society," Aberdeen, 1922, p. 46 et seq.

to the Infirmary and a physician in Aberdeen. Prior to being made Professor of Chemistry, he and Dr. Livingston, afterwards Professor of Medicine, had proposed, in 1786, to give a six months' course of clinical lectures at the Infirmary. He was succeeded in 1833 in the Chair of Chemistry by Professor Thomas Clark, an M.D. of Glasgow. Clark's health broke down in 1843, and his class was conducted by a number of substitutes, one of whom, James Smith Brazier, lectured to the class from 1852, and also conducted that of Professor Fyfe at King's College in 1854, becoming later Professor of Chemistry in the University of Aberdeen in succession to Professor Fyfe, in 1862.[1]

Dr. Macrobin, as professor of medicine, and Dr. Thomas Clark, as Professor of Chemistry, appear to have been active teachers, and, in the year 1839, two new Chairs were founded by Queen Victoria, that of anatomy, to which Dr. Allen Thomson was appointed, and that of surgery, of which Dr. Pirrie was made professor. Professor Pirrie was the author of a treatise on " Principles and Practice of Surgery " (1852), and in 1860 he became Professor of Surgery in the University of Aberdeen.[2] In the Chair of Anatomy, Allen Thomson, who resigned the Chair at Marischal College in 1841 to take up the professorship of physiology at Edinburgh, was succeeded by Alexander Jardine Lizars, previously an Edinburgh lecturer and author of " Elements of Anatomy " (1844), who continued in office as Professor of Anatomy in the University of Aberdeen after 1860.[3]

In 1857, a Chair of Medical Logic and Medical Jurisprudence was founded, Francis Ogston, who had been lecturing on medical jurisprudence since 1839, was appointed. He was the author of " Lectures on Medical Jurisprudence " (1878), and, in 1860, he continued in office as Professor in the University of Aberdeen.[4]

The following is a list, so far as known, of lecturers in connection with the Medical School at Aberdeen up to the year 1860. Some of these were connected with King's College, others with Marischal College, while some were independent :—

1758 Dr. David Skene	Midwifery	
(In 1759, the Kirk Session of Old Machar published a recommendation of Dr. Skene's midwifery class, animadverting upon the ignorance of midwives)		
1786 Dr. French and Dr. Livingston	Clinical Lectures at the Infirmary.	
1790 Mr. James Russel	Clinical surgery at the Infirmary.	
1802 Dr. Charles Skene	Anatomy	
1811 Dr. William Dyce	Midwifery	

[1] p. 58, [2] p. 61, [3] p. 62, [4] p. 64 : " Records of Marischal College," Vol. II.

1818	George Barclay	Surgery
	William Henderson	Materia Medica
	(The proprietor of Caskieben, near Aberdeen)	
	Alexander Ewing	Physiology
	(This was the first year of the joint school)	
1819	Robert White	Institutes of Medicine
1820	Patrick Blaikie	Surgery
1823	Alexander Ewing	Anatomy
1826	Alexander Fraser	Midwifery
1827	William Knight	Botany

(Dr. Knight had conducted a botany class
at intervals for several years before this time.
In 1780, Rev. Robert Memis had been granted
£6 per annum by the Town Council towards
the formation of a Botanic Garden, and, in
1787, had taught a class in botany.   From
1792 to 1799, Rev. Alexander Smith had
conducted a class, and, from 1801 to 1810,
Professor James Beattie had conducted a
class of ten to twenty students)

1828	James Torrie	Institutes of Medicine
1830	Alexander Ewing	Surgery
	William Pirrie	Anatomy and Physiology
	William Laing	Clinical Medicine
1831	John Geddes	Institutes of Medicine
1834	William Laing	Surgery
1837	Alexander Murray	Clinical Medicine
	William Laing	Clinical Surgery
1839	William Henderson	Materia Medica
	Francis Ogston	Medical Jurisprudence
	Alexander Harvey	Institutes of Medicine
	William McKinnon	Comparative Anatomy
	James Jamieson	Midwifery
1840	John Shier...	Botany
1841	Robert Dyce	Midwifery
1845	Robert Jamieson	Mental Diseases
1849	George Ogilvie	Institutes of Medicine
	John Forbes Ogilvie	Insanity
1853	Wyville Thomson	Botany
1854	William Rhind	Botany
1855	Robert Beveridge	Botany

A severe blow had been dealt to medical studies connected with the Aberdeen Colleges by an occurrence known as " the burning of the burking-house," in 1831. Early in the 19th century, before the passing of the Anatomy Act (1830), the supply of bodies for dissection had been very difficult to obtain and had only been made possible by the enthusiastic though often ill-directed " Resurrectionist " activities of the Aberdeen medical students in the surrounding country churchyards, which vied with those recorded of Liston and other surgeons in Edinburgh. The terror inspired by the Burke and Hare affair of 1828 in Edinburgh had spread to Aberdeen, where Andrew Moir was lecturer on anatomy in 1831. The anatomist was apparently not too careful in his work, and one day a dog scraping in the open ground behind the anatomical theatre in St. Andrew Street revealed a dissected human limb to some women passing to the bleach-green. A crowd gradually collected, and it was found that the fragments of a dead body had been carelessly buried. The theatre appears to have had a sinister appearance, with three false windows to the front and receiving its lighting from behind. An excited and furious mob gradually collected, broke into the theatre and found three bodies laid out ready for dissection, which were borne off through the streets in triumph. The place was ransacked, instruments and furnishings destroyed and the mob, swelled to thousands, filled the neighbouring streets. Among them were jostled the protesting Provost of Aberdeen, members of the Town Council, policemen, and soldiers from the barracks, incapable of any action amid a mob of twenty thousand howling people. Andrew Moir, appearing on the spot, was pursued by a section of the crowd, thirsting for his life, but finally managed to conceal himself beneath a tombstone in the churchyard of St. Nicholas. Tar barrels and other combustible materials were brought and set on fire, the walls of the building were undermined, and in an hour literally not one stone was standing upon another of the blazing theatre. So ended this extraordinary example of mob law, which formed a serious setback to medical study in Aberdeen.[1]

An important event in the Aberdeen Medical School towards the end of the 18th century was the foundation of the Aberdeen Medical Society. The prime mover in this was James McGrigor, who, with his companion, James Robertson, after completing his studies at Marischal College, had travelled to Edinburgh and spent a year at this University. In Edinburgh the Royal Medical Society, managed by students, had enjoyed over fifty years of flourishing existence, and on their return to Aberdeen, McGrigor and Robertson, together with ten other medical students from Marischal College, determined, in 1789, to found a debating society for mutual benefit, under the name of The Aberdeen Medical Society. The Society met once a week in the Greek Class-room for papers, criticism and discussions on the lines of the Edinburgh Students' Society. In 1790, twelve more names were added, and in 1791 several more joined. James McGrigor was first Secretary of the Society till 1790, and was evidently its moving spirit.

[1] E. H. B. Rodger: " Aberdeen Doctors," 1893, p. 240 et seq.

Among the first honorary members of the Society was Mr. Wynne, private chaplain to the Prince of Wales, afterwards George IV. His support was secured in a somewhat amusing manner. A dispute arose as to how the letter offering him honorary membership should be worded. It was thought improper that it should be too curt, and to terminate by wishing him the compliments of the season appeared to some members impertinent, so that these difficulties were finally overcome by the appointment of a committee to write the letter in Latin. James McGrigor, who happened to be leaving for London to try his fortunes, agreed to deliver the letter in person in order to save the postage. McGrigor's early energy was continued in later life, so that he became Director-General of the Army Medical Service in the Peninsula, and, as Sir James McGrigor, was one of Wellington's most trusted advisers.

Sir James McGrigor continued to take a close and practical interest in the affairs of the Society and later, when, in 1820, the Society built a Hall, he was largely instrumental in the successful issue of the project. This building, situated in King Street, and still the home of the Society, was the first work in beautifully-dressed white granite of Archibald Simpson (1790–1847), Aberdeen's most notable resident architect, who erected the Royal Infirmary and other principal buildings in the first half of last century, and gave a new character to Aberdeen as the " Granite City." As the student members of the Society graduated, those who lived in Aberdeen or its neighbourhood continued to attend its meetings, and the Society, before 1820, was divided into two classes—a senior class, consisting of medical practitioners, who met in the Hall, and a second or junior class consisting of medical students or apprentices, who had their own President and Secretary, and met in the Library. The junior class gradually languished, and eventually came to an end, but the senior class, under the title of the Aberdeen Medico-Chirurgical Society, a name adopted about 1812, continued to flourish, and made itself one of the most important influences in the developing medical school of Aberdeen.[1]

The Commissioners, appointed by the Act of 1858 to improve and regulate the course of studies in the Universities of Scotland, united in 1860 the two foundations of King's College and Marischal College, as the University of Aberdeen. Henceforth, the Faculty of Medicine in this University was lodged in Marischal College, which was more favourably placed than King's College for a medical school. For one thing, it was situated in the new town of Aberdeen, and was nearer to the Infirmary, which had been founded in 1739, and in which clinical teaching had gradually been established. In King's College there was only one professor, the mediciner, other subjects being represented by lecturers. The re-organisation of the Medical School approximated closely with the passing of the Medical Act of 1858. Regius Chairs in physiology, materia medica and midwifery were founded at the same time, while a Chair in pathology was added in 1882, and other Chairs and lectureships have gradually followed, as at other Universities.

---

[1] J. Scott Riddell: " Records of the Aberdeen Medico-Chirurgical Society," Aberdeen, 1922, pp. 23–28.

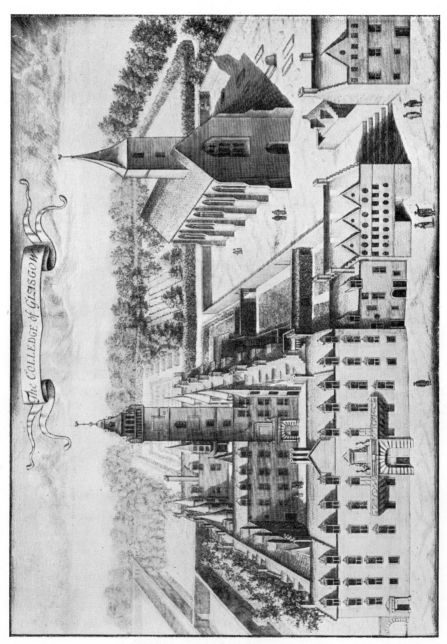

The Colledge of Glasgow

THE OLD COLLEGE OF GLASGOW AND BLACKFRIARS CHAPEL

(From engraving by Slezar about 1650)

The buildings were demolished about 1874. The front entrance is preserved as the lodge at Gilmorehill

CHAPTER X

THE EARLY MEDICAL SCHOOL OF GLASGOW

GLASGOW, until the early part of the 19th century, was not a town of great size. About the middle of the 16th century it seems to have occupied only the eleventh place in size among the Scottish towns, with a population of between four and five thousand,[1] and even at the beginning of the 17th century it occupied about the same relative position. It consisted practically only of the High Street,

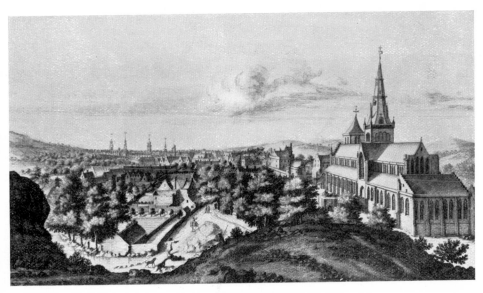

GLASGOW IN THE 17TH CENTURY, FROM THE EAST

The Bishop's Castle, upon the site of which the Royal Infirmary was built, is shown beyond the Cathedral.
The College is in the centre of the spires to the left

(Engraving by Slezer)

crossed at its upper end by Rotten Row, and at its southern end by the Trongate, with a few straggling houses between this and the Clyde, and numerous narrow wynds branching off from both sides of the main streets. The College was in the High Street not far from the Cathedral. Most of the houses had gardens behind, and in the 16th and 17th centuries Glasgow must have been a pleasant little town.

---

[1] Gibson: "History of Glasgow," p. 78.

L

In the early part of the 12th century, David I. settled a Bishop at Glasgow, and in 1175 William the Lion granted to the Bishop the right of having a burgh of barony, although the place was not a Royal Burgh.   In these surroundings a " *studium generale* " was founded at the instance of Bishop Turnbull by a Bull of Pope Nicholas V., in 1451, and this, in a letter of James II., under the Great Seal in 1453, is called the University of Glasgow.   Medicine does not, however, appear to have been actively taught in this University for a long time after its foundation.   In 1469, Andrew de Garleis, *Doctor in Medicinis*, seems to have been admitted to the University, but there is no further trace of him.   In 1536, Andrew Borde speaks of studying and practising medicine in Glasgow, where his services were in request and countenanced by the University.   He was an agent of Thomas Cromwell, maintaining communication with the political party favourable to England.[1]

In the 16th century barber surgeons or physicians probably came from other places and settled in Glasgow, and it appears from records of the Town Council, mentioning regulations directed against plague, leprosy and other diseases, that the Council had the benefit of expert advice in these matters.

Plague was a serious and destructive disease to the early inhabitants of Glasgow. It appeared several times during the 14th century.[2]   In the 15th century and 16th century, the city was four times ravaged by the plague : namely, in 1455, 1501, 1515 and 1545,[3] and at this time Glasgow was a place of suspicion to the neighbouring authorities of Edinburgh.   In 1584 and 1588, when plague was present in the burghs of the Fife coast and in Paisley, the Glasgow authorities established a rigid quarantine against the infected districts, and the danger was averted.   The most serious epidemic of the plague which visited Glasgow was that of 1645–1646, when a house-to-house visitation was adopted, daily reports sent to the Magistrates regarding the sick, and an old expedient, which had been previously tried, of transporting the plague-stricken out of town to the muir, was practised. At this time the Principal, regents and other members of the College were transferred to the town of Irvine.   Long before 1665, however, when the plague made its memorable visitation of London, Glasgow had been freed by these means from the dreaded disease.[4]

To compensate for the scanty inducements to ordinary practice, the Town Council of Glasgow, at an early period, began to offer salaries to doctors whom they invited to settle in the place.   There is a minute of the Town Council of 17th May, 1577, to the effect that " Allexander Hay, chirurgiane," was granted a yearly pension of ten merks, to be paid by the Treasurer of the town, while at the same time, he was made a burgess and freeman of the burgh, and to be free from taxes, conformably to the privilege held by James Abernethie, his master,

¹ Buist : " Andrew Borde," *Caledonian Med. Journ.*, June, 1921.
² Gibson : " History of Glasgow," pp. 72 and 73.
³ James Coutts, M.A. : " History of the University of Glasgow," Maclehose, Glasgow, 1909, p. 3.
⁴ Duncan : " Memorials of the Faculty of Physicians and Surgeons of Glasgow, 1599–1850," Glasgow, 1896, pp. 10 and 11.

previously.[1]   In 1589, it is recorded that Thomas Myln, a salaried surgeon, was brought up before the Council for speaking slanderously of the town, calling it the "hungrie toun of Glasgw." For this offence, the culprit was ordained to forfeit his pension for one year, the money to go to the improvement of the burgh.[2] Allaster M'Caslan was another surgeon men-

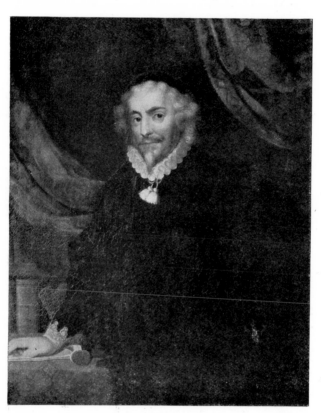

PETER LOWE
(Original picture in the Hall of the Royal Faculty of Physicians and Surgeons of Glasgow)

tioned as being paid by the baillies for "curing of sindry puir anes in the towne" in 1596.[3] At the end of the 16th century, the number of surgeons practising in the town probably did not exceed six, and there appears to have been only one physician. There were however, in addition, at least two midwives, who transacted most of the obstetric practice of the burgh.[4] In the year 1598 the Kirk Session appears to have taken an active interest in medical life, for it sent a deputation to the Town Council representing that an enquiry should be made as to those practising within the town, who pretended to have skill in medicine and had not the same, and that those who had skill should be retained and the others rejected. In April, 1599, the Town Council took action by appointing three baillies, three city ministers, and three University officers, with other men skilled in the art, to examine for the future those who practised medicine in the town. This committee had, however, hardly got to work, when the matter was settled from another direction. King James VI.

[1] "Extracts from the Records of the Burgh of Glasgow, 1573-1642," Glasgow, 1876, p. 58.
[2] Ibid., p. 138.
[3] Ibid., p. 178.
[4] Duncan : "Memorials of the Faculty of Physicians and Surgeons of Glasgow, 1599-1850," Maclehose, Glasgow, 1896, p. 18.

granted, in November, 1599, letters under the Privy Seal empowering Peter Lowe and Robert Hamilton, " professoure of medecine and their successouris indwelleris of our Citie of Glasgow," to examine and try all who professed or practised the art of surgery, to license those whom they adjudged fit, and to exclude the unqualified from practice, with power to fine those who proved contumacious. These " visitors," as Lowe and Hamilton were called, reported to the city Magistrates in cases of death by accident, violence or poison, and were empowered to exclude from the practice of medicine all who could not produce a testimonial of a famous University where medicine was taught. These extensive powers of licensing for medical practice extended over the burghs of Glasgow, Renfrew and Dumbarton, and the Sheriffdoms of Clydesdale, Renfrew, Lanark, Kyle, Carrick, Ayr and Cunningham, thus covering the greater part of the south-west of Scotland. This was the beginning of the Royal Faculty of Physicians and Surgeons at Glasgow.

Maister Peter Lowe probably arrived in Glasgow about the beginning of 1598, and the fact of his selecting Glasgow for his residence when he returned from the Continent raises the presumption that he belonged to the west of Scotland. From his use of the descriptive title " Arellian," it is possible that he may have been born at Errol or at Ayr. He was undoubtedly a Scot, because he appends the title " Scottishman " almost every time he writes his name, and he probably left Scotland for the Continent after the middle of the 16th century and about the time of the Reformation. He was a friend of Gilbert Primrose, Deacon of the Incorporation of Surgeons in Edinburgh, to whom, along with James Harvie, Surgeon to the Queen, he dedicates his " Chyrurgerie." He speaks of having had occasion to use remedies on service "in France, Flaunders and else-where, the space of twenty-two yeares : thereafter being Chirurgian-Major to the Spanish Regiments at Paris, two yeares: next following the French King my Master in the warres six yeares, where I tooke commoditie to practise all points and opera- tions of Chyrurgerie." [1]   As the Spanish regiments were assisting to hold Paris in 1588–1590 against Henry IV., this fixes the dates of his service on the Continent as lasting from 1566 to 1596. The period included such memorable historical events as the Massacre of St. Bartholomew and the Revolt of the Netherlands. From the side on which Lowe was serving, it appears that he was then a Catholic ; and as he was later " ordinary Chyrurgion to the French King and Navarre," he must have changed sides about 1590, and probably at the same time changed his religion. He also described himself as " doctor in the facultie of Chyrurgerie at Paris," and was therefore apparently a master surgeon of the Collège de St. Côme. His return to Britain was probably made in 1596, for in this year his book on " The Spanish Sicknes " was published in London. In the following year, 1597, his " Chyrurgerie " appeared, being dated from London, although the materials for the book had been collected abroad, and he made his appearance in Glasgow

---

[1] Peter Lowe : " Chyrurgerie," Edn. of 1612 ; address to the reader.   See also for full account, Finlayson : " Account of the Life and Works of Maister Peter Lowe," Glasgow, 1889.

in the early part of 1598.   He was not long in coming into collision with the power of the Kirk, for on 8th August, 1598, there is a minute of the Presbytery indicating that he had been condemned to stand on the " piller " for three Sundays, apparently for some offence against ecclesiastical discipline, and to pay a fine.   Mr. Peter Lowe had apparently treated the punishment with ridicule, but whether he ever " made his repentance as ordanit " is a matter of which there is now no record.

A book which must have been used to a considerable extent by Scottish practitioners, especially those in the west of Scotland, was the " Chyrurgerie " of Peter Lowe, first published in 1597, with later editions in 1612, 1634 and 1654.   This little treatise was the outcome of Lowe's experience in France.   It is essentially practical, and its descriptions of operations indicate by their accuracy of detail, his personal knowledge and practical experience of the things of which he wrote.   The earlier part of it deals with the theory of surgical treatment, and takes the form of a dialogue between Peter Lowe and his son John, in which the latter is questioned and answers, somewhat after the manner of a catechism.   The follow-

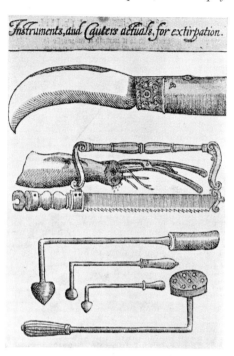

FIGURE OF 16TH CENTURY AMPUTATION
(From Peter Lowe's " Chyrurgerie")

ing extract gives a good example of Lowe's style, and describes the method used in the 17th century for an amputation of the leg :—

" The usage of this ribben or band is divers.   First, it holdeth the member hard and fast, so that the instrument or incising knife may cut more surely.   Secondly, that the feeling of the whole parts may be stupified, and rendred insensible.   Thirdly, that the fluxe of bloud may be stayed.   Fourthly, it holdeth up the skinne and muscles which must cover the bone after it be cut, and so it maketh it more easie to heale.   The bandage then being thus made, wee cut the flesh with a rasor or incising knife, which must be somewhat crooked to the forme of a hooke or halfe moone.

" The flesh then being so cut to the bone, the said bone must be diligently rubbed and scraped with the backe of the sayd knife, which backe must be made purposely for that effect, to the end the periost which covereth the bone, may be lesse painfull in cutting of the bone.   Otherwise it teareth and riveth with the same, so causeth great dolour : Also letteth [*hinders*] the cutting, although the bone have no feeling of it selfe.   This being done, you must saw the bone with a sharpe sawe: then loose the ligatour, draw downe the skin, and cover the bone in all the pares ; and if there be great putrifaction, let it bleed a little, for that dischargeth the part, and so is lesse subject to inflamation ; then one of the Assisters shall put the extreamities of his fingers on the great vaine & artiers, to stay them from bleeding, till the Chyrurgion either knit or cauterize them one after another."

The following is Peter Lowe's description of his operation for the relief of hernia, especially when it is strangulated, and of the truss which should be worn by elderly persons or by persons in whom the hernia is so great as to make operation unsuitable :—

" Of the Herne intestinall, called by the Greekes *Interocele*.   This kinde of rupture is when the guts fall downe in the cods, either through ruption or enlarging of ye Periton where the spermaticke vessels doe passe, and where the muscles *Cremastres* doe end, and the membraines *Dartos* and *Erethroides* begin, wherein the gut Call or both doth fall. . . . . If the fecall matter let [*hinder*] the reduction of it, you must use such remedie as is set downe in the last Chapter, with glisters to discarge the intestine.   If by those remedies the intestine do not reduce, but the matter fecall doe waxe hard with great dolour, you shall make incision in the upper side of the codde, eschewing the Intestine.   Thereafter put a little piece of wood up by the production of the Periton, neere unto the hole.   Of dissent[1] the piece of wood must be round on the one side and flat on the other, whereon you shall make the rest of your incision, then rubbe the inticed part & whole of dissent with a little oyle of Cammomill, or Lyllies, which will make it lubricke, and cause it to reduce more easily. . . . This operation must not be used but in great necessity, and the sicke strong prognosticating of the daunger, *Ne fefellisse aut ignorasse videæris:* being reduced, it must with bandages and astringent fomentations be contained, with this emplaister upon Leather . . . and keepe the bed for the space of fortie dayes . . . using in the meane time good dyet and of light digestion.   Abstaine from strong drinke, weake, and windie meats, from hoysting [*coughing*], crying, or other violent motion, so farre as the patient may.   In the meane time, keepe open the wombe [*bowels*], and lye in such sort, that the head and shoulders be lower than the hanches and fundament : by these meanes sundry doe heale, when the dilation or ruption is not great.   In great dilations and people of elder age, I find no remedie, save onely the bandage made of cloth with Cotton, Iron or Steele, as shall be most meete :   such people as doe ryde great Horses and are armed, are much subject to this disease, as I have often seen amonst the French, Almaine, or Ryfters Horse-men :   who for the most part have their bandages of Iron, eyther for one side or for both."[2]

As a result of the report by Peter Lowe to the Privy Council upon the abuses of medical practice in Glasgow, he got a privilege under the Privy Seal to " try and examine all men upon the Art of Chirurgerie, and to discharge, and allow in the West parts of Scotland, who were worthy or vnworthy, to professe the same." In 1601, he accompanied the Duke of Lennox, Lord Great Chamberlain of Scotland, who was appointed special ambassador for the Scottish King at the Court of France, upon an embassy to that country.   For this purpose he obtained leave of absence from his duties in Glasgow with a continuation of his salary for a year.[3] In 1602, he was back again in Glasgow, and there are numerous other references

---

[1] The two words " of dissent " belong to the previous sentence, but are printed here as in the original.
[2] Peter Lowe : " A Discourse of the whole art of Chyrurgerie," 3rd edition, 1634, pp. 90 and 91, 247-249.
[3] " Extracts from the Records of the Burgh of Glasgow, p. 223.

to him in the minutes of the Faculty and those of the Town Council. He published a second edition of his " Chyrurgerie," dated 20th December, 1612, and died apparently in the next year.

The great work of Peter Lowe was the establishment of the Faculty of Physicians and Surgeons, which embraced within its powers the regulation of the practice of medicine, surgery and pharmacy in the west of Scotland. The Charter instituted medico-legal examiners who reported to the authorities, thus forming in 1599 a very early example of State medicine. It was the duty of the Faculty to examine and license surgeons, but physicians were only to be called upon to produce the diploma from their University. As none of the Scottish Universities at this time granted degrees in medicine, this presumably refers to graduates of foreign Universities, who might be expected to settle in Glasgow. The Faculty also at a very early date undertook the gratuitous medical visitation and treatment of the sick poor. This practice was apparently taken by Peter Lowe from one of the regulations of the Collège de St. Côme at Paris.

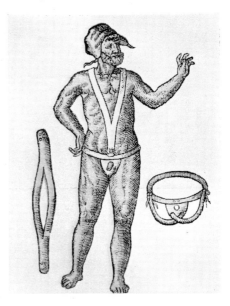

FIGURE OF 16TH CENTURY TRUSS
(From Peter Lowe's "Chyrurgerie")

The fact that physicians and surgeons were both included in the operation of the original Charter, and that they have remained united in this body to the present day, has had a great deal to do with moulding the character of the Glasgow Medical School. Although the University did not establish a Medical Faculty till the beginning of the 19th century, the rapid rise of this school and its celebrity as a training-place for efficient general practitioners, has probably been largely due to the fact that its surgeons have always possessed a good knowledge of medicine, while many of its physicians have been competent practitioners of surgery. This Charter is of so much inportance for the influence which it has had on Scottish medicine that it is given here in full :—

" JAMES, be the Grace of God, King of Scottis, to all Provostis, baillies of burrowis, scheriffs, stewartis, baillies of regalties, and otheris ministeris of justice within the boundis following, and their deputis, and all and sundrie otheris ouir leigis and subditis, quhom it efferis, quhase knawledge thir our letteris sal cume, greiting, WIT ZE WE, with auise o oure counsall, understanding the grit abuisis quhilk hes bene comitted in time bigane, and zit daylie continuis be ignorant, unskillit and unlernit personis, quha, under the collour of Chirurgeanis, abuisis the people to their plesure, passing away but [*without*]

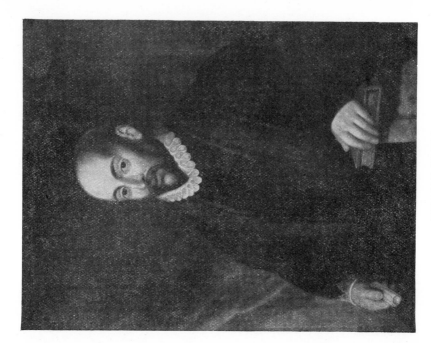

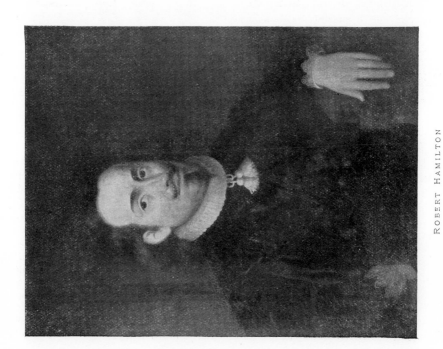

ROBERT HAMILTON   WILLIAM SPANG

(Original pictures in the Hall of the Royal Faculty of Physicians and Surgeons of Glasgow)

tryel or punishment, and thairby destroyis infinite number of oure subjectis, quhairwith na ordour hes bene tane in tyme bigane, specially within oure burgh and baronie of Glasgow, Renfrew, Dumbartane, and oure Sheriffdomes of Cliddisdale, Renfrew, Lanark, Kyile, Carrick, Air and Cunninghame ; FOR avoiding of sik inconvenientis, and for gude ordoure to be tane in tyme cuming, to have made, constitutit and ordanit, and be the tenoure of thir oure letteris, makis, constitutis, and ordinis Maister Peter Low, our Chirurgiane and chief chirurgiane to oure dearest son the Prince, with the assistance of Mr. Robert Hamiltone, professoure of medecine, and their successouris, indwelleris of our Citie of Glasgow, GEVAND and GRANTAND to thaime and thair successoures, full power to call, sumonnd, and convene before thame, within the said burgh of Glasgow, or onie otheris of ouir said burrowis, or publict places of the foirsaids boundis, all personis professing or using the said airt of Chirurgie, to examine thame upon thair literature, knawledge and practize ; gif they be fund wordie, to admit, allow, and approve thame, give them testimonial according to the airt and knawledge that they sal be fund wordie to exercise thareftir, resave thair aithis, and authorize thame as accordis, and to discharge thame to use onie farder nor they have knawledge passing thair capacity, laist our sub-jectis be abusit ; and that every ane citat report testimonial of the minister and eldris, or magistratis of the parochin quhair they dwell, of thair life and conversatione ; and in case they be contumax, being lauchfullie citat, everie ane to be unlawit in the soume of fortie pundis, toties quoties, half to the judges, other half to be disponit at the visitoures plesure ; and for payment thairof the said Mr. Peter and Mr. Robert, or visitoures, to have oure uthere letteris of horning [*outlawry*], on the partie or magistrates quhair the contemptuous personis duellis, chargeing thame to poind thairfoire, within twentie four houris, under the pain of horning ; and the partie not haveand geir poindable, the magistrate, under the same pain, to incarcerate thame, quhill cautioun responsall be fund, that the contumax persone sall compir at sik day and place as the saidis visitouris sall appoint, gevan trial of thair qualifications :

" *Nixt*, that the saidis visitouris sall visit everie hurt, murtherit, poisonit, or onie other persoun tane awa extraordinarly, and to report to the Magistrate of the fact as it is :

" *Thirdlie*, That it sall be leisum to the said visitouris with the advice of their brethren, to mak statutis for the comoun weill of our subjectis, anent the saidis artis, and using thairof faithfullie, and the braikeris thairof to be punshit and unlawit be the visitoures according to their falt :

" *Fordlie*, It sall not be leisum to onie mannir of personis within the foresaidis boundis to exercise medicine without ane testimonial of ane famous universitie quhair medecine be taught, or at the leave of oure and oure dearest spouse chief medicinarie ; and in case they failzie, it sal be lesum to the said visitouris to challenge, perseu, and inhibite thame throu using and exercing of the said airt of medicine, under the pain of fourtie poundis, to be distributed, half to the Judges, half to the pure, toties quoties they be fund in useing and exercing the same, ay and quhill they bring sufficient testimonial as said is :

" *Fythlie*, That na manir of personis sell onie droggis within the Citie of Glasgow, except the sam be sichtit be the saidis visitouris, and be William Spang, apothecar, under the pane of confiscatioune of the droggis :

" *Sextlie*, That nane sell retoun poison, asenick, or sublemate, under the pane of ane hundred merkis, excep onlie the apothecaries quha sall be bund to tak cautioun of the byaris, for coist, skaith and damage :

" *Seventlie*, Yat the saidis visitouris with thair bretherene and successouris, sall convene every first Mononday of ilk moneth, at sum convenient place, to visite and give counsell to pure disaisit folkis gratis : and *last of all*, Gevand and grantand to the saidis visitouris

indwellers of Glasgow, professouris of the saidis airtis, and thair bretherene, p'nt and to
cum, imunite and exemptioune from all wappin shawengis, raidis, oistis, beiring of armour,
watching, weirding, stenting taxationis, passing on assises, inquestis, justice courtis,
scheriff or burrow courtis, in actiounes criminal or cival, notwithstanding of oure actis,
lawis, and constitutionis thairoff, except in geving yairr counsall in materis appertaining
to the saidis airtis : ORDAINING you, all the foresaidis provestes baillies of borrowis,
sheriffis, stewartis, baillies of regalities, and otheris ministeris of justice, within the saidis
boundis, and zoure deputis, to assist, fortifie, concur and defend the saidis visitouris, and
their posterior, professouris of the foresaidis airtis, and put the saidis actis maid and to be
maid to executioun ; and that our otheris letteris of our sessioun be granted thereupon
to charge thame to that effect within twentie four houris nixt after they be chargit thairto.
GEVIN under oure previe seill, at Haliruid house, the penult day of November, the zeir
of God jmvc. and fourscore ninetein zeiris, and of oure regun the threttie thre zeir."[1]

An early act of the Incorporation was to adopt the barbers in June, 1602,
as " a pendecle of Chirurgerie." The barbers were apparently adopted as a
necessity of the times, but on a distinctly inferior plane. The barber was to be
" free of his ain calling " but not of the Incorporation as a whole, and the barber
was to " medill with simple wounds allenarlie." This position continued for about
a century till, in 1703, the barbers appealed their grievances to the Town Council,
and applied to be disjoined from the chirurgeons. In 1708, the Magistrates
effected this separation, the barbers taking one-fifth of the property of the
Incorporation, and being re-incorporated by themselves under a Letter of
Deaconry. It may be added that in Edinburgh the union between the surgeons
and barbers came to an end in 1719.

Another early activity of the Faculty was the enactment of a code of rules
in regard to the education of the members. In 1602, it was ordained that
apprentices must be entered for seven years, although in the last two they were
to receive board and fee. The apprentice was to pay five pounds for entry money,
was to be examined at the end of three years, giving a dinner at the time to his
examiners, and again to be examined at the end of five years and at the end of
seven years. The examinations were apparently to be partly written and partly
practical, and at the end of his term of apprenticeship, before passing as master,
he was to pay ten pounds. Finally, if he intended to practise in Glasgow, he had
to be enrolled as a burgess of the town at a further fee, and he had to pay to the
Faculty a quarterly subscription, which was rigorously exacted.

Individuals seem to have been licensed in the early days to practise limited
parts of the art of medicine. Thus, in 1668, Matthew Miller was licensed for the
" applicatione of coulters & ventosis [*cupping*], the cuiring of simple woundes, and
embalming of corpes," with the proviso that if he should be found afterwards
to attain more knowledge and skill of his calling, and found qualified by the
Faculty, he should be admitted thereto. Again, from the city records of
21st March, 1661, it was decided by the Magistrates and Council to pay yearly

---

[1] Duncan : " Memorials of the Faculty of Physicians and Surgeons of Glasgow, pp. 217 and 218."

to Evir M'Neill "that cutis the stone, ane hundreth markis Scotis, and he to cut all the poor for that freilie." This salary was apparently paid to him for many years, as he retired in 1688 in favour of Duncan Campbell. Evir M'Neill had been licensed by the Faculty in 1656, on the strength of ten years or thereby of experience " in cutting of the stone," to practise this department only within the bounds of the Faculty's supervision. Again, in 1654, Mr. Arch. Graham was licensed to practise " pharmacie and medicine," but was forbidden to exercise any point of " Chirurgerie."

In 1656, the Faculty made a closer rapprochement with the Town Council by obtaining in favour of the chirurgeons and barbers a Letter of Deaconry or Seal of Cause. In 1672, the Faculty obtained from the Scottish Parliament a ratification of this municipal charter, drawn in favour of the surgeons, apothecaries and barbers.

In 1645, one of the provisions of the original Charter was carried out by the admission to the Faculty, without examination, of Mr. Robert Mayne, the first Professor of Medicine in the University of Glasgow, and Mr. James Dwining, who were both doctors of medicine. Dr. Mayne's activities as a professor in the University were short-lived. He was one of the Regents in the Faculty of Arts, and became Professor of Medicine in 1637. He apparently lectured in the University on Fridays and other convenient occasions, dealing with medicine, although he had no other colleagues in the Medical Faculty. A Commission appointed by the General Assembly, in 1642, to hold a visitation of the Scottish Universities, reported that medicine was not necessary for the College in Glasgow, although they recommended that Mr. Robert Mayne should continue in his post during his time. He died, however, in 1646, and the Chair lapsed for over a century.[1]

Until the latter part of the 17th century the Faculty does not appear to have felt itself strong enough to extend its operations beyond the town of Glasgow, although it had been given a purview over medical practice in a much wider area. In 1673, however, examiners were appointed in Ayr and Kilmarnock to examine applicants for entrance to the Faculty. These were the times of the Covenanting troubles, and some of the Faculty were enthusiastic Covenanters, though most of them tempered piety with prudence. In 1677, the Faculty had the misfortune to have a Treasurer, Mr. Thomas Smith, who attended conventicles, and who had been denounced and called before the Lords of Secret Council. Having some fear that the Corporation might be fined for his misdemeanours, his fellow-members summarily ejected him from office and appointed a successor *ad interim.* On the other hand, the Faculty had much trouble with the impious barbers, who acted as "prophaners of the Sabath by barborizing of persons yt day."

---

[1] Duncan : " Memorials of the Faculty of Physicians and Surgeons of Glasgow," p. 111.

This practice was found by the Faculty, in 1676, to be "contrair to the word of God, and to all lawes both humane and divyne." A resolution was therefore passed that any member of the Faculty convicted of plying his craft of barber on the Sabbath day should be fined forty pounds Scots, and, upon refusal to pay the same, be ejected from the Faculty.[1]

About this time the Faculty seem to have been extraordinarily busy in the prosecution of quacks and other unlicensed practitioners within their area, and the records are filled with cases of unqualified persons brought up before the Faculty in its judicial capacity. These were either fined or forbidden under penalty to practise further.

In 1697, the Faculty acquired a property contiguous to the Tron Church, where the members set up a hall and commenced the formation of a medical library, for up to this time they had been without a meeting-place, holding their meetings usually either in the Crafts' Hospital or Hutchesons' Hospital. In 1791, the Faculty moved its hall to the east side of St. Enoch Square, and, in 1860, sold this site to the Railway Company with advantage and moved to its present premises in St. Vincent Street.

In the 18th century it appears that the term of apprenticeship for surgeons was five years, although apprenticeships of four years and three years were also recognised when this apprenticeship was supplemented by attendance on lectures at a Medical School. In 1785, the Faculty established a licentiateship, which gave to country surgeons the power of practising in a limited area on payment of a reduced admission fee.

Several men eminent in medicine were members of the Faculty during the 18th century. Dr. Matthew Brisbane, in the end of the 17th century, had been several times elected Rector of the University, the only medical man in that century to attain the distinction. In common, however, with the general opinion of the times, he apparently had some sympathy with the idea that witchcraft was a possible practice, for in 1696 he made a lengthy report upon a girl, Christian Shaw, daughter of the Laird of Bargarran, whom he had seen to bring hair, straw, coal, cinders and such-like "trash" out of her mouth without its being wet. The case at the present day would unhesitatingly be attributed to hysteria and imposture, but, for the alleged crime of bewitching this wretched girl, four persons were burned at Paisley.[2]

As a pioneer in surgery, much credit is due to Mr. Robert Houston, for whom a claim is made of being the first ovariotomist, by reason of an operation which he performed in 1701, more than a century before the celebrated operations of Dr. Ephraim McDowell, of Kentucky.[3] The case concerned a woman,

---

[1] Duncan : "Memorials of the Faculty of Physicians and Surgeons of Glasgow," p. 72.
[2] Duncan : "Memorials of the Faculty of Physicians and Surgeons of Glasgow," pp. 112 and 113.
[3] "Philosophical Transactions," London, 1733. Vol. XXXIII.

Margaret Millar, whom, in August, 1701, he found to have the abdomen distended to an enormous size. Being pressed by Lady Anne Houston, who took a great interest in the patient, and by the patient herself, to do what he could to relieve the condition, he, with very ineffective instruments, opened the abdomen, removed some nine quarts of gelatinous fluid and numerous cysts, and, after dressing the wound for three weeks, had the satisfaction of seeing the patient again at work, and later of recording her survival for thirteen years in perfect health.

A well-known member of the Faculty about the middle of the century was Dr. John Gordon, to whom Tobias Smollett served an apprenticeship. The latter puts into the mouth of one of his characters, Mr. Bramble, the following appreciation of his old master, who, outside of medicine, conferred upon the city the great benefit of introducing linen manufacture there : " I was introduced to Mr. Gordon, a patriot of a truly noble spirit, who is father of the linen manufactory of that place, and was the great promoter of the city workhouse, infirmary, and other works of public utility. Had he lived in ancient Rome, he would have been honoured with a statue at the public expense." Another friend of Dr. Gordon was Dr. William Smellie, the obstetrician, also a member of the Faculty, who practised in the town of Lanark, and afterwards went to London, where he composed his celebrated " Midwifery," which was revised by Tobias Smollett. Dr. John Gordon lectured for a time in the College on Anatomy, and other lecturers on this subject at various periods between 1730 and 1750, were Mr. John Paisley, Mr. John Love, Dr. Robert Hamilton and Mr. John Crawford.

Other celebrated members of the Faculty were William Cullen and Joseph Black, whose lives and work are mentioned in connection with the Medical School of Edinburgh. Until the early part of the 18th century, Glasgow medicine had busied itself mainly with the improvement of medical and surgical practice, and the few attempts at teaching which have been mentioned had proved abortive. During the second decade of the 18th century, however, the University began to bestir itself for the erection of a Medical School. The Chair of Medicine, which had been abolished by the Commissioners of Assembly in 1646, was revived in 1714, and Dr. John Johnstoun, who had graduated in medicine at Utrecht five years previously, was appointed professor. Dr. Thomas Brisbane, son of Dr. Matthew Brisbane, was next appointed professor of anatomy and botany in 1720. It appears, however, that neither of these professors lectured, and that they regarded their appointments as merely titular.[1] In 1744, Dr. William Cullen, who had moved from Hamilton into Glasgow, began to deliver a course of lectures on medicine outside the University, and in 1746, by an arrangement with Professor Johnstoun, he began to lecture in the University. He persuaded the University also to fit up a chemical laboratory in 1747, and began to teach that subject with the help of Mr. John Carrick, assistant to Dr. Hamilton, now professor of

---

[1] Thomson : " Life of Cullen," Vol. I, p. 24.

anatomy. In 1748 Cullen also began to teach materia medica and botany. In 1750, Dr. Johnstoun resigned the Chair, and Cullen was appointed his successor in January, 1751.

Cullen was one of the first persons in Britain to treat chemistry as a scientific subject apart from its connection with pharmacy. He also stimulated his pupil, Joseph Black, to take up the subject from the same aspect. Black went to Edinburgh as a student in 1751, and here he accomplished the brilliant feat of isolating " fixed air " (carbonic acid gas), which inaugurated a new era in chemistry. In 1755, Cullen left Glasgow to take up the Chair of Chemistry at Edinburgh ; at the same time, Dr. Robert Hamilton, the professor of anatomy, was transferred to the Chair of Medicine, and Dr. Joseph Black succeeded Hamilton as professor of anatomy for one year. Dr. Hamilton having died in 1757, Dr. Joseph Black succeeded to the Chair of Medicine and Chemistry, but in 1766 he again resigned this to succeed Cullen in the Chair of Chemistry at Edinburgh, when the latter was transferred to the Chair of Medicine in that University.

To Cullen and Black the foundation of the Glasgow School of Medicine may reasonably be credited. Black was succeeded in 1766 in the Chair of Medicine and Chemistry by Dr. Alexander Stevenson, and he in turn by his nephew, Dr. Thomas Charles Hope, in 1791. After Black left Glasgow, Mr. John Robison was appointed a lecturer in chemistry, and Dr. William Irvine a lecturer in materia medica. Professor Hope succeeded Joseph Black in the Edinburgh Chair in 1795. It was unfortunate for the developing school at Glasgow that all these men of ability were transferred to other spheres of activity almost as soon as they had made their mark.[1]

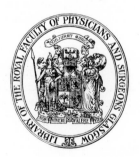

SEAL

ROYAL FACULTY OF PHYSICIANS AND SURGEONS

GLASGOW

---

[1] Duncan : " Memorials of the Faculty of Physicians and Surgeons of Glasgow," pp. 129-132.

CHAPTER XI

THE EARLY MEDICAL SCHOOL OF ST. ANDREWS

THE University of St. Andrews was the first of the Scottish seats of learning to be instituted. From its beginning in the year 1411, when it was founded by Henry Wardlaw, Bishop of St. Andrews, the institution was a " *studium generale*," or " *universitas studii*," and as such it was entitled to include all the faculties in theology, canon and civil law, arts and medicine. The foundation of Universities in Scotland was somewhat late as compared with those in other countries, despite the fact that many Scotsmen sought learning at foreign Universities. The War of Independence with England was largely responsible for this, although a pious Scottish lady, Dervorguilla, Countess of Galloway, and widow of John de Baliol, had founded a College at Oxford in 1269, probably moved to this step in large part by the desire to encourage young Scotsmen to travel and familiarise themselves with the manners of the wealthier southern country.

St. Andrews from early times had been a resort of pilgrims, because of the relics supposed to have been brought by St. Regulus to that town, and for the reception and succour of these pilgrims, there was a hospital associated with the Church of St. Leonard.[1] This hospital, along with the associated Church, was incorporated in the College of St. Leonard in 1512. At this time Archbishop Alexander Stewart, in his charter, mentioned that " miracles and pilgrimages . . . had in a measure ceased, so that the hospital was without pilgrims, and the Priors did set therein certain women, chosen by reason of old age, who did give little or no return in devotion or virtue." In a deed of 1529, a reference is made to Mr. George Martine as Preceptor, Master and Possessor of the Hospital and Leper-house beside the city of St. Andrews, founded for the honour and worship of St. Nicholas.[2] Little else, however, appears to be available in the way of information regarding early medical activities at St. Andrews.

The foundation of the University was sanctioned in 1413 by a Papal Bull from Pope Benedict XIII., and, in the succeeding century, the University showed considerable development till it came to include three separate Colleges. These were as follows :—

(1) St. Salvator's College, was founded in 1450 by James Kennedy, Bishop of St. Andrews.

(2) St. Leonard's College, was founded in 1512 by Alexander Stewart, Archbishop of St. Andrews, and John Hepburn, Prior of the Metropolitan Church.

---

[1] Herkless : " Votiva Tabella," Maclehose, Glasgow, 1911, p. 31.
[2] Buist : " Votiva Tabella," p. 197.

It received in the same year the Royal confirmation of James IV., and was intended for twenty-six students.

(3) St. Mary's College, was founded in 1537 by Archbishop James Beaton, on the site of the " Pedagogium," the original academical building. It was further endowed by Archbishop John Hamilton in 1553, and reconstituted by him under a Papal Bull, being intended for twenty-four students.

In 1579, soon after the Reformation, the constitution of the University was changed. The College of St. Mary was now reserved for theology, while the Colleges of St. Salvator and St. Leonard were restricted to the teaching of philosophy, law and medicine. The Act of 1579 was partially repealed in 1621, but, in 1747, the two Colleges of St. Salvator and St. Leonard were finally joined by Act of Parliament, and have since been known as the United College of St. Salvator and St. Leonard. University College, Dundee, was founded and endowed, in 1880, by Miss Baxter, of Balgavies, and Dr. John Boyd Baxter, and was opened in 1883.[1]

There seems already to have been some teaching in medicine, for when John Major came to be Principal of St. Salvator's College, he brought with him William Manderston, who had been a student of Montaigu College in Paris and was a doctor of medicine. William Manderston, according to the fashion of the times, in his " Bipartitum in Morali Philosophia," published in 1523, includes a commendation received from " *Robertus Gra. medicinae amator*," who refers to William Manderston as " *praeceptori suo apollonie artis professori peritissimo*." Robert Gray had apparently been a pupil of Manderston in Paris, and as there are not likely to have been two *amatores medicinae* named Robert Gray at the time, this is probably the same Robert Gray who was appointed mediciner at King's College, Aberdeen, in 1522. Gray, at all events, refers to Manderston as a leader in medicine (without which the State would be altogether poor), and speaks of him as being recalled by Archbishop James Beaton to his native soil as desired for his high reputation *(spectatum et desideratum)*.[2]

In the re-organisation of Scottish education which followed the Reformation, under the personal direction of John Knox, a definite scheme took form, that, of the three Scottish Universities, St. Andrews should be the school where medicine was to be taught. The plan is laid down in the Buke of Discipline of 1560, where it is said :—

" . . . nixt we think it necessarie thair be three Universities in this whole Realme, establischeit in the Tounis accustumed. The first in Sanctandrois, the secound in Glasgow, and the thrid in Abirdene.

And in the first Universitie and principall, whiche is Sanctandrois, thair be thre Colledgeis. And in the first Colledge, quhilk is the entre of the Universitie, thair be four classes or saigeis [*chairs*] : the first, to the new Suppostis, shalbe onlie Dialectique ; the nixt, onlie Mathematique ; the thrid of Phisick onlie ; the fourt of Medicine. . . . .

---

[1] " St. Andrews University Calendar, 1926–1927," pp. 26 and 27.
[2] Manderston : " Bipartitum in Morali Philosophia Opusculum," 2nd Edn., Paris 1523.

" In the fourt classe, shall be ane Reidar of Medicine, who shall compleit his course in five years: after the study of the whiche tyme, being by examinatioun fund sufficient, thei shall be graduat in Medicine. . . . .

" *Item,* That nane be admittit to the classe of the Medicine bot he that shall have his testimoniall of his tyme weall spent in Dialecticque, Mathematique, and Phisicque and of his docilitie in the last."[1]

As to the salary of the teacher, the provision was made " for the Stipend of everie Reader in Medicine and Lawis, ane hundreth threttie thre pundis, vi. s. viii. d."[2]

At the same time, it was intended that Glasgow University should teach Arts only, and Aberdeen Laws and Divinity. Nevertheless, the scheme never came into operation, and Gilbert Skeen continued as mediciner at King's College, Aberdeen, for fifteen years, when he betook himself to practice in Edinburgh. Twenty-two years later the Town Council of Edinburgh also disregarded the general plan of the Reformers for Scottish education by establishing their Town's College.

The failure of Knox's plan for a medical school at St. Andrews is readily

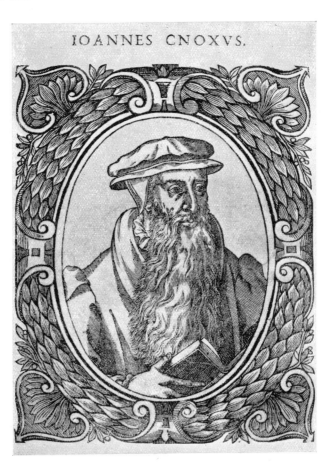

IOANNES CNOXVS.

JOHN KNOX (1505-1572)
(From the contemporary engraving by Beza)

understood when one reflects that a living study like that of medicine can hardly flourish save in a centre of population, and can certainly never bear fruit in the output of practitioners skilled in the knowledge of human beings, and capable

---

[1] " Works of John Knox," edited by David Laing, Edinburgh, 1848, Vol. II, pp. 213–215.
[2] Op. cit., p. 218.

M

of treating their disorders, unless associated with other forms of intellectual and social endeavour.   St. Andrews had never been a great centre of commerce, and after the Reformation it ceased to be even a centre of religious activity and resort of pilgrims.

In the report of the Commission appointed by King James VI. to visit the University in 1579, it was provided that the Principal of St. Salvator's should be professor in medicine, and should read this subject four times in the week. Another report, in 1588, mentions that " The Provest, sin the reformatioun, affirmis he teichis tuyis [*twice*] ilk oulk [*week*], the Aphorismes Hippocrates, quhill [*until*] October last ; sensyne [*since then*] he hes teichit na thing ; the Maisteris sayis he nevir teichis, skantlie anis [*hardly once*] in the moneth."[1]

The teaching of law at St. Andrews laboured under much the same difficulties as that of medicine, for the Provost reported of the reader in law, Mr. William Walwood, that "he neglectis oft," and on one occasion, the Provost came to his school " and commandit him to come doun, for he wald teich himselff at that hour ; quhairupoun great slander followit," and at a later date it was found " that the Professioun of the Lawes is na wayes necessar at this tyme in this Universitie."[2]

A Commission of 1642, after prescribing certain books which should be studied at St. Andrews, added to the list, "if so much tyme may be spared, some compend of Anatomy." In 1649, there was a provision that one of the Masters of St. Salvator's College should teach medicine twice a week.   In all these regulations for teaching medicine, however, this subject was simply a part of the Arts curriculum, taught to students as a valuable part of general knowledge. Nevertheless, the University still held to the privilege conferred by its Bull of foundation in granting degrees in medicine.   These were sometimes given *honoris causa*, frequently *in eundem gradum*, and sometimes, unfortunately, *in absentia*, in return for a payment.   The most frequent condition was that of giving the degree *in eundem gradum*, which meant that an applicant already a graduate of some foreign University, desired to add to his qualifications the degree of M.D. from a Scottish University, and this was granted on production of the foreign diploma, which thus offered a certain amount of protection to the University.   It appears, from the report of a Committee in 1747, that the fee for a degree was £10 sterling, of which the professor of medicine received £3.[3]

In the 18th century the University appears to have obtained an opportunity of gratifying its long-cherished wish to have a professorship of medicine.   Prior to 1722, the Duke of Chandos, through his son's tutor, Dr. Charles Stuart, offered the University £1000, with the suggestion that it should be employed for the

---

[1] Buist : " Votiva Tabella," p. 201.
[2] Buist : " Votiva Tabella," p. 202
[3] Buist : " Votiva Tabella," p. 216,

establishment of a Chair of Eloquence.   The University, however, decided that
it should be used for the foundation of a Chair of Medicine and Anatomy.
A letter from Dr. Stuart, dated 28th November, 1720, gives an amusing criticism
upon what he regards as a useless proposal :—

> " . . . ye Theory and Practise of Medicine are not only considered as distinct Professions
> in some of ye Universitys abroad, but there are likewise other Sciences such as Anatomy,
> Chimistry and Botany, which are unseparable retainers to that Science and absolutely
> necessary to ye study of it : now there are no foundations in your University for any
> of these Sciences, nor perhaps will be for these hundred years to come, and as one man
> can hardly be sufficient for more than one or at most two of them, I can not see of what
> great use a Professor of Medicine wou'd be at St. Andrews, where an Anatomist may be ten
> years in looking for a body to dissect ; I think I plainly forsee that this Profession wou'd
> quickly fall into ye hands of some young Physitian who, wanting imployment, should
> have interest enough to get himself chosen to it, for a livelyhood to him, without having
> so much as one scholar to teach. . . . ."[1]

Nevertheless, the University persisted in its intention, and Thomas Simson
(1696–1764) was appointed first Chandos Professor of Medicine in 1722.   He
had graduated M.D. at Glasgow in 1720, and on his introduction to the Chair at

St. Andrews, delivered an oration : " De
Erroribus tam veterum quam recentiorum
circa Materiam Medicam." He also published a treatise, " De Re Medica," in 1726,
concerning the need of investigating the
laws under which the human machine acted,
and of studying the natural history of disease
by experiment, and a treatise on " A System
of the Womb," at Edinburgh, in 1729. He
lectured in English instead of the Latin,
which was then commonly employed, and he
appears to have thrown himself into the
duties of his post with considerable ardour.
He was succeeded by his son, James Simson,
who had graduated M.D. at St. Andrews in
1760, with a dissertation, " De Asthmate

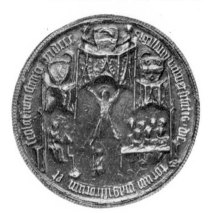

SEAL OF THE UNIVERSITY OF
ST. ANDREWS

Infantium Spasmodico," which is to be   found   in   the   " Miscellanies "   of
Andrew Duncan.   He in turn was succeeded by James Flint in 1770, but there is
no evidence that either James Simson or James Flint delivered any lectures.

After the death of James Flint, Robert Briggs was appointed to the Chair
in 1811, and the University before his appointment saw fit to enact that the
Chandos Professor should be a teaching professor, and should open classes to be
regularly taught during the session of the United College for the instruction of

---

[1] Buist : " Votiva Tabella," p. 209.

any students, who might apply to him, in the principles of medicine, anatomy and chemistry. This is the first mention of chemistry in connection with the Chair, and the University further provided apparatus for practical work, which was successful, and was continued till the death of Professor Briggs in 1840.

In 1808, Dr. John Gray, of London, had left a sum of money to found a special professorship of chemistry. The funds were allowed to accumulate until

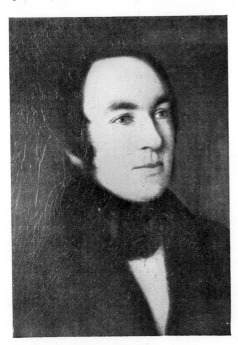

JOHN REID. M.D. (1809-1849)
(Original in the University of St. Andrews)

1840,[1] when the Chair of Chemistry was inaugurated, and Arthur Connell was appointed professor. He held the Chair till 1862, when he was succeeded by Matthew Forster Heddle.

After the death of Professor Briggs, the Chandos Chair again became one of medicine only, and John Reid (1809–1849), a man of much finer qualities than his predecessors, was elected professor in 1841. Reid was a native of Bathgate, and had studied medicine at Edinburgh University, where he graduated M.D. in 1830. After a period of study in Paris, he returned to Edinburgh in 1832, and was one one of a committee of investigation who went to Dumfries to enquire into an outbreak of cholera. He had been a demonstrator of anatomy at Surgeons' Hall, had joined the College of Surgeons as Fellow in 1836, and in the same year had become lecturer there on physiology. He was also greatly interested in pathology, and, between 1838 and 1841, acted as pathologist to the Royal Infirmary at Edinburgh. Immediately on his appointment as Chandos Professor, he began a course on comparative anatomy and physiology at St. Andrews, which proved attractive to students and successful. In 1848 he published a well-known collection of papers entitled " Physiological, Anatomical and Pathological Researches," a volume remarkable for originality and accuracy of observation. One of the papers contained in it was " An Investigation of the Epidemic Fever of Edinburgh in the Years 1836, 1837 and 1838." It is a remarkable fact, as illustrative of the changes which have taken place in the incidence of certain

---

[1] Anderson : " The Matriculation Roll of the University of St. Andrews, 1747–1897," Edinburgh, 1905, p. xxx.

diseases, that 2037 patients were treated during fifteen months for this fever in the Royal Infirmary of Edinburgh, with a mortality of over 13 per cent. Reid clearly described in this disease the pathological changes characteristic of typhoid fever. He was thus one of the first to differentiate between typhoid and typhus fevers. The University of St. Andrews suffered a great loss when Reid died from cancer of the tongue in 1849.

After the death of Reid, George Edward Day (1815–1872) was appointed Chandos Professor. He had already made a reputation by translating Simon's " Animal Chemistry," for the Sydenham Society, and later he translated for the same series the fourth volume of Rokitansky's " Pathological Anatomy." Immediately after his appointment he published " A Practical Treatise on the Domestic Management and Most Important Diseases of Advanced Life," and, in 1860, a work on " Chemistry in its Relation to Physiology and Medicine." He worthily continued the reputation which Reid had gained for this Chair, both in teaching and in publication. He resigned the Chair in 1863, when Oswald Home Bell was appointed, to be succeeded in 1875 by J. Bell Pettigrew. Under Bell and his successors, the Chandos Chair became a professorship of physiology.

The desire of the University to establish a Faculty of Medicine was again evinced in a somewhat curious way in connection with the Chair of Civil History. A professorship of Civil History had existed from 1747, and an experiment had been made in 1825 by the appointment of Mr. J. G. Macvicar as lecturer on natural history, which had proved that the latter subject was one in which a successful course could be held. In 1850, when Dr. William Macdonald was appointed professor of Civil History, it was made a condition of his appointment that he should be able and willing to teach natural history, although this was a totally different subject. The Chair was thereafter continued as a professorship of natural history, and Macdonald was succeeded in 1875 by Professor Henry A. Nicholson.

It was not till the establishment of University College in the neighbouring city of Dundee, in the year 1880, that the design which St. Andrews University had entertained for several centuries, of establishing a full medical school, succeeded in taking definite shape. This College was opened in 1883, with Chairs of Chemistry and Biology in addition to other subjects. The incorporation of University College with the University of St. Andrews was accomplished in 1897, and by this time Chairs of Physics, Botany, Anatomy, Physiology and a lectureship on surgery had been set up. Finally, in 1898, the University Medical School was inaugurated, on the basis of teaching the preliminary subjects both in Dundee and St. Andrews, and conducting the subjects of the final three years, which are chiefly of a technical and clinical nature, in the city of Dundee.

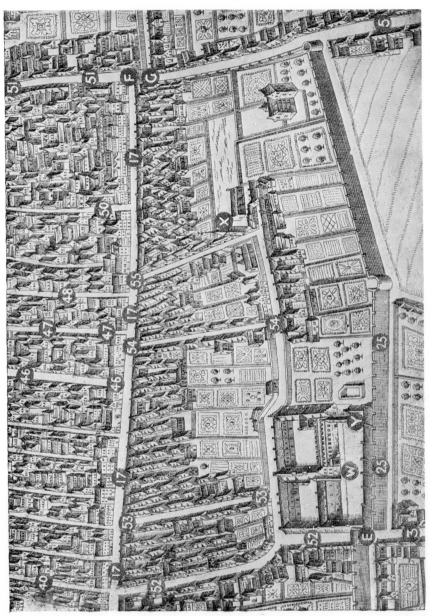

THE TOWN'S COLLEGE IN 1647

From Gordon of Rothemay's Plan of Edinburgh

E Potter-row port.   F Cowgate port.   G St. Mary's port.   O The College   W The High School   X The Kirk o' Field   3 Potter-row.   5 Pleasance.
17 Cowgate.   25 Town Wall.   40 Borthwick's Close.   46 Niddrie Wynd.   47 Dickson's Close.   48 Blackfriars' Wynd.   50 Gray's Close   51 St. Mary's Wynd.
52 Horse Wynd   53 College Wynd   54 Robertson's Close.   55 High School Wynd

(Compare with view on page 30)

Chapter XII

Foundation of the College of Physicians and of the Faculty of Medicine at Edinburgh

THE regulation of surgical practice at Edinburgh by the Guild of Surgeons and Barbers, and their increasing efforts to develop a knowledge of anatomy, have been already described. The regulation of medicine was another important step necessary before a Medical School could be constructed. The early Edinburgh physicians had mostly obtained a knowledge of medicine on the Continent, and during the 17th century several capable and distinguished physicians practised in Edinburgh. As early as 1617, when James I. re-visited Scotland, an attempt had been made to found a College of Physicians at Edinburgh, but it had been opposed by the Universities and the Bishops. A second attempt to push the matter was made in 1630, and a third attempt was made, in 1656, to obtain Cromwell's support of the proposal, which was to give powers of supervision for the whole of Scotland. By this time the surgeons had adopted the work of apothecaries as part of their practice, and the attempt was therefore naturally opposed by them, so that Cromwell was dissuaded from signing the proposed Charter. About 1670, the leading physicians of Edinburgh, moved by a desire to reform medicine, set themselves to lay out a Physic Garden and to obtain a Charter for the institution of a College of Physicians. The men chiefly concerned in this movement were Sir Robert Sibbald, Dr. Archibald Pitcairne, Sir Andrew Balfour, Sir Thomas Burnet and Sir Archibald Stevenson (father-in-law of Dr. Pitcairne).

The study of botany was then considered along with anatomy the most important preliminary to a scientific knowledge of medicine. The surgeons, as we have seen, had already made provision for anatomy, and thus it lay with the physicians to cultivate botany. Dr. Balfour had settled as a physician in Edinburgh in 1667, and in the small garden attached to his house had raised many plants never before seen in Scotland. His friend, Mr. Patrick Murray, of Livingstone, had also developed at his country seat a botanic garden containing over 1000 specimens of plants. Sibbald and Balfour determined to establish a regular Physic Garden, and Sibbald gives the following account of the way in which this project started :—

" Dr. Balfour and I first resolved upon it, and obtained of John Brown, gardner of the North yardes in the Abby, ane inclosure of some 40 foot of measure every way. We had, by this tyme, become acquaint with Master James Sutherland, a youth, who, by his owne industry, had attained great knowledge of the plants and of medals, and he undertook the charge of the culture of it. By what we procured from Leviston (*i.e.*, Patrick Murray, Laird of Livingstone) and other gardens, and brought in from the Country, we made a collection of eight or nyne hundred plants ther.

" We got several of the Physitians in town to concur in the designe, and to contribute so much a yeer for the charge of the culture and importation of foreigne plants.

" Some of the Chirurgeon Apothecaryes, who then had much power in the town, opposed us, dreading that it might usher in a Coledge of Physitians, bot, by the care and dexterity of Doctor Balfour, these were made friends to the designe, and assisted us in obtaining of the Counsell of Edinburgh ane leese to Mr. James Sutherland, for nynteen years, of the garden belonging to Trinity Hospitall, and adjacent to it.   And Doctor Balfour and I, with some others, were appointed by the Town Counsell visitors of the garden." [1]

These two early Physic Gardens were situated, the first north-east of Holyrood Abbey, on a spot occupied at present by a small stretch of turf ;   the second is shown

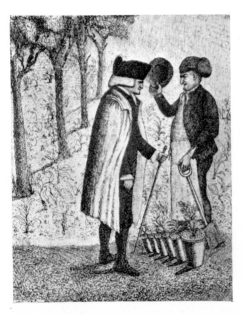

JOHN HOPE (1725-1786)
(From Kay's " Portraits ")

as the Garden of Trinity Hospital in Gordon of Rothemay's plan of Edinburgh.   Here, in 1676, James Sutherland was established as Professor of Botany, and in 1683 published his " Hortus Medicus Edinburgensis."   He had a salary of twenty pounds from the city, and taught the science of herbs to students for small fees.   In 1689, during the siege of the Castle, it was thought necessary to drain the North Loch, and the water for several days ran over the Physic Garden at Trinity Hospital, completely spoiling it.   Sutherland, therefore, in 1695, extended his Garden at Holyrood, which seems to have become a very fine place. Sutherland died in 1705, and was succeeded by Dr. Charles Preston, and he in turn by his brother George Preston, in the Chair of Botany.   The latter did much to improve the Garden, and built a green-house therein, for which he received an allowance of ten pounds yearly from the Town Council.   He also kept a shop on the north side of the High Street, opposite the head of Blackfriars Wynd, where he sold " all sorts of spices, sugars, tea, coffee, chacolet, etc." [2]

The Prestons were succeeded by Charles Alston as Professor of Medicine and Botany, and he in turn by John Hope in 1761.   Finding that the Garden was unsuited for the development which had taken place, Hope obtained a grant from the Treasury and removed the Garden to a site on the west of Leith Walk, near

---

[1] " The Autobiography of Sir Robert Sibbald, Knt., M.D." printed 1833, pp. 21 and 22.
[2] Bower : " History of the University of Edinburgh," Vol. II, p. 121.

the present Gayfield Square.   The old Garden at Trinity College disappeared about 1770.[1]

Professor Hope was succeeded by Daniel Rutherford in 1786, who, although Professor of Botany and Medicine, was much more of a chemist, and was the discoverer of nitrogen gas.   Subsequent professors were Robert Graham and John Hutton Balfour, known to his students as " Old Woody Fibre." The present Botanic Garden in Inverleith Row was formed in 1822–1824, and the adjoining Arboretum was opened in 1881.

To return to Sibbald, Pitcairne and the others, who, about 1670, were laying out the Physic Garden and considering the formation of a College of Physicians at Edinburgh, we find that the state of medicine at this time in other places was as follows.   Sydenham was practising in London.   Harvey's discovery had been published over forty years previously, and was still disputed, though Borelli, by his laborious mathematical investigations, had developed its principles into the Iatro-mechanical School of Thought.   Boyle, Mayow, Willis, and kindred spirits of the Royal Society of London were studying various problems of life and disease. Malpighi and Leeuwenhoek were using the earliest microscopes to investigate the structure of the bodily fluids and tissues.   Sylvius, at Leyden, was founding physiological chemistry and introducing the new idea of instruction in the wards of his hospital as a part of medical education.

Dr. Archibald Pitcairne (1652–1713) was perhaps the most celebrated Scottish physician of the time, and he more than anyone else may justly be regarded as the founder of the Edinburgh Medical School.   Beginning the pursuit of Law, he went to study in Paris, and there took to medicine.   From 1675 to 1680, he studied medicine in that city, and in the latter year became M.D. of Rheims. On the inducement of his friend, David Gregory, Professor of Mathematics at Edinburgh, he devoted himself with great assiduity to mathematics, becoming later, like Borelli in Italy, one of the founders of the Iatro-mechanical or Iatro-mathematical school of thought.   The system developed from Harvey's demonstration of the circulation ; for when the importance of this dynamic principle was grasped, in contradistinction to that of the leisurely ebb and flow of humours, its adherents attempted to prove that all the bodily activities, including even those of the nervous system and of digestion, were mere mechanical exercises. Although this idea could not persist for long, it formed for the century after Harvey a fruitful working hypothesis.   Pitcairne threw himself into this controversy with zest, and his attitude is indicated by the title of an attack made on him by Sir Edward Eizat in " Apollo Mathematicus, or the Art of Curing Diseases by the Mathematics " (1695).   Pitcairne was one of the original members of the Royal College of Physicians in 1681, and in 1685 he, Sir Robert Sibbald and Dr. James Halket were made the first three Professors of Medicine in the Town's College,

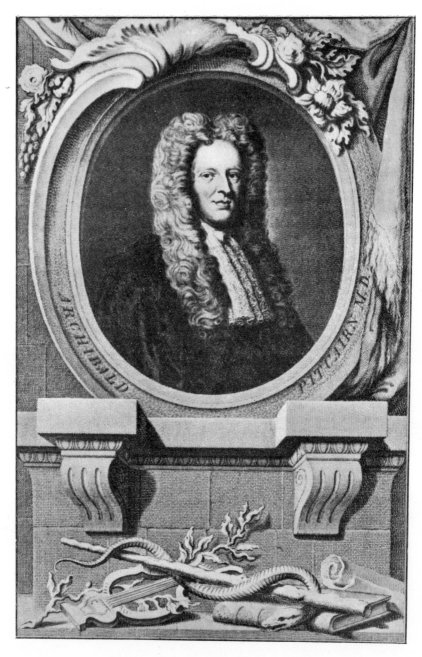

ARCHIBALD PITCAIRNE (1652–1713)

or, as it now began to be called, the University of Edinburgh. The professors of medicine were unsalaried, and although they probably lectured from time to time (Pitcairne certainly did), they do not appear to have delivered any regular course. Dr. Halket seems to have been a well-known physician of his time, but has left no literary remains. The only reference to him that I have been able to find is the following account of a consultation between him, Robert Clerk, surgeon, and Mr. Hamilton, regarding the illness and death of Lady Clerk of Penicuik :—

> " We had called for one of the chief Physitians in Town, one Doctor Hackete, and two of the chief chyrurgeons, my unckle Robert Clerk, and one Mr. Hamilton, a man much emploied in Midwifery. They took all the pains about her they cou'd think of, but I am afraed they were too hasty in their operations, by which she lost a vast deal of blood. The placenta, it seems, was adhering to the uterus, and this they thought themselves oblidged to bring away by force."[1]

Pitcairne's eminence, as one of the protagonists of the Iatro-mathematical School, procured for him, in 1692, an invitation from the University of Leyden to assume the Chair of

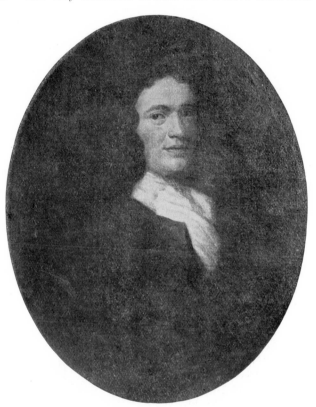

ROBERT CLERK

Flourished about 1689. He was father of Dr. John Clerk later President of the Royal College of Physicians
(*Original in the Royal College of Surgeons, Edinburgh*)

Medicine at that celebrated University, which he accepted. There he lectured till 1693, when he returned to Edinburgh for family reasons. The fact that the infant school of Edinburgh furnished a Professor to the old-established chair in Leyden must have given a great uplift to the former, still more the fact that Pitcairne had among his pupils many men who afterwards rose to fame, notably Mead and Boerhaave. Pitcairne's writings included

---

[1] " Sir John Clerk's Memoirs, 1676-1755," Scottish Hist. Soc., Edinburgh, 1892, p. 40.

numerous polemical pamphlets, poems, and dissertations on medical subjects, as, for example, on the " Quantity of the Blood," the " Motion of the Stomach," and especially a dissertation upon the " Cure of Fevers." This was an important contribution to the medicine of that day, when fevers formed two-thirds of all diseases.

Pitcairne's appointment, in 1692, as Professor of Medicine at Leyden, was largely due to the prominence which he had obtained as a controversialist on the discovery of the circulation of the blood made by Harvey some fifty years previously. Before Malpighi and Leeuwenhoek had demonstrated the capillaries and blood corpuscles, Pitcairne, by a kind of mathematical reasoning similar to that adopted by Harvey, had indicated the nature of the minute vessels through which the fine particles of blood must pass, and, in particular, he had established the view that there existed no gross anastomosis between the arteries and the veins, for which many persons contended, even of those who adopted Harvey's principle of circulation in a general way.[1]

Sir Robert Sibbald (1641–1722) had gone through a theological course in Edinburgh, and in 1660 proceeded to Leyden to study medicine. In his autobiography, he says :—

" I stayed at Leyden ane yeer and a half, and studied anatomie and chirurgie, under the learned Professor Van Horne. I studied the plants under Adolphus Vorstius, who had been then Botanick professor 37 yeers, and I studied the institutions and practice, under Sylvius, who was famous then. I saw twentye-three human bodies dissected by him in the Hospitall which I frequented with him. I saw some dissected publickly by Van Horne. I was fellow student with Steno, who became famous afterwards for his wrytings. He dissected in my chamber sometymes, and showed me there, the ductus salivalis superior, he had discovered. I frequented ane apothecaryes shop, and saw the materia medica and the ordinary compositiones made. I studied Chimie, under a German called Witichius, and after he went away, under Margravius, brother to him who wrott the naturall history of Brasile. Sometyme I heard the lessons of Vander Linden, who was famous for critical learning.

" I composed ther (the last summer I stayed ther,) Theses de variis Tabis speciebus. Sylvius was praeses when I defended them publickly in the schools. . . . In September, 1661, I went from Leyden for Paris. . . .

" I stayed some nyne moneths at Paris, where I was well acquainted with the famous Guido Patin, who lent me bookes, and gave me for a tyme the use of his manuscript written for the direction of his two sons, Robert and Charles (who were then Doctors of the Faculty of Paris,) in their studies. I studied the plants under Junquet in the King's Garden, and heard the publick lessons of Monsieur de la Chambre the younger, and Monsieur Bazalis, and I frequently was present at ther publick disputes, and visited then the Hotel de Dieu, and the Hospital of the Charity.

" From Paris I went to Angiers with letters of recommendation from Guido Patin to Bailif Sentor, the Dean of Faculty. I stayed a moneth ther, and was examined by his son, by Ferrand Joiselin and Boisenute, and gott my patent of Doctor ther."[2]

---

[1] Pitcairne : " A Dissertation upon the Circulation of the Blood through the Minutest Vessels of the Body." Works, Translated, London, 1715.

[2] " The Autobiography of Sir Robert Sibbald, Knt., M.D.," 1833, pp. 16 and 17.

Such was a medical course in the 17th century.   Sibbald had a large and influential practice in the neighbourhood of Edinburgh, was appointed by Charles II. Geographer Royal for Scotland, and left considerable literary remains, dealing especially with the natural history and archæology of Scotland.

Sir Robert Sibbald gives an account of the help afforded by Prince James, Duke of York, and his physician, Sir Charles Scarborough, in obtaining a patent for the erection of the College of Physicians at Edinburgh. After much opposition from the surgeons and the Town Council of Edinburgh, as well as the Universities and the Bishops, and after many conferences, the patent finally received the King's signature and the Great Seal upon the 29th November, 1681, and the College of Physicians was then established. In the following year, Drs. Sibbald, Stevenson and Balfour were knighted by the Duke of York.

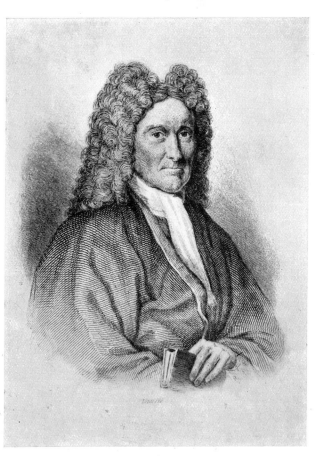

SIR ROBERT SIBBALD (1641-1722)

In 1686, Sir Robert Sibbald was persuaded by the Earl of Perth to embrace the Roman Catholic faith, but having been hunted out of his house by the Edinburgh mob, and having thereafter made a visit to London, where, as he says, " I perceaved, also the whole people of England was under a violent restraint then, and I foirsaw they would overturne the Government," he resolved to return to the Church in which he was born, and, as he quaintly remarks : " After my returne, it pleased God the popish interest decayed dayly, and good men thought I by my returne had

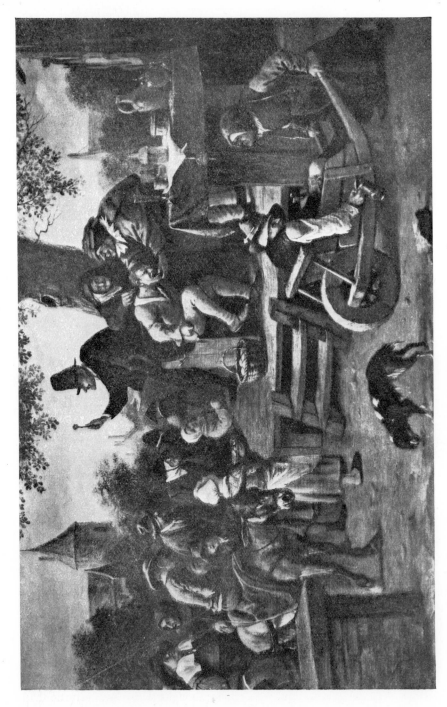

A TRAVELLING MOUNTEBANK OF THE 17TH CENTURY

Illustrating a class of men who invaded Scotland in the 17th and 18th Centuries (*see page* 191)

(*From the original picture by Jan Steen of Leyden, 1626–1679*)

done it more damage then my joining had profited them."[1]   The Revolution occurred two years later.

Other important physicians in Edinburgh at this time who were associated with Pitcairne and Sibbald in founding the College of Physicians were Sir Thomas Burnet, author of a highly popular compendium of medicine, the " Thesaurus Medicinae " (1673), and Sir Archibald Stevenson.

The necessity for a supply of good doctors in Edinburgh, as in other parts of Scotland, and the further necessity for a controlling influence, such as that exerted by the College of Physicians, is demonstrated by the frequency with which strolling mountebanks appeared, even in the capital city.   In 1672, Joannes Michael Philo, physician, and " sworn operator to his majesty," petitioned the Privy Council for permission to erect a public stage in Edinburgh for the practice of his profession, which was allowed, though he was forbidden " to have any rope-dancing."   He was reported later to have " thereon cured thretteen blind persons, several lame, and cut several cancers, and done many other notable cures, as is notourly known, and that out of mere charity."   The Privy Council, after he had been three months in Edinburgh, gave him a warrant " to go and do likewise in all the other burghs of the kingdom," for six months, and recommended him to the help and countenance of the Magistrates of the burghs.[2]

Again, in 1677, there is notice of a travelling doctor styling himself Joannes Baptista Marentini, who with the permission of the Edinburgh Town Council, erected a stage in the city for practising his skill in physic and otherwise.   Marentini had a servant, Monsieur Devoe, about whom James Baynes petitioned the Privy Council because he, while " servant to the mountebank who was lately in this place, hath, by sinistrous and indirect means, secured and enticed the petitioner's daughter and only child to desert her parents, and to live with him upon pretence of a clandestine marriage."   The Council issued a warrant to have the offender imprisoned in the Tolbooth, but he appears afterwards to have settled down in Edinburgh as a dancing-master.[3]

Again, in 1684, Cornelius a-Tilbourne, a German mountebank, applied to the Privy Council for license to erect a stage in Edinburgh.   The College of Physicians was now in existence, and opposed the application, which, nevertheless, was granted.   He had previously made a successful experiment upon himself in London by taking poisons administered by the physicians there, after he had drunk an antidote, and the King had granted him a medal and chain.   In Edinburgh he expressly excluded mercury, aqua fortis and other corrosives from the trial, but carried out the experiment on his servant.

---

[1] " The Autobiography of Sir Robert Sibbald, Knt., M.D.," printed 1833, pp. 35–41.
[2] Chambers : " Domestic Annals of Scotland," Vol. II, Edinburgh, 1859, p. 347 ; [3] pp. 383 and 384.

The Edinburgh poisons were apparently more effective than those of London, and the servant died.[1]

During the time of Sir Robert Sibbald's presidency of the College of Physicians the Pharmacopœia was completed.   The first Pharmacopœia to appear in Britain had been that of London in 1618, but its formulæ were not binding upon the apothecaries of Scotland.   From 1699, when the Edinburgh Pharmacopœia first appeared, its successive editions were in general use throughout Scotland until the British Pharmacopœia of the General Medical Council was issued in 1864. Another important activity of this College consisted in the provision of a Dispensary for attendance and supply of medicines to the sick poor, and a Repository for furnishing medicines to the sick poor was set up in 1708.   The design of founding an Infirmary in Edinburgh, where clinical instruction could be furnished, was next mooted by the College about 1725, and the College thereafter took effective steps to carry out this project. At an early stage of its existence, on 5th February, 1683, the College had agreed to the formula for a licentiate's diploma, and in order to prevent irregular practice in Edinburgh and its neighbourhood, the College insisted that all persons desiring to practise as physicians in Edinburgh and its vicinity should first be recognised by them. In 1683 also, the formation of a Library occupied the attention of the Fellows, and this Library has steadily grown, till at the present time (1927) it includes some 100,000 volumes.

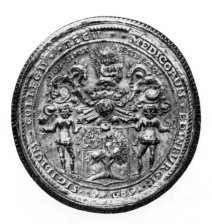

SEAL OF THE ROYAL COLLEGE OF PHYSICIANS OF EDINBURGH

The meetings of the Fellows of the College of Physicians were at first held in the private houses of the officials, but on 17th April, 1698, the College resolved to buy a house of its own, and, in 1704, it acquired the house and grounds of Sir James Mackenzie in Fountain Close, between the High Street and Cowgate.   Seven years later, the College acquired the neighbouring land belonging to Baillie Jeffrey, and laid out a garden and shrubbery, extending down to the then fashionable Cowgate. This was the envy of the neighbouring peers, to whom in several cases the privilege of walking in the garden was permitted as a favour.   About the same time, the College converted certain ruinous buildings bordering on the Cowgate into a bath-house, which was open to the inhabitants generally at a charge of twelve shillings Scots, and one penny to the servant, for each ablution, or at an annual charge of one guinea.   The bath, however, was let in 1714, and shortly after abandoned.

---

[1] p. 458, Chambers: "Domestic Annals of Scotland," Vol. II, Edinburgh, 1859.

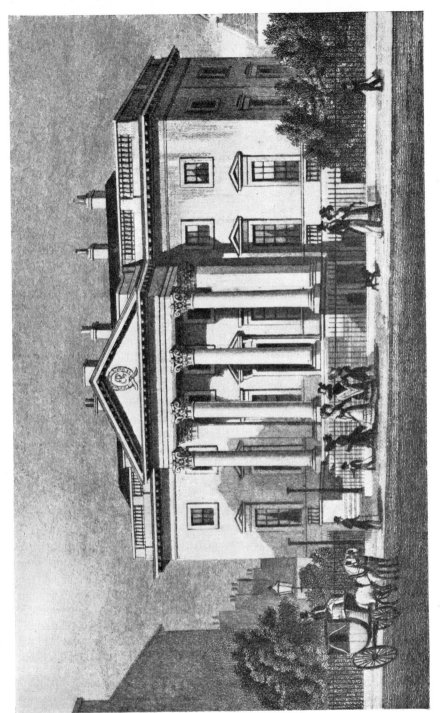

HALL OF THE ROYAL COLLEGE OF PHYSICIANS IN GEORGE STREET, EDINBURGH, FROM 1775 TO 1843

In 1722, a new Hall was erected in the garden, but the building appears to have been unsatisfactory, for, in 1766, it became necessary to apply to the Managers of the Royal Infirmary to deposit the Library in a spare apartment of that building, and to hold the meetings of the College in the Managers' Board-room.   These requests were granted, and the privilege was continued to the College for fifteen years.   In 1781, the premises in Fountain Close were sold, and the Library and meetings of the College were transferred to a new Hall near the east end of George Street.   The foundation stone of this Hall had been laid on 27th November, 1775, by the President, Dr. William Cullen.   In 1843, the George Street Hall, which had been a very fine building, was sold to the Commercial Bank for £20,000, and from this transaction, the prosperity of the College dates. The present Hall was occupied in 1846.[1]

The first important step in the foundation of a Medical School at Edinburgh had been the early development of anatomical instruction in the hands of the surgeons from the beginning of the 16th century.   The physicians of Edinburgh, in the 17th century, had developed the teaching of botany in the Physic Gardens. The next department of knowledge with a bearing upon medicine which received attention was chemistry, in which a professorship was founded in 1713. Van Helmont, who may be regarded as the last of the alchemists, had died in 1644, and Glauber, who is usually looked upon as the first of the chemists, had died in 1688.   Sylvius, at Leyden, about the middle of the 17th century, had been one of the first to see the importance of the relationship between chemistry and medicine, and he and his pupils, De Graaf, Stensen, etc., had investigated the secretions of the glands.   Boerhaave's " Elementa Chemiæ," published in 1732, was one of the first text-books on this subject, so that the Town Council of Edinburgh were very early in the field of chemistry with their professorial appoint-ment.   Dr. James Crawford was elected professor of physic and chemistry to the University of Edinburgh on 9th December, 1713, after a testimonial as to his fitness for the post had been furnished by the College of Physicians to Principal Carstares.   Crawford had followed the usual custom in studying under Boerhaave, at Leyden, and two rooms in the University were allotted to him for teaching, although he received no salary.[2]

On 12th August, 1724, the Town Council, on the recommendation of the Royal College of Physicians, " considering the great benefit and advantage that would accrue to this city and kingdom, by having all the parts of medicine taught in this place," decided to appoint Mr. William Porterfield, doctor of medicine in Edinburgh, to teach the institutes and practice of medicine.   Porterfield had graduated at Rheims in 1717, and had received a licence to practice from the Royal College of Physicians in 1721.   He is now best known by an excellent treatise on the eye, which he published in 1759.   The Town Council appear to

---

[1] " Historical Sketch and Laws of the Royal College of Physicians of Edinburgh," pp. 39 et seq.
[2] Bower : " History of the University of Edinburgh," Vol. II, Edinburgh, 1817, p. 126.

have considered that Porterfield's lectures on institutes and practice of medicine would be sufficient to cover the whole of medicine, and Bower is inclined to think that he never delivered a course of lectures.[1]

On 11th November, 1724, the same year that Porterfield was appointed, a memorial was presented to the Town Council by Drs. Rutherford, Sinclair, Plummer and Innes, showing that they had "purchased a house for a chemical elaboratory, adjoining to the college garden," and craving that they might be allowed the use of the garden for supplying chemical medicines and instructing students of medicine.   On 9th February, 1726, it was reported to the Town Council that Rutherford, Sinclair, Plummer and Innes had, under the Council's protection, undertaken the professing and teaching of medicine in the city; and the Council, considering that these men had given the clearest proof of their capacity and ability to teach, appointed Sinclair and Rutherford to be professors of the theory and practice of medicine, and Plummer and Innes professors of medicine and chemistry.[2]   This is the date from which the Medical Faculty of Edinburgh University actually begins.

The University had, prior to this time, exercised the right of conferring medical degrees, and had remitted the examination of candidates to two members of the College of Physicians, whose certificate, when presented to the University, was sustained and the degree conferred.[3]   Dr. Sinclair appears to have lectured upon the theory of medicine (physiology) by explaining the "Institutiones Medicæ" of Boerhaave, while Dr. Rutherford dealt with the practice of medicine. Dr. Rutherford has a special claim to remembrance as having been the first professor who delivered clinical lectures in the Infirmary, commencing these immediately after the disturbance caused by the Rebellion had passed off in 1746, when his class was attended by a great many students.   His lectures appear to have been greatly appreciated, and a pupil, the celebrated Dr. William Buchan, said of him: "Rutherford is slow but absolutely sure."[4]   John Rutherford was the maternal grandfather of Sir Walter Scott, and his son, Dr. Daniel Rutherford, at a later date, acted as professor of botany, and was celebrated as the discoverer of nitrogen gas.

Dr. Andrew Plummer had commenced study at the University of Edinburgh, and afterwards repaired to Leyden, where he studied medicine under Boerhaave, and took the degree of M.D. in 1722.   He was specially interested in chemistry, and a great part of his course consisted in showing "a variety of useful and amusing processes," but a considerable portion of the course also consisted in teaching pharmacy.   His name is preserved in a pill of antimony and mercury still known as "Plummer's Pill," and he was the first person to analyse the water of Moffat Spa, and to recommend patients to betake themselves to that health resort.[5] Little is known of Dr. Innes.

---

[1] pp. 201–203, [2] pp. 204–208, [3] p. 210 : Bower : "History of the University of Edinburgh," Vol. II, Edinburgh, 1817.
[4] pp. 213–215, [5] pp. 215–216 : Bower : "History of the University of Edinburgh," Vol. II, Edinburgh, 1817.

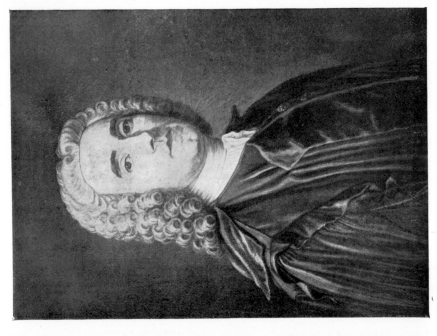

ANDREW PLUMMER (Died 1756)

(Original picture in the possession of Major C. H. Scott Plummer)

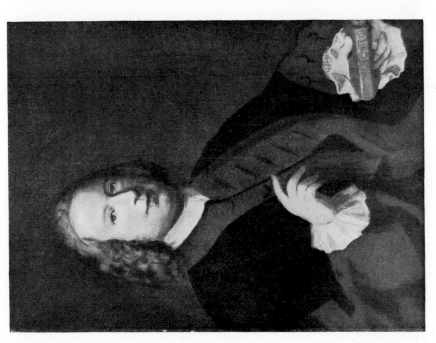

JOHN RUTHERFORD (1695-1779)

(Grandfather of Sir Walter Scott)

(Original picture by Allan Ramsay, in the possession of Miss Russel)

Another very important step in the development of the Medical School was taken on 9th February, 1726, when the Town Council considered a petition received from Mr. Joseph Gibson, a practitioner in Leith,[1] supported by a declaration under the hands of four doctors of medicine, that he should be appointed a professor of midwifery.   The practise of this art in Scotland at that time was entirely in the hands of female practitioners, and the somewhat opprobrious term of " man midwife " was generally applied in Britain to physicians who specialised in this branch of practice.   This appointment was the first of its kind in the kingdom, and Professor Gibson taught classes both of midwives and of medical students.   He was succeeded in 1739 as professor of midwifery in the Town's College by Mr. Robert Smith, who held the professorship for seventeen years, till 1756, when Dr. Thomas Young was appointed professor and first delivered a systematic course of lectures upon the subject.[2]   Dr. Young's important step, taken on his appointment in 1756, of fitting up a ward in the attic storey of the recently-erected Royal Infirmary for the reception of lying-in women, and his clinical instruction there, have been already mentioned.

The requirements for the degree of M.D. at Edinburgh, when the Medical Faculty was founded in 1726, were as follows :   The student was required to have studied medicine during at least three years at Edinburgh or some other University, and must have attended during this time lectures on anatomy and surgery, chemistry, botany, materia medica and pharmacy, theory and practice of medicine and clinical lectures in the hospital.   He was then required to compose a dissertation in Latin upon some medical subject, and to submit it to one of the medical professors two months before the day of graduation.   The dissertation was next submitted to the whole Faculty, a question was proposed to the candidate, and he was afterwards examined by two professors as to the proficiency he had made in his medical studies.   If his answers were satisfactory, his test was finished.   If not, one of the aphorisms of Hippocrates was assigned to him by one of the professors, and a medical question by another.   He had to illustrate the former by a commentary, and to answer the latter with proper arguments before the Medical Faculty.   Two histories of diseases accompanied with questions were also given to him in writing, and he had to give his opinion on them before the Faculty.   If he now gave satisfaction, he had to print his thesis and defend it publicly, this, however, being apparently a matter of form. Thereafter, he received the degree of doctor of medicine.   All these proceedings were conducted in the Latin tongue.[3]

---

[1] Bower : " History of the University of Edinburgh   ol. II, p. 254.
[2] Op. cit., Vol. III, p. 5.
[3] Bower : " History of the University of Edinburgh,' Vol. II, pp. 216-220.

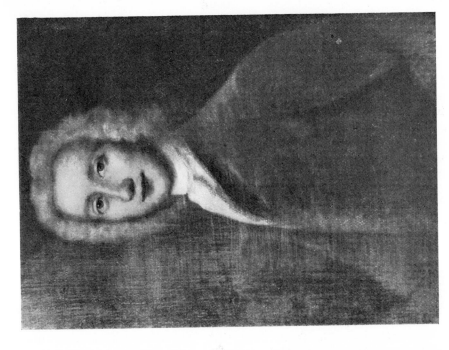

ROBERT WHYTT (1714–1766)

(Original by Belluci, preserved at Mount Melville, Fifeshire)

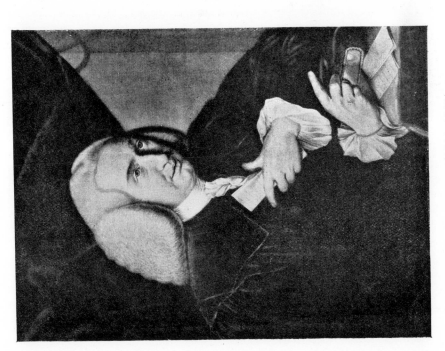

WILLIAM CULLEN (1710–1790)

(Original picture by Cochrane, in Hunterian Museum, Glasgow)

Chapter XIII

Medicine at Edinburgh in the Latter Half of the Eighteenth Century

THE Rebellion of 1745 produced great confusion in the arrangements for medical teaching, as well as in other departments of social activity throughout Scotland. By the winter of 1746–1747, however, affairs had settled down, and various re-arrangements took place in the Medical Faculty. Dr. Innes had in the meantime died, and it became necessary to appoint a successor. The Town Council accordingly elected Dr. Robert Whytt to succeed Dr. Innes as professor of the institutes of medicine, and at the same time he was elected professor of the practice of medicine on 26th August, 1747. Dr. John Rutherford had been lecturing on the practice of medicine for over twenty years, and it is not quite clear why Dr. Whytt now took over these duties. The reason is probably to be found in the fact that Dr. Rutherford began in the winter session of 1746–1747 to deliver clinical lectures in the Infirmary, and that these occupied a great deal of his time and energy. He still, however, nominally lectured on the practice of physic for another twenty years, when he resigned, and he died in 1779. Andrew Sinclair, before this time, seems to have fallen out of notice as a lecturer, and Andrew Plummer, the fourth of the original professors, devoted himself latterly entirely to chemistry.

John Rutherford, in commencing his clinical lectures, described his plan as follows :—

> " I shall examine every Patient capable of appearing before you, that no circumstance may escape you, and proceed in the following manner. 1st, Give you a history of the disease. 2ndly, Enquire into the Cause. 3dly, Give you my Opinion how it will terminate. 4thly, lay down the indications of cure yt arise, and if any new Symptoms happen acquaint you them, that you may see how I vary my prescriptions. And 5thly, Point out the different Method of Cure. If at any time you find me deceived in giving my Judgement, you'll be so good as to excuse me, for neither do I pretend to be, nor is the Art of Physic infallible, what you can in Justice expect from me is, some accurate observations and Remarks upon Diseases."[1]

Robert Whytt received his early education at Kirkcaldy, and later went to St. Andrews University, where he graduated in Arts in 1730. The next four years he spent in Edinburgh, studying medicine at the school which Monro *(primus)*, Sinclair, Rutherford, Innes and Plummer had done much to develop in the previous decade. In 1736, he graduated M.D. at Rheims, and, returning to Scotland next year, received the degree of M.D. also from St. Andrews University. In 1737, he

---

[1] MS. Notes of Rutherford's Clinical Lectures in the Royal College of Physicians' Library, Edinburgh, p. 7.

joined the Edinburgh College of Physicians as a Licentiate, started medical practice in Edinburgh, and became a Fellow of the College in the following year.

About the time that Whytt commenced to practise, great public interest was manifested in the search for substances which would dissolve stones in the bladder. This was probably due to several well-known persons having suffered from calculus about the period, but the condition seems in any case to have been commoner then than now.   Whytt had taken a great deal of interest in this subject, and carried out an elaborate series of experiments in the Royal Infirmary of Edinburgh with lime-water made from calcined egg-shells, cockle-shells, oyster-shells, etc., which he found had a considerable power in disintegrating calculi.   Not only had he tried the effects of the solvent *in vitro*, but he had carried out courses of injections into the bladder of various patients in the Infirmary who were suffering from vesical calculus.   His " Essay on the Virtues of Lime-water and Soap in the Cure of the Stone " was first published in 1743.   The treatment upon which he finally settled was to administer daily, by the mouth, an ounce of alicant soap and three pints or more of lime-water.

Whytt was one of the first doctors in Scotland to devote himself to medical research in the modern connotation of this term, and he busied himself, for some years after his appointment as Professor in the University of Edinburgh, chiefly with physiological researches.   To this period belong " An Essay on the Vital and other Involuntary Motions of Animals," first published in 1751 ; and two " Physiological Essays " published in 1755.   Of these, the one was " An Inquiry into the Causes which promote the Circulation of the Fluids in the very small Vessels of Animals."   The other was entitled " Observations on the Sensibility and Irritability of the Parts of Men and other Animals : occasioned by M. de Haller's late Treatise on these Subjects."

The Essay on Vital and Involuntary Motions contains a record of numerous experiments dealing especially with the reflex movements.   Whytt was the first to localise a reflex by showing that lasting dilatation of the pupil might be due to compression of the optic thalamus.[1]   He also showed that the brain is unnecessary for reflex action, and that a portion of the cord suffices for this, for in a brainless frog the reflexes of the upper and lower limbs are in different parts of the cord.[2]   These were the first attempts, I believe, since the time of Galen, to localise the seat of reflex acts.   They preceded by nearly a century the important memoir presented to the Royal Society by Marshall Hall (1833) on " The Reflex Function of the Medulla Oblongata and Medulla Spinalis."

One of the Essays published in 1755, " On the Sensibility and Irritability of the Parts of Men and Animals," brought Whytt into conflict with Albrecht von Haller, and so gained for him prominent notice in Germany, Switzerland and

---

[1] " Works of Robert Whytt, M.D.," published by his son, 1768, p. 71.
[2] Op. cit., p. 203.

France.   The whole dispute, both on the side of Haller and on that of Whytt, was of a dialectic character, and tended rather to involve the names of things than actual facts of nature.   It must be remembered, too, that the dispute took place between sixty and seventy years before the experiments of Bell (1811) and Magendie (1822) showed the separate existence of motor and sensory nerve paths. Whytt advanced some telling arguments in support of his contention that all muscular action was governed by nervous control.

Of much more permanent interest, however, is Whytt's " Observations on the Nature, Causes and Cure of those Disorders which are commonly called Nervous, Hypochondriac, or Hysteric."   This was published in 1764.   It shows great clinical acumen and is well worth reading still, particularly for the vivid accounts that Whytt gives of a great number of cases of hysteria and similar conditions.   He refers to " a particular sympathy between the nerves distributed to the teguments of the abdomen and those of the intestines."[1]   He also mentions the pain felt in the groins and down the thighs in scirrhus of the uterus.

Whytt's chief claim to lasting remembrance, however, lies in the fact that he was the first to give a clear description of tuberculous meningitis, or, as he called it, " Observations on the Dropsy in the Brain."   This is a short treatise of twenty-three quarto pages, included in the collected works published after his death.   The disease is still described according to the three stages into which Whytt divided its symptoms, and even at the present day there is little to add to his description from the clinical aspect.

Monro *(secundus)*, who acted as Professor of Anatomy at Edinburgh from 1754 to 1798, and whose name is familiar to medical students in connection with the foramen connecting the lateral and third ventricles of the brain, has an interesting point of contact with Whytt in this connection.   The foramen was first observed greatly dilated in a case of hydrocephalus which Monro and Whytt saw in consultation in the year 1764.[2]

To continue the facts of Whytt's life, in 1752 he was elected a Fellow of the Royal Society of London as the result of the reputation gained by his " Essay on the Vital and other Involuntary Motions of Animals."   Several short communications were addressed to this Society.   In 1761, he was made Physician to the King in Scotland, and in 1763 he was elected President of the Royal College of Physicians at Edinburgh.   He had many friends and correspondents in various parts of the world, and in particular he maintained a close friendship with Sir John Pringle, who had been a fellow-student. He died in 1766.[3]

William Cullen, who had come from Glasgow to be professor of chemistry at Edinburgh in 1755, succeeded Whytt as professor of institutes of medicine

---

[1] " Works of Robert Whytt, M.D.," published by his son, 1768, p. 542.
[2] Alexander Monro : " Observations on the Nervous System," 1783, Plate III, Fig. 4.
[3] See further, Comrie : " An 18th Century Neurologist," *Edin. Med. Journ.*, November, 1925.

in 1766. At the same, time John Gregory, who had been mediciner at King's College in Aberdeen, succeeded Whytt as professor of practice of medicine. The developing medical school at Edinburgh thus had, at an early stage, important connections with Glasgow and Aberdeen.

William Cullen (1710–1790) was born at Hamilton, his father being factor to the Duke of Hamilton and proprietor of Saughs, a small estate near Bothwell. William Cullen was the second of a family of nine, and on the death of his father and elder brother, at an early age, Cullen assumed the responsibility for the education of the younger members of the family. His preliminary education took place at the Grammar School at Hamilton, and at the age of seventeen he went to the University of Glasgow to study those subjects which were then considered part of an education in polite letters.

At this time, although there were several medical professors in that University, they were professors in title only and delivered no lectures, so that after Cullen had been for two years apprentice to Mr. John Paisley, a surgeon of Glasgow, he went, in 1729, to London to further his education and prospects. Obtaining a position as ship's surgeon, he sailed from London to the West Indies on a two years' voyage, and, on his return, spent a few months with Mr. Murray, an apothecary in Henrietta Street.

Towards the end of 1731, he returned to Scotland, set up in practice for some months at the village of Shotts, and afterwards commenced a practice at Rothbury in Northumberland. This somewhat varied experience is a good example of the type of medical education which was in vogue in the early part of the eighteenth century, and is reminiscent of the career of Smollett's "Roderick Random" in Glasgow and elsewhere.

Cullen, however, aspiring to a status above the average in his profession, determined to take the degree of M.D., and betook himself in the year 1734 to Edinburgh, where he attended the medical school in the sessions 1734–1735 and 1735–1736. This was some eight years after the foundation of the Medical Faculty in the University. During his stay in Edinburgh he joined himself, in the year 1735, to a private debating club of students, from which later developed the Royal Medical Society.

Returning again to Hamilton in 1736, Cullen became medical attendant to the Duke and Duchess of Hamilton, a position which he mentions that he held at a financial loss to himself, although that aristocratic connection proved of great value to his subsequent advancement. Very shortly after settling in Hamilton, he took as apprentice a youth from the neighbouring village of Longcalderwood, who afterwards became the celebrated physician William Hunter, and with whom Cullen maintained friendly intercourse to the end of Hunter's life.

In the year 1740, Cullen took the M.D. degree at Glasgow University with the intention of limiting his practice to that of a physician, and in November,

1741, he married.   In 1744, he removed his practice to Glasgow, and two years later he formed a teaching connection with this University by obtaining permission from Dr. Johnstoun, then titular Professor of Medicine, who, however, had never delivered lectures, to give a six months' course of lectures on Practice of Medicine.

Next year he joined Mr. Carrick, a practitioner of the city, in giving a course of lectures on Chemistry, and in the following year added Materia Medica and Botany.   Carrick having died in 1750, Cullen continued to give lectures on Medicine and Chemistry for the rest of his stay in Glasgow.   The interest which he succeeded in creating for the subject of Chemistry is shown by the fact that the University of Glasgow, in 1747, sanctioned the spending of £52 in order to fit up a chemical laboratory.   Later the amount was raised to £136, and a grant of £20 annually was made for the maintenance of the laboratory.   The apparatus must have been of a somewhat elaborate type, because considerable difficulty was experienced in procuring part of it even in London.   In this chemical class Cullen had another pupil, Joseph Black, who subsequently attained great fame as a chemist.   Black remained his pupil for six years in Glasgow, went to Edinburgh in 1751, where Dr. Plummer was then lecturer in Chemistry, and three years later graduated M.D.

In 1751, Cullen succeeded Dr. Johnstoun as Professor of Medicine in the University of Glasgow, and continued to give lectures upon chemistry and medicine for four years until 1755, when he secured an appointment as Joint Professor of Chemistry with Plummer in the University of Edinburgh. Plummer died of apoplexy some months later, and under Cullen the class of Chemistry prospered greatly, rising from seventeen students in the first session to fifty-nine in the second, and gradually developing into a class of 145.

Teaching chemistry did not, however, satisfy Cullen's medical ambitions, and in 1757 he undertook to deliver clinical lectures in the Royal Infirmary of Edinburgh, a new type of lecture upon the cases of patients, which had been commenced by Dr. Rutherford ten years earlier on the model of lectures that he had heard given in the Hospital at Leyden.   In 1766, Cullen became Professor of Institutes or Theory of Medicine (Physiology), and, in 1769, an arrangement was effected with Dr. John Gregory by which Gregory and Cullen gave alternate courses in Practice of Medicine.   Cullen became sole Professor of this subject when Gregory retired in 1773, and by this time he had also developed a large, lucrative and aristocratic consulting practice in Edinburgh.

It is interesting to note that Cullen did not succeed to the professorship of medicine till he was 63 years old, an age at which many men of the present day are preparing to retire.   Throughout his professional life Cullen lived and saw his patients in a small house in Mint Close or South Gray's Close, which, despite its confined character, was one of the principal residential districts of the day.   In 1778, however, the cares of practice were decreasing, and he purchased Ormiston Hill House, near Kirknewton, some nine miles west of Edinburgh, where he spent much time in laying out a garden and sylvan retreat.   Here, after resigning his Chair in 1789, he died in 1790.

Cullen's reputation in his own day, and his subsequent fame, rest almost entirely upon his skill as a teacher and sagacity as a consultant.   With regard to research, as the term is understood at the present day, his only work was a short pamphlet recording experiments " On the Cold produced by Evaporating Fluids."   He took an active part in preparing the new edition of the " Edinburgh Pharmacopœia," issued in 1774, and in obtaining a new hall for the College of Physicians.   In 1783 his persevering endeavours secured the incorporation of the Philosophical Society as the Royal Society of Edinburgh.

His works were all text-books elucidating various departments of medicine, and included " Lectures on Materia Medica," which was at first pirated and published without his consent in 1771, but subsequently issued as a " Treatise on Materia Medica " by him in 1789 ; and " First Lines on the Practice of Physic," published in 1776–1784, and in numerous subsequent English, French and German editions.   But the work which brought him the greatest measure of fame was his " Nosology," published in 1769, a small pamphlet which aimed at a rigid classification of diseases by their symptoms on the same arbitrary principle as Linnæus had adopted for classifying plants.   It arranges all diseases by classes, orders, genera and species and, regarding them as fixed entities, makes in a sense a system of the whole of medicine. Although up to a certain point logical, such a system is unnatural, and while Cullen's classification greatly simplified medicine and established his reputation during his lifetime, it fell into complete disuse half a century after his death.[1]

The influence that he exerted on the public mind, and the great attraction that he exercised in bringing students from a distance, were due to his clearness of perception, sound reasoning and judgment, more than to any originality.   As a lecturer, he had powers of interesting his students and inspiring them with enthusiasm.   One of his pupils highly commended his excellent arrangement, his memory of facts, and the ease, variety, vivacity and force of his lectures.   He lived at a time when medical practice was driven hither and thither by conflicting theories and systems, which his clear mind and power of expression enabled him to codify and set in their proper places.   In his day, theories as to the nature of life and vital processes were considered all-important, a matter which is difficult to understand in the present age, when the human mind accepts the mystery of life as a fact, and inquires only into the ways in which it is manifested.

Cullen adopted a standpoint somewhere between the views of his immediate predecessors, Stahl and Boerhaave.   Stahl had explained all vital phenomena by

---

[1] See Thomson : "Life, Lectures, and Writings of William Cullen, M.D.," Edinburgh, 1859.

reference to the activity of a "sentient soul," while Boerhaave, the great upholder of the iatro-mechanical school of thought, was purely materialistic in regard to the action of the nervous system.   Cullen adhered to the views of his predecessor in the Chair of Medicine, Robert Whytt, who maintained a " sympathetic " action of all parts of the body connected by nerves and vessels ; but he also supported the views of Haller, who pos-
tulated a *vis insita* in the individual tissues which rendered them excitable for independent action.

Out of the question of "excitability" arose a great deal of trouble, about the year 1778, between Cullen and a rival lecturer, Dr. John Brown.   Brown revived the ancient methodism of Asklepiades and pro-mulgated a simple idea with regard to the nature of vital processes and disease, which is known as the "Brunonian Theory," and which attributed disease pro-cesses to a state of too great or too little excita-bility of the tissues. All therapeutic measures, therefore, resolved them-selves into stimulation if the excitability was lessened, and soothing remedies if the excita-bility was too great. Brown's system, which

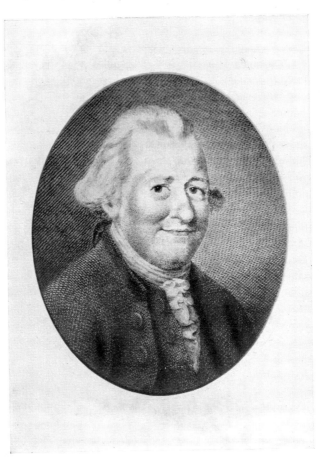

JOHN BROWN (1735-1788)

was both easy to understand and required very little knowledge of medicine, not only appealed strongly to the Edinburgh students, but secured him a great following among scientific men all over Europe.   He and Cullen engaged in much polemic writing on the subject, but Brown ultimately died from a practical application of his theories to his own person, by alternate recourse to stimulants and sedatives, and the dispute, so far as Edinburgh was concerned, ended.

Another link with the Glasgow Medical School is formed by Joseph Black (1728–1799), who may be described as the first of the scientific chemists as distinguished from medical chemists.   He was born at Bordeaux, of Scottish parents, and, in 1746, commenced the study of medicine at Glasgow, where he had William Cullen for his teacher in chemistry. A close friendship sprang up between the two, which continued when Black went to Edinburgh in 1751 to continue his medical studies.

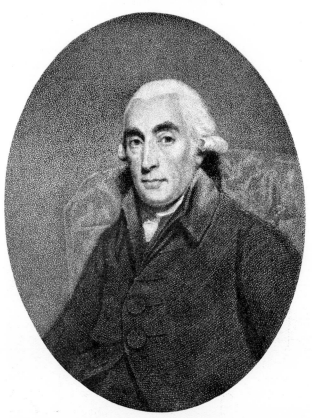

JOSEPH BLACK (1728-1799)

During 1752 – 1753, Black busied himself in research for a solvent of urinary calculi.   In the course of his experiments he discovered that the difference between calcareous earth (limestone) and quicklime was produced by the expulsion of a "fixed air," and that by the action of slaked lime upon the mild alkalies these were in turn rendered caustic by the transference of their "fixed air" to the slaked lime, whereby the latter again became mild. By quantitative experiments he found further that instead of gaining something from the fire (phlogiston) as was then the general view, the limestone had sustained a substantial loss owing to the escape of a gas to which, therefore, he gave the name of "fixed air."

This discovery of carbon dioxide was embodied in his thesis submitted in 1754 for the degree of M.D., entitled " De Humore Acido a Cibis Orto, et Magnesia Alba."   He seems to have had some modest doubts as to whether this discovery was sufficient for an M.D. thesis.   A fuller account in English of his experiments was published next year under the title " Experiments upon Magnesia Alba, Quicklime, and some other Alcaline Substances."

Black suggested to his friend Professor Cullen the investigation of the effects in producing cold by evaporating fluids, upon which Cullen subsequently published a short treatise. In the same connection Black, in 1762, discovered the principle of latent heat, which was described in a paper to the Philosophical Club of Glasgow, but was not published till it appeared in Black's " Lectures," edited by Robison, in 1803.

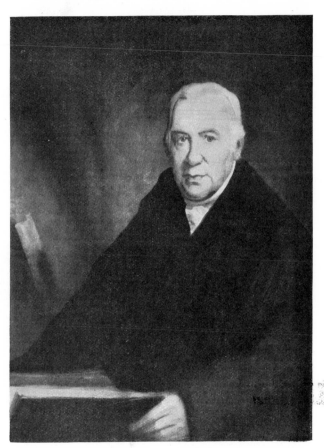

DANIEL RUTHERFORD (1749-1819)

The practical importance of Black's discovery was at once recognised by James Watt, through whose genius latent heat was transformed into useful mechanical work in the invention of the steam engine.

Black and Cullen were two active early members of the Royal Society of Edinburgh, which was re-organised from the Philosophical Society with a Royal Charter in 1783. In 1757, Black was appointed professor of chemistry and medicine at Glasgow on the death of Professor Hamilton. In 1766, when Cullen was transferred from the Chair of chemistry at Edinburgh to that of institutes of medicine, he was succeeded by his friend Joseph Black. Black had engaged during his time at Glasgow in busy practice as a physician, but on coming to Edinburgh he devoted himself to research, mainly on the subject of latent heat, and to teaching. In 1795, Thomas Charles Hope was appointed joint professor of chemistry with him, and Black died in 1799. After his death, his lectures, expanded from his own notes, were published by his friend and colleague, Professor John Robison, in 1803, as " Lectures on the Elements of Chemistry, delivered in the University of Edinburgh."

A younger contemporary of Joseph Black was Daniel Rutherford (1749–1819), the son of Dr. John Rutherford.   In 1772 he submitted for the degree of M.D. a thesis entitled " De Aere Fixo Dicto, aut Mephitico."   In this he pointed out that after Black's " fixed air " had been removed from respired air by caustic lye, the air still extinguished both flame and life no less than before, although it produced no precipitate with lime-water.   This was the discovery of nitrogen gas.   Although Daniel Rutherford's inclinations lay towards chemistry, he was later appointed professor of medicine and botany in 1786.

The professorship of botany had been separated from that of materia medica in 1768, when Dr. Francis Home, an army surgeon, was appointed to fill the Chair of Materia Medica.   In 1798 he retired, and was succeeded by his son, Dr. James Home.   Dr. Francis Home wrote several treatises of great importance on the virtues of the water of Duns, on bleaching, on agriculture, and on croup, as well as a text-book, the " Principia Medicinæ," published in 1758.[1]

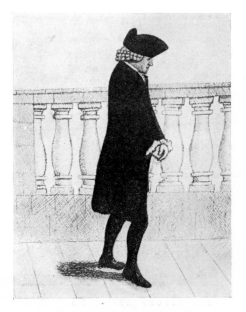

FRANCIS HOME (1719-1813)
(From Kay's " Portraits ")

The comprehensive course of lectures on anatomy begun by Professor Monro in 1720 was continued every winter for nearly forty years, a period during which the numbers of students attracted to Edinburgh yearly increased.   His best-known work is a " Treatise on Osteology," which went through many English editions, and which was translated into French and published as a large folio volume with magnificent copper-plates by M. Sue, Demonstrator of Anatomy to the Royal Schools of Surgery at Paris (1759).   Besides this he published some fifty short papers, some anatomical, some surgical, not of any great importance or permanent interest.

His son, Alexander Monro (secundus) (1733–1817), was educated with a view to succeeding his father in the Chair of Anatomy, and at the age of twenty-one was elected Conjoint Professor, taking full charge of the department at the age of twenty-five, in 1758, when the first Monro restricted himself to teaching clinical medicine.   Placed in easy circumstances from the outset, and provided with

[1] Bower : " History of the University of Edinburgh," Vol. III, p. 120.

a class which came to him independently of any attractions he had to offer, Monro *secundus* might well have failed to reach the success as a teacher and as a citizen to which the first Monro had by his efforts attained.   Yet the second Monro showed himself the greater man, both as a teacher and investigator, and, among more brilliant colleagues than those with whom his father had had to compete, he maintained an easy equality and was the acknowledged head of the developing medical school.

It is useful, as showing the progress of the Edinburgh Medical School, to consider the number of students attending the Anatomy class during the decennial periods throughout the regime of the first two Monros.[1]

In 1720	.	.	.	.	57	Average 1760–1770 .	. 194
,, 1730	.	.	.	.	83	,, 1770–1780 .	. 287
,, 1740	.	.	.	.	130	,, 1780–1790 .	. 342
,, 1750	.	.	.	.	158	After 1800 over .	. 400

A short account of the lectures delivered by Monro *secundus* is given in the Memoir of his son.   Monro was accustomed, after very careful preparation, to lecture in an extempore manner from headings, but a manuscript copy in excellent handwriting, taken down by one of his students, is preserved in the Library of the Edinburgh College of Physicians, and another in the Museum of the College of Surgeons.

With regard to the contributions made by Monro *secundus* to the increase of anatomical knowledge, it is a striking fact that none of the great works on which his reputation chiefly rests was published till after he was fifty years of age. These were " Observations on the Structure and Functions of the Nervous System " (1783), " The Structure and Physiology of Fishes explained, and compared with those of Man and other Animals " (1785), " Description of the Bursæ Mucosæ of the Human Body " (1788), and " Treatise on the Brain, the Eye, and the Ear " (1797).

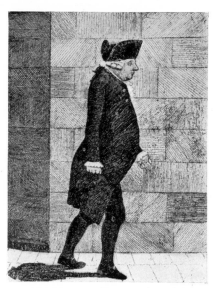

ALEXANDER MONRO (*secundus*)
(1733-1817)
(*From Kay's " Portraits "*)

One of Monro's earliest fields of inquiry was on the function of the lymphatic vessels, and his dispute with William Hunter for priority in the elucidation of their nature was one of the celebrated medical controversies of the eighteenth century.   Nobody up to 1755 had supposed that the lymphatic vessels were more than a class of very small

---

[1] J. Struthers : " The Edinburgh Anatomical School," Edinburgh, 1867, p. 23

veins originating like the " red veins " from the arteries.   Monro *secundus*, while in Berlin in 1757, published a Latin thesis, " De Venis Lymphaticis Valvulosis," in which he deals with their origin from spaces in the connective tissues.   Hunter had mentioned the same thing in his lectures, and suggested that the lymphatics are the absorbents of the body, and Monro charged Hunter with having adopted the idea from him.

He supported his contention by a letter from Joseph Black, dated 24th March, 1758, in which Black states that Monro had shown him a paper in 1755 in which he maintained that the lymphatics " are a distinct

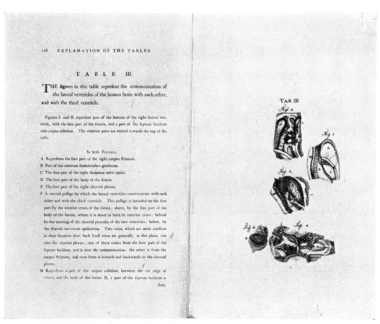

PAGES FROM MONRO "ON THE BRAIN"
Showing his original description and figures of the "foramen of Monro"

system of vessels, having no immediate connection with the arteries and veins, but arising, in small branches, from all the cavities and cells in the body, into which fluids are thrown ; and that their use is to absorb the whole, or the thinner parts, of these fluids, and restore them to the mass of circulating humours."[1]   Monro's main method of proof had been by injecting the arteries in such a way as to rupture them, when he found that the injection fluid passed from the alveolar spaces into the neighbouring lymphatics, and, on the balance of probability, the original discovery that the lymphatics form an independent absorbent system is really his.

[1] Monro : " Observations, Anatomical and Physiological," 1758, p. 27.

A similar controversy was later raised with Hewson, who had been a pupil of Monro in Edinburgh and of Hunter in London, and who published in 1774 his celebrated " Description of the Lymphatic System in the Human Subject and in other Animals."   The dispute this time was whether he or Monro had first discovered lymphatics in birds, amphibians, etc.[1]   It is quite clear that Monro had shown injections of the lymphatics in these animals to his class before Hewson became a medical student, but he certainly never described and figured them with the fullness and accuracy of the latter's work.

Monro's " Observations on the Structure and Functions of the Nervous System " (1783) not only summarised and illustrated by admirable plates the current knowledge of the time, but contained numerous additions from his own observation.   Among the new points described may be mentioned the foramen connecting the lateral and third ventricles, which has made his name familiar

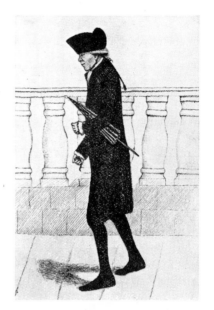

ALEXANDER WOOD
("Lang Sandy Wood") (1725-1807)
(From Kay's "Portraits")

to every medical student.   Monro's description runs :—

" So far back as the year 1753, soon after I began the study of Anatomy, I discovered, that the Lateral Ventricles of the Human Brain communicated with each other, and, at the same place, with the Middle or Third Ventricle of the Brain. And, as a passage from the Third Ventricle to the Fourth is universally known, it followed, that what are called the Four Ventricles of the Brain are in reality different parts of one cavity."[2]

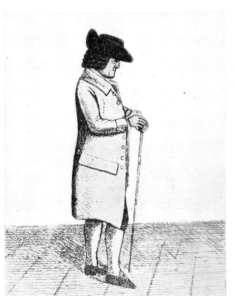

JAMES RAE
Deacon of Surgeons, 1764
(From Kay's " Portraits ")

---

[1] Monro : " Structure and Physiology of Fishes," 1785, p. 39.
[2] Monro : " The Brain, the Eye and the Ear," 1797, p. 9.

The first observation of this foramen was made on a case of tuberculous meningitis seen in consultation with Robert Whytt, which also furnished the latter with part of the material for his original description of this disease.[1]

" The Structure and Physiology of Fishes" (1785) was the first important work on Comparative Anatomy in Edinburgh, and founded in Scotland a taste for that branch of Science which had been recently introduced and elaborated by the Hunters and their pupils in London. Monro's "Description of the Bursæ Mucosæ of the Human Body" (1788) was of a more practical type, and of great importance in relation to surgery.

The development of the Faculty of Medicine in the University during the first three-quarters of a century of its existence was chiefly along the lines of medicine, although several important representatives of surgical practice were found in the College of Surgeons. The subject of surgery was treated simply as an appendix to the lectures on anatomy delivered by the first two Monros, of whom the second was a consulting physician with a large practice. Efforts were made to bring about more thorough teaching of surgery, but were resisted as an infringement of the interests of the Monro family, until the College of Surgeons, by an amusing expedient which will be mentioned later, forced the appointment to the University of a professor of surgery in 1831.

One of the best known of the 18th century Edinburgh surgeons was Alexander Wood (1725–1807), known to his contemporaries as " Lang Sandy Wood," and greatly respected for his dexterity in practice, which did much to raise the reputation of the surgical department in the Royal Infirmary, as well as beloved for his amiable social qualities. The general opinion of him, in a day when Edinburgh doctors were celebrated for disputation and bickering, is summed up in a couplet by the writer of a parody on Byron's " Childe Harold " :—

> " Oh, for an hour of him who knew no feud—
> The octogenarian chief, the kind old Sandy Wood."[2]

John Kay has represented him in wig and cocked hat with an umbrella under his arm, in allusion to the fact that he was the first person in Edinburgh to make use of the latter article. At a time when personal peculiarity was widely affected by Edinburgh people, Wood specially distinguished himself by going to see his patients accompanied by a pet sheep and raven.

James Rae was Deacon of the Incorporation of Surgeons in 1764, and was one of the first to urge that surgery deserved to be taught in a complete course of lectures apart from anatomy. For some years he conducted a private course in surgery and attracted a considerable number of students. He also gave lectures on diseases of the teeth and, in connection with his course in surgery, held lectures

---

[1] " Works of Robert Whytt," 1768, p. 728.
[2] " Fragment of a Fifth Canto of Childe Harold's Pilgrimage," Blackwood's Magazine, May, 1818.

on clinical surgery in the Infirmary.   He may, therefore, be regarded as the first teacher in clinical surgery at Edinburgh.[1]   He died in 1791.

Benjamin Bell (1749–1806) was a native of Dumfries, where he served an apprenticeship to Mr. James Hill, surgeon.   At the age of seventeen, he came to Edinburgh to attend the medical classes, and afterwards spent two years in the great surgical school of Paris and in London, where he studied under William Hunter.   His reason for going abroad indicates the character of the Edinburgh Medical School in 1770. He said : " Had I been now entering to the world as a physician, I should never have thought of going further than where I have been ; but for a *surgeon*, I assure you Edinburgh comes greatly short of either Paris or London, and for that reason, Dr. Monro and any others that I have spoke to here upon the subject, approve of the scheme very much."[2]

Benjamin Bell should be regarded as the first of the Edinburgh scientific surgeons.   He was one of the first to seek for some means of preventing or diminishing pain in surgical operations, and, in his " System of Surgery," described several methods for effecting this, which, however, were superseded sixty years afterwards

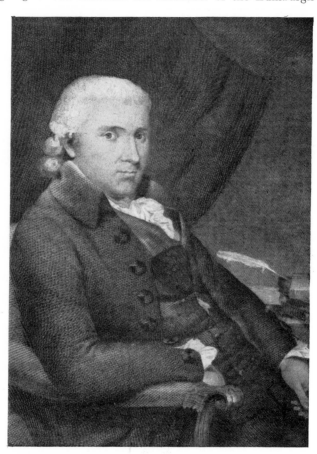

BENJAMIN BELL (1749-1806)

by the introduction of   ether and chloroform.   In his paper, " On the Chirurgical Treatment of Inflammation " (1777), he described the use of the seton, a practice recommended thirty years earlier by James Rae.   His most important

[1] Alexander Miles : " The Edinburgh School of Surgery before Lister," London, 1918, p. 79.
[2] " The Life, Character and Writings of Benjamin Bell," by his Grandson, Benjamin Bell, Edinburgh, 1868, p. 23.

contribution to surgery was his "Treatise on Gonorrhœa Virulenta and Lues Venerea," published in 1793, in which, for the first time, he distinguished clearly between these two diseases. His "System of Surgery," in six volumes, was an attempt to rival Heister's "System of Surgery," the great surgical text-book of that time, and though it was unfavourably criticised, both by his contemporary John Bell and by Sir Benjamin Brodie, it went through seven editions and was translated into French and German.[1]

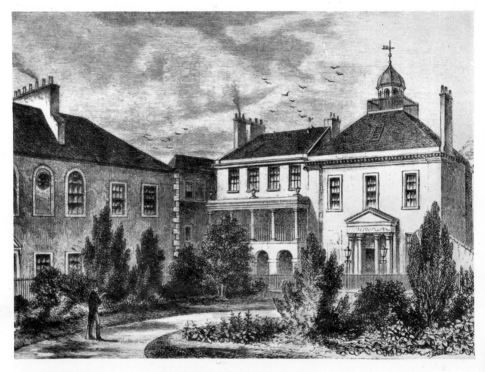

SURGEONS' SQUARE IN 1829
Showing from left to right, Surgeons' Hall of 1697, Gordon's class-room, Royal Medical Society's Hall, and Knox's (formerly Barclay's) class-room

An important part in the educational advantages of the Edinburgh Medical School has been played almost since its beginning by a Medical Society of students which commenced in the year 1734. In August of that year, six men studying medicine at Edinburgh—Dr. Cleghorn, Dr. Cuming, Dr. Russel, Dr. Hamilton, Mr. Archibald Taylor and Dr. James Kennedy—who were in the habit of spending social evenings together at a tavern, decided that this little society should meet regularly once a fortnight at their respective lodgings, when

---

[1] Miles, Op. cit., p. 59.

a dissertation in English or Latin on some medical subject should be read by each of the members in rotation and criticised by the other five.   In 1735, Cleghorn, who later became professor of anatomy in Dublin, was the only member left in Edinburgh.   He and some other students, including William Cullen, who had come to Edinburgh as a student, and John Fothergill, continued the meetings, and the Society was definitely constituted as the Medical Society of Edinburgh by ten members towards the end of the year 1737.

The meetings took place in a tavern until the year 1763, when the Society obtained permission from the Managers of the Royal Infirmary to hold the weekly meetings in a room of the hospital.   At the same time, the Society began to collect a library, which, by 1778, amounted to about 1500 volumes. A proposal was made about this time to build a hall for the meetings, which was warmly supported by various friends among the professors and the practitioners of Edinburgh, particularly by Doctors Cullen, Hope and Duncan.   Finally, under the presidentship of Mr. Gilbert Blane, the foundation stone of the Medical Hall was laid by Dr. Cullen, and the Hall on the west side of Surgeons' Square was opened on 26th April, 1776.

The Society has included in its list of members the names of many men who afterwards attained eminence, and among those in the early days are the names of Mark Akenside (1740) and Oliver Goldsmith (1752).   From its list of annual Presidents, many have become teachers in the Edinburgh School or have attained distinction in other places.   In the present Hall are two memorial tablets to Presidents of the Society, Jacob Pattisson and Francis Foulke, who died during their term of office.   The latter was killed in a duel on 22nd December, 1789.   A quarrel with an officer, Mr. G., having occurred, a challenge ensued, and the two met on Seafield Sands attended by their seconds. At the third discharge of pistols, Foulke fell with a bullet in his heart.[1]

A Royal Charter was obtained for the Society from King George III. in December, 1779, largely by the exertions of Dr. Andrew Duncan.   At this time there was a kind of obsession for the foundation of societies, both among the students and the practitioners of the town.   These included the Medico-Chirurgical Society (founded in 1767), the Physico-Chirurgical Society (1771), the Chirurgo-Physical Society, the American Physical Society, the Hibernian Medical Society, the Chemical Society, the Natural History Society and the Didactic Society.   All of these waned and were one by one absorbed by the Royal Physical Society, which was incorporated in 1788 after erecting a hall in immediate proximity to the Royal Public Dispensary in 1784.

The Royal Medical Society, however, continued to flourish as a meeting-place for students.   Its objects, in the words of an early President, were " mutual improvement and the investigation of truth ; the development of the seeds of

[1] Grant : " Old and New Edinburgh," Vol. III, p. 266.

genius, and the detection of falsehood ; the emancipation of the mind from the fetters of prejudice, and the cultivation of true friendship by social and liberal intercourse." At its weekly meetings during the winter session, the plan proposed at the beginning of the Society was followed, by which the members in turn submitted a dissertation on some prescribed subject, which was discussed by the Society, with occasional addresses from former members, and debates.

In the middle of the 19th century, partly in consequence of the Society having outgrown its premises at Surgeons' Square, partly because these premises were showing signs of decay, and partly because the character of the locality at Surgeons' Square had changed, the present Hall at Melbourne Place was opened on 7th November, 1852.[1]

During the latter half of the 18th century, Edinburgh was the great medical resort of all the Britons beyond the seas, much as Leyden had been the resource for those who wished to take a medical degree half a century earlier. The number of graduates is not, however, an indication of the number of students, for many men who studied medicine at Edinburgh took the qualification of the College of Surgeons, while right up to the passing of the Medical Act, in 1858, a large number of students were content to learn their profession as apprentices to some practitioner, and to take a few classes at some medical school, such as Edinburgh, without proceeding to graduation. Out of thirteen graduates in 1765, five belonged to Scotland, five were American, two English and one Irish. In 1787, after the troubles connected with the War of American Independence had subsided, out of forty-four graduates, nineteen were Scottish, nine English, six came from America, and ten were Irish.

Several of the most distinguished pioneers of American medicine graduated at Edinburgh : for example, William Shippen (with a thesis entitled " De Placentæ cum Utero Nexu," 1761), John Morgan (" De Puris Confectione," 1763), Samuel Bard (" De Viribus Opii," 1765), Benjamin Rush (" De Coctione Ciborum in Ventriculo," 1768), and Philip Syng Physic (" De Apoplexia," 1792).[2] Ephraim McDowell, the Kentucky ovariotomist, studied in Edinburgh (1793–1794), though he did not graduate.

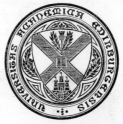

SEAL, EDINBURGH UNIVERSITY

---

[1] Stroud : " History of the Royal Medical Society," Edinburgh, 1820.
[2] " Edinburgh Medical Graduates, 1705–1866," Edinburgh, 1867.

CHAPTER XIV

The Glasgow School in the First Half of the Nineteenth Century

ONE of the most important steps in connection with the development of the Glasgow Medical School was the foundation of a hospital where clinical teaching could take place. Glasgow, in 1712, was a small burgh with a population of 14,000,

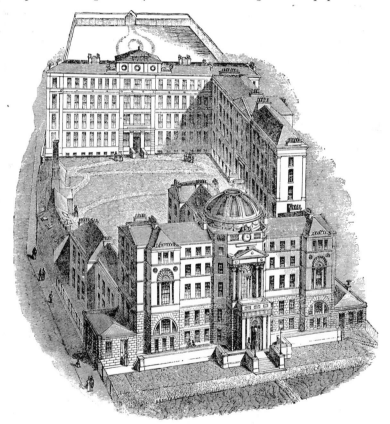

GLASGOW ROYAL INFIRMARY IN 1861

The original Adams building (medical house) is to the front: the fever-house (later surgical) to the right: and the newly-erected surgical block to the rear. Lister's Wards are those on either side of the door in the rear building: the male ward on the ground floor, to the left, and the female ward on the first floor up, to the right

but during the 18th century, in consequence of the development of trade with the American colonies, the population rose rapidly, and in 1801 had reached 83,000, while thirty years later a still more rapid rise brought the number of inhabitants of the city and its suburbs to about 200,000 in the year 1831.   Situated in the Old Green, the Town's Hospital, which corresponded very much to a modern workhouse, subserved the needs of the city in the early part of the 18th century. A movement, begun in 1787, to provide a general hospital, which was an indispensable adjunct to a medical school, took shape, so that in December, 1794, the Royal Infirmary was formally opened for the reception of patients.   The site of this hospital was that of the old Archbishop's Castle, adjoining the Cathedral and close to the University buildings in the High Street, and, as originally built, its capacity was for 150 patients.[1]   The Western Infirmary was not inaugurated until 1874, when another hospital became necessary, partly because of the increase of the population in the city and partly because of the migration of the University to Gilmorehill in the western part of Glasgow.   The Victoria Infirmary was not instituted until 1887.

By the beginning of the 19th century, the Faculty of Physicians and Surgeons had been engaged for two hundred years in maintaining and improving the standard of practice in the west of Scotland, but it had done little or no teaching. The prosecution of quacks had by this time become less necessary, and it was falling into desuetude.   Its gradual abandonment was due to two factors : in the first place, the summary powers conferred in the 16th century by which the Faculty summoned delinquents before them and fined them forty pounds Scots, could hardly be exercised in the 19th century ; and, secondly, a penalty of forty pounds Scots, in its modern equivalent of two pounds sterling, held no terrors, in fact, provided a useful advertisement, for a successful quack.   The early part of the 19th century saw a still more serious invasion of the Faculty's privileges by the developing University of Glasgow.

There had always been a doubt whether the doctors in medicine whose diplomas were inspected and who were then sanctioned to practise by the Faculty, could also practise surgery.   It had been the habit for any doctors of medicine who wished to practise surgery in or near Glasgow to submit to examination in that craft by the examiners of the Faculty.   A decision of the Court of Session was obtained by the Faculty in 1815 that a degree in medicine did not entitle the holder to practise surgery within the bounds of the Faculty.   Accordingly, in 1816, the University of Glasgow astutely resolved to add to its list of degrees that of Chirurgiæ Magister (C.M.).

By 1826 there were twenty-three persons in the western counties practising surgery by virtue of holding the C.M. of Glasgow, and against the whole of these the Faculty raised an action of interdict in the Court of Session.   This action dragged on with various suits, counterpleas and appeals until 1840, when judgment was given by the House of Lords in favour of the Faculty.   This

---

[1] John Fergus, M.D. : " Glasgow Royal Infirmary : Past, Present and Future," Glasgow, 1927.

judgment was, however, practically nullified by the Medical Act of 1858, when all territorial restrictions regarding medical practice were abolished.

The rise of the Glasgow Medical School is well seen from the number of students enrolled in the anatomy class between 1790 and 1860. The statistics were made up by the late Professor Allen Thomson :—

YEAR	NUMBER
1790	54
1800	113
1810	232
1820	162
1830	167
1840	61
1850	130
1860	256

Various causes operated to produce the great fluctuations in the numbers of students. Immediately after the battle of Waterloo there was a great diminution in the number of students, who had been steadily increasing during the French Wars with the demand for surgeons which they occasioned. From 1797 to about 1828, there were several private lecturers on anatomy who went by the general name of the College Street School, and who attracted large numbers of students to their dissecting rooms. Also, Anderson's College taught anatomy to steadily increasing numbers of students till about the 'forties, when its numbers were almost double those of the University. From 1830 to 1844, there was also a school in Portland Street with a considerable number of students. In the University, from 1790 to 1848, Professor James Jeffray held the Chair of Anatomy and although he had been successful as a teacher during the earlier part of his tenure, the failing health and lack of energy of his later years were probably largely responsible for the diminution in the numbers of students. Immediately on Professor Allen Thomson's appointment, in 1848, the numbers of the University class rose again.

An important factor in the development of the Glasgow Medical School was the bequest of Dr. William Hunter, who died on 30th March, 1783, and directed by his will that his Museum should be made over to the University of Glasgow, together with a sum of £8000 to erect a building at Glasgow for the reception of the Museum and to keep the collection in proper order. In early life, Hunter had taken a course in languages and philosophy at Glasgow University, had been apprenticed to William Cullen at Hamilton, and had studied medicine for one session at Edinburgh. He had afterwards gone to London, where he rose to eminence as a practitioner in medicine and obstetrics and a teacher of anatomy, and where he gained great wealth. His Museum was transferred to Glasgow in 1807, at the time

---

[1] Duncan : " Memorials of the Faculty of Physicians and Surgeons of Glasgow." pp. 172 and 173.

when great efforts were being made to develop the medical school in this city. This Museum included specimens of geology and natural history, pictures, valuable manuscripts, paintings, coins and archæological relics, as well as a great collection of carefully prepared and mounted anatomical specimens, partly collected by himself and partly presented to him by former pupils. As this collection was a life-long work, the Museum is of great value, and when Hunter died in March 1783, he directed that it should ultimately be given to the University of Glasgow, when his nephew Dr. Matthew Baillie, and his partner in the anatomical class, William Cruikshank, should have finished with it.

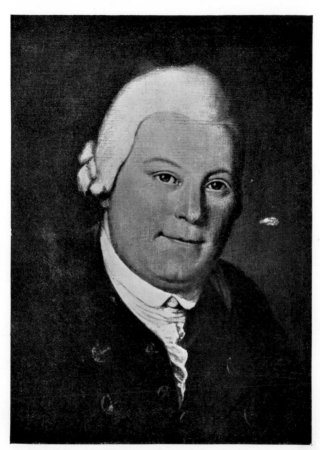

JOHN ANDERSON (1726-1796)
(Original in the Royal Scottish National Portrait Gallery)

His younger and more famous brother, John Hunter, was ten years younger than William, and the youngest of a tolerably large family. Somehow, his early education was neglected, and he, unlike his cultured brother William, was at the age of seventeen able neither to read nor write. His boyhood was entirely spent in his native parish of Long Calderwood, near Glasgow,[1] where his father was a small landed proprietor. In early manhood he settled in London as assistant to his brother William, and, afterwards becoming one of the greatest anatomists of Europe, attained a last resting-place in Westminster Abbey. His collection, as is well known, is preserved at the Royal College of Surgeons in London.

[1] Freeland Fergus: "Origin and Development of the Glasgow Medical School," *Glasgow Medical Journal,* November, 1911, p. 9.

A profound influence was exerted upon the Glasgow Medical School during the 19th century by the Andersonian College. This institution was founded on the death of Professor John Anderson in 1796 as an educational establishment, designed to supply courses and means of instruction in general and scientific branches of study, and to be a rival to the University. Various scientific departments originally included in it have been merged in the Glasgow and West of Scotland Technical College founded in 1886, but the Medical School of Anderson's College is still conducted separately.

John Anderson (1726–1796) was appointed Professor of Oriental Languages in 1755. In 1757 he was appointed Professor of Natural Philosophy, which he taught with great acceptance to the students and to his fellow-townspeople.[1] He was an ingenious man, and, as an example of his inventive skill, he presented to the French National Convention, in 1791, a gun, of which the recoil was absorbed by an air-chamber. In his zeal for reforming abuses in the University, he quarrelled with most of his fellow-professors. Failing in an attempt, made in 1784, to obtain a Royal Visitation of abuses in the University, with a view to reform, which seems to have been very necessary, he conceived the idea of leaving his property to found the College which bears his name, as an opponent and stimulus to the University. Anderson's College Medical School has proved a valuable training-ground for young lecturers, from which the professoriate in Glasgow University has been to a large extent recruited. In the century and a quarter of its existence, it has also frequently provided competent instruction in various departments, when the professors of corresponding subjects in the University happened to be inept.

Another important factor in the development of the Glasgow Medical School early in the 19th century, was the foundation, in 1802, of the Glasgow University Medico-Chirurgical Society for undergraduates. This Society, formed on the plan of the Royal Medical Society of Edinburgh, has had a long and prosperous existence. A little later, on 27th October, 1814, three physicians and three surgeons of the city met for the purpose of forming a Society, which they agreed to call the Glasgow Medical and Surgical Society. The Faculty of Physicians and Surgeons immediately granted the use of its hall for the meetings of the Society, which at first met twice in each month throughout the year. At a later date, the meetings of the Society were held on the second Tuesday of each month from March to October. In 1866, the Society amalgamated with another medical society and changed its name to the Medico-Chirurgical Society of Glasgow, of which Dr. Allen Thomson was the first President. An important meeting was held on 17th April, 1868, at which Professor Joseph Lister described the results of his investigations on the treatment of wounds with antiseptic dressings, this being believed to be the first occasion on which Lister gave a public

---

[1] Addison : " Roll of Graduates of the University of Glasgow. 1727–1897," p. 18.

demonstration of his researches on this subject. The Society continued to prosper, and has had an important influence on the development of medical opinion and teaching in the Glasgow Medical School.[1]

Provision for botanising and instruction in botany had been made in Glasgow from an early date. In 1704, it had been decided that a portion of the great garden of the College should be converted into a Physic Garden, and John Marshall, a surgeon in the city, was appointed as keeper of the garden, and to give instruction in botany to students at an annual salary of £20. In 1708, Queen Anne allocated a sum of £30 a year to the Professor of Botany. This Botanic Garden existed in the grounds of the University for a century.[2] The gardener who looked after the plants in the Physic Garden held the rest of the College garden rent free on condition of keeping both in order. Professor William Hamilton, from 1784, took great interest in the Botanic Garden, stocking it with new plants, erecting a conservatory at his own expense, and teaching in the garden. Professor Jeffray also taught here, and, in all probability, William Cullen.[3]

After 1800, Dr. Thomas Brown and Dr. Robert Graham successively taught the class of botany, and the latter in 1818, when the Chair was instituted, was made Professor of this subject. In 1820, Professor Robert Graham was elected by the Town Council of Edinburgh Professor of Botany in this University, and he superintended the transfer of the Edinburgh Botanic Gardens from Leith Walk to their present site in Inverleith Row. The next Professor of Botany at Glasgow was William Jackson Hooker, who afterwards became Director of the Botanic Gardens at Kew in 1841, when he was succeeded at Glasgow by John Hutton Balfour, who four years later succeeded Graham as Professor of Botany in Edinburgh. Professor Balfour was succeeded in Glasgow by George Arnott, who held the Chair till 1868.[4]

In 1789, Professor Thomas Charles Hope, son of John Hope, the Professor of Medicine and Botany at Edinburgh, and a nephew of Professor Stevenson, became assistant to the latter in the professorship of medicine and succeeded him in 1791.[5] While Hope was in Glasgow, he published his important research dealing with the maximum density of water, but in 1795 he was transferred to Edinburgh to succeed Joseph Black in the Chair of Chemistry. He is thus regarded as an Edinburgh professor (see page 207). In the Glasgow Chair of Medicine he was succeeded, at the beginning of 1796, by Dr. Robert Freer, an Edinburgh physician. In 1791, Robert Cleghorn, who had been lecturer on Materia Medica since 1788, was appointed lecturer in Chemistry, a post which he held till the institution of a professorship in Chemistry in 1818. Cleghorn was an Edinburgh graduate, who had started practice in Glasgow, and he was one of the first two physicians to the Royal Infirmary of Glasgow.

[1] Downie: "The Medico-Chirurgical Society of Glasgow," 1908.
[2] p. 483, [3] p. 502, [4] pp. 531–533, Coutts: "History of the University of Glasgow," Glasgow, 1909.
[5] Coutts: Op. cit., p. 496.

In 1790, James Towers, surgeon, who had studied obstetrics at the Royal Infirmary of Edinburgh, and also in London, asked to be allowed to lecture upon midwifery in the University of Glasgow.[1] He was appointed year by year till 1815, when he was made Professor of Midwifery, enjoying a salary of £45 per annum. He was succeeded in 1820 by his son, John Towers, who died in 1833. Robert Lee, an obstetric physician and lecturer in London, was appointed Professor of Midwifery in 1834, but resigned office almost immediately, and William Cummin, a son of the Professor of Oriental Languages, who had been a surgeon in the Army, and afterwards Professor of Botany in Anderson's College, was appointed Professor of Midwifery. Although he expended about £200 in the purchase of preparations, drawings, casts and models from Paris, London and elsewhere, he held the Chair only for six years, and was succeeded in 1840 by John MacMichan Pagan, an Edinburgh graduate, who held the Chair till 1868.[2]

The year 1815 was an important one for the School of Medicine at Glasgow. In addition to the Chair of Midwifery, a Chair in Surgery was also established in that year, and, three years later, in 1818, Chairs of Botany and Chemistry were founded by the Crown, and a salary of £50 per annum was granted from the Treasury to each of the four new professors.[3]

The first professor of surgery was John Burns, son of a Glasgow minister, who had been educated at the Universities of Glasgow and Edinburgh, and who had already taught anatomy, surgery and midwifery for some time in connection with Anderson's College. He had also, as surgeon to the Royal Infirmary, taken to giving clinical lectures there in the session 1797–1798. He was the author of two books, " The Principles of Midwifery " and " The Principles of Surgery," which attained great success. As a teacher he was highly popular and successful, his class at times exceeding 200 students. Professor Burns occupied himself much with Parliamentary and other business connected with the University, and in 1850, when returning to Glasgow, he was a passenger on the steamer " Orion," which was wrecked near Portpatrick, and he was drowned.[4] He was succeeded as professor of surgery, in 1850, by James Adair Lawrie, who had graduated at Glasgow in 1822, served in the East India Company, and subsequently lectured in Anderson's College. He died in November, 1859.[5]

On 28th January, 1860, Queen Victoria issued a commission to Joseph Lister, Esq., who was at the time a lecturer on surgery in Edinburgh, to be Professor of Surgery at Glasgow. He was admitted to office as Professor of Surgery on 9th March, 1860, after reading, according to the fashion of the time, a Latin dissertation, " De Arte Chirurgica Recte Erudienda."[6]

In 1818, a Chair of Chemistry was founded, and Dr. Thomas Thomson received the appointment of professor from the Crown. In the time of Joseph Black,

---

[1] p. 500, [2] pp. 526–528, [3] p. 526, [4] pp. 528–530, [5] pp. 530 and 531, [6] p. 582, Coutts : Op. cit.

the Chair had been one of medicine and chemistry, and in the interval the subject of pure chemistry had been taught by lecturers. Thomson had acted as editor of the third edition of the "Encyclopædia Britannica." He had published a "System of Chemistry," in 1802, which went through several editions, and was the author of numerous works dealing with history of chemistry, history of the Royal Society, and outlines of mineralogy and geology. He had graduated in 1799 as M.D. at Edinburgh, and he had been a student under Joseph Black. He is perhaps best known as the inventor of the oxy-hydrogen blow-pipe, and as the introducer of symbols in chemistry. The number of students and of persons doing research whom he attracted made it necessary to obtain a new chemistry department, and this was erected in Shuttle Street, a short distance from the University, and opened in 1831.

This laboratory is generally stated to be the first laboratory in the world devoted to research in chemistry, although Cullen and Black had previously had laboratories where they carried out their individual researches. In 1848, his failing health made it necessary that he should obtain permission from the Senatus that his nephew, Dr. Robert D. Thomson, should conduct the class for him, and this arrangement was continued till 1852, when Professor Thomson died, and was succeeded by Thomas Anderson, an Edinburgh graduate. Anderson took over the department in October, 1852, and held the Chair for twenty-two years, till his death in November, 1874.[1]

As regards anatomy, James Jeffray had been appointed professor of anatomy and botany in 1790, and he held the Chair of anatomy for fifty-eight years, which is the record for tenure of a Medical Chair in a Scottish University. Beginning as a student under Cullen at Edinburgh, where he graduated M.D. in 1786, he lived to see anæsthetics established in surgery. He began, immediately on his appointment, to improve the conditions under which anatomy was taught, by obtaining increased accommodation for the dissecting room and by establishing a library for his students. He was not unmindful that botany formed a part of the subjects to which his Chair was devoted, and he lectured for several years on this subject in the garden established by William Hamilton. From 1800, however, the subject of botany was treated by lecturers till a professor of botany was appointed in 1818.

The students in Glasgow appear to have participated only to a very slight extent in the Resurrectionist activities which were a notable feature of other schools, although in 1803 a party of soldiers had to be requisitioned for the protection of the College, in fear of an attack by the mob. The Medical School of Glasgow was, however, very well supplied with anatomical material, due, no doubt, to the easy means of communication with Ireland. A memorial, drawn up by Professors Jeffray and Burns in April, 1830, was largely instrumental in

[1] Coutts : Op. cit., pp. 533–535.

effecting the passing of the Anatomy Act of 1832.[1] Professor Jeffray was assisted by his son during the last ten years of his life, and during this time took little part in the teaching of the class.

He was succeeded in 1848 as Professor of Anatomy by Allen Thomson, the son of John Thomson, who held various Chairs in the University of Edinburgh. Allen was brother of William Thomson, who was Professor of Medicine at Glasgow from 1841 to 1852. Allen Thomson had studied at Edinburgh, graduated M.D. in 1830, and acted as an extra-mural lecturer upon physiology. From 1839 to 1841 he had been Professor of Anatomy at Marischal College, Aberdeen, and, from 1842 to 1848, Professor of Physiology at Edinburgh University. He held the Glasgow Chair of Anatomy till 1877, when he was succeeded by John Cleland. By the time he came to Glasgow, Thomson had made a large collection of material for anatomical and physiological teaching, and this was added to the Hunterian Museum. The number of students increased greatly under his regime,

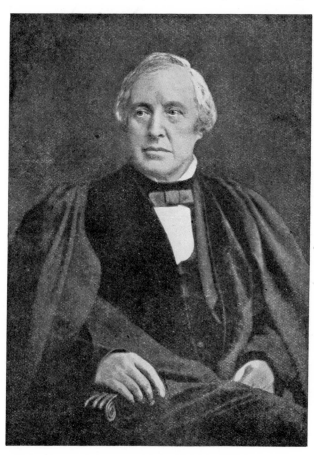

ALLEN THOMSON (1809-1884)

but, in addition to the arduous work of teaching, he was able to devote much time to University management and to anatomical research. He was a skilful draughtsman, and many sketches by his hand still appear as illustrations in text-books of anatomy. He was one of the editors of the seventh and eighth editions of Quain's "Anatomy," and carried out important researches in embryology.[2]

---

[1] pp. 518 and 519, Coutts: Op. cit. ; [2] pp. 519-521, Coutts: Op. cit.

Dr. Robert Freer had succeeded Hope in the Chair of Medicine in 1796, and continued to act as Professor of Medicine till he was eighty years of age, though this long continuance in office cannot have been a good thing for the Glasgow Medical School.　On his death in 1827, Charles Badham, F.R.C.P., was appointed by the King to be Professor of Medicine, and the Crown, on his appointment, reserved power to appoint a fellow professor to teach the theory or practice of medicine, both of these subjects up to this time having been taught from the same Chair.[1] Badham's tenure of the Chair does not appear to have been a success for he had numerous disputes with the Faculty, appears to have neglected his duties, and in 1841, after having been absent in the south of Europe for over two years, he resigned his Chair to the Home Secretary, ignoring the Senatus of the University altogether.

The Crown now appointed William Thomson to be Professor of Medicine. He was brother of Allen Thomson, professor of anatomy, and had studied medicine both in Edinburgh and Glasgow, as well as taking

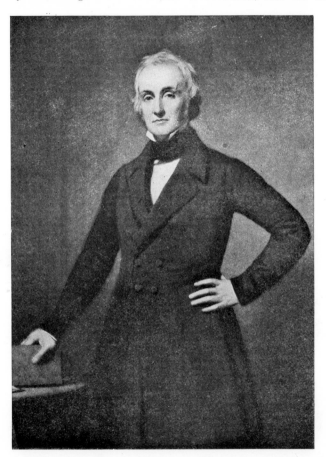

HARRY RAINY (1792–1876)

the M.D. degree at Marischal College, Aberdeen.　At Edinburgh he had been a lecturer both on theory and practice of medicine, and had also acted for his father in the Chair of Pathology.　On his appointment to the University of Glasgow, he became one of the physicians to the Royal Infirmary, and did a great deal of administrative work for the University, especially in connection with the proposed

---

[1] p. 522, Coutts : Op. cit.

removal from the buildings in the High Street to the west side of the city. He died in 1852, and was succeeded by John Macfarlane, who had graduated M.D. at Glasgow, and had been a surgeon to the Royal Infirmary.

This professor held the Chair for only ten years, retiring in 1862, and being succeeded by Dr. (later Sir) William Tennant Gairdner.[1] Gairdner had graduated M.D. at Edinburgh in 1845 with a thesis " On Death," and was a physician of philosophic mind who contributed a great deal to the high reputation of the Glasgow Medical School in the latter part of the 19th century. He was affectionately known to many generations of students as " Old G."

During Professor Badham's tenure of the Chair of Medicine, he announced, in 1832, that he was unable to give his course of lectures on the theory of medicine in addition to his course on practice of medicine, and Dr. Harry Rainy was appointed to give a course of lectures on the theory of medicine, and, in 1833, was re-appointed to give a full course. In 1839, on account of Badham's absence, Rainy was appointed for two years to lecture on practice of medicine.[2]

In this year, 1839, the Queen founded Chairs in Theory of Physic or Institutes of Medicine (Physiology) and Forensic Medicine. Dr. Andrew Buchanan, who had graduated M.D. at Glasgow in 1822, and had lectured on materia medica in Anderson's College, was appointed professor in the new Chair of Theory of Physic. Buchanan, who was one of the first to investigate the subject of coagulation of the blood, held the Chair till 1876.[3]

The other Chair founded by the Queen in 1839, was that of Forensic Medicine, to which Robert Cowan, who had graduated M.D. at Glasgow in 1834, and had been both physician and surgeon to the Royal Infirmary, was appointed. Cowan died after two years' tenure of the Chair, and in December, 1841, Dr. Harry Rainy was appointed Professor of Forensic Medicine by the Crown. He had graduated M.D. at Glasgow in 1833, having already been in practice in medicine with a licence from the Faculty of Physicians and Surgeons, and, as mentioned above, he had acted for Badham during the absence of the latter. He continued in office until 1872.[4]

A Chair of Materia Medica was established by the Crown in 1831, and its first incumbent was Dr. Richard Millar, who had taught this subject as a lecturer since 1791. He had virtually been professor since 1819, when he had been made lecturer for life with a salary of £70 in addition to the class fees paid by the students, a scale of remuneration very much the same as that of the other professors. On his resignation in 1833, he was succeeded in the Chair by Dr. John Couper, who held the Chair until 1855, when he in turn was succeeded by John Alexander Easton, who had graduated M.D. at Glasgow in 1836, and had already taught materia medica in Anderson's College for some fifteen years. His name has attained a permanent record in that of a preparation introduced by him

---

[1] pp. 524 and 525, [2] p. 523, [3] p. 540, [4] pp. 537–540, Coutts : Op. cit.

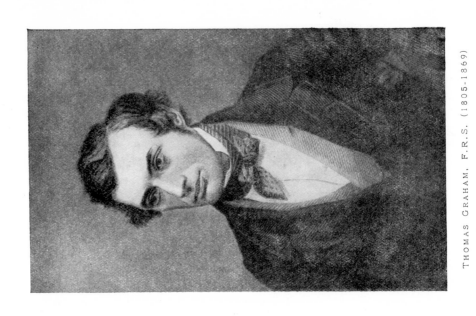

THOMAS GRAHAM, F.R.S. (1805–1869)

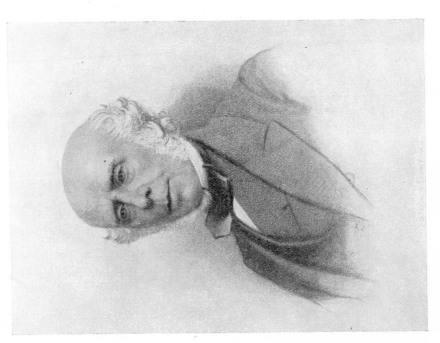

WILLIAM MACKENZIE (1791–1868)

and still known as " Easton's Syrup."   He held the Chair till his death in 1865.[1]

Although many of the lecturers in the Portland Street School and Anderson's College figured at a later date as professors in the Medical School of the University, several left Glasgow to attain distinction in other places, and a large number devoted most of their energies to practise of various specialities in the city.

In 1828, Thomas Graham (1805–1869), who had been a pupil of Thomas Thomson, professor of chemistry, and had spent some time in Edinburgh studying under Thomas Charles Hope, began to lecture on chemistry in the Portland Street School.   Two years later he transferred to the Andersonian College, and in 1837 he was appointed professor of chemistry in University College, London, a post which he held till 1855, when he became Master of the Mint.   He was one of the most distinguished chemists of the 19th century, and to his Glasgow period belongs his elaborate series of experiments upon the diffusion of gases, which he published about 1834.   His researches on osmosis and the diffusion of crystalline and colloid substances through membranes also belong to the same time.   While professor of chemistry at University College, Graham was the teacher and friend of Joseph Lister, and it was on the recommendation of this teacher, as well as of Professor Sharpey, that Lister decided to go to Scotland in order to study surgery under Syme.

When Thomas Graham left the Andersonian College, he was succeeded by William Gregory, who became professor of chemistry in Edinburgh in 1839, when he in turn was succeeded by Dr. Frederick Penny.

William Mackenzie (1791–1868) was in his day perhaps the most distinguished ophthalmic surgeon in the United Kingdom, and attracted patients from all over the world.   He studied for a time in London, but, returning to Glasgow, he became professor of surgery and of anatomy at the Andersonian College in 1819. In 1824, he and Dr. Monteath founded the Glasgow Eye Infirmary, the first hospital for this speciality in Scotland.   His practical treatise on " Diseases of the Eye " was translated into German, French and Italian, and he made many contributions to the clinical side of ophthalmology, being the first to give a clear and definite clinical picture of glaucoma, and of sympathetic ophthalmitis.[2]

Robert Watt (1774–1819) was the son of a small farmer in Ayrshire, and began life as a ploughman and road-maker.   At a later date he joined his brother as a cabinet-maker, and in his spare time studied Latin and Greek, entering Glasgow University in 1793.   In 1795–1796 he also attended philosophy classes at Edinburgh and taught in a private school.   After a winter's study of anatomy at Edinburgh in 1796, he finished his medical studies at Glasgow in 1799.   Obtaining the licence of the Faculty, he began practice in Paisley in the same year.   He found time to make numerous contributions to the "London Medical and Physical Journal" from 1800 onwards, especially one giving a

---

[1] pp. 535-537, Coutts : Op. cit.
[2] Fergus : " The Origin and Development of the Glasgow School of Medicine," 1911, p. 26.

description of diabetes.   As he had a strong inclination to teaching, he took the M.D. degree of Aberdeen in 1810, and immediately afterwards removed to Glasgow, where he began to lecture on medicine in 1811. For the use of his students he formed a medical library, of which, in 1812, he printed a catalogue with subject-index.   The utility of this impressed him so forcibly that he set about enlarging his catalogue so as to embrace all the medical works published in the United Kingdom, and to these he finally added those on law, divinity, and the whole round of science and literature.   In this way the " Bibliotheca Britannica " of this talented man evolved.

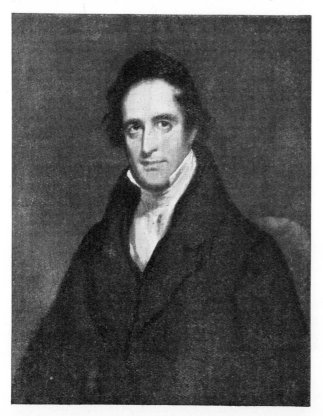

ROBERT PERRY (1783-1848)

Robert Perry (1783–1848) was for some years surgeon, and later (1834–1848) physician to the Glasgow Royal Infirmary. He is often stated to have been the person who originally distinguished between typhus and typhoid fever. These two diseases, along with relapsing fever, were hopelessly confused with one another and, indeed, in the early part of the 19th century, more than one of them probably often affected a patient simultaneously.   In January, 1836, Dr. Robert Perry published a paper in which he correctly described many of the distinctions between typhus and enteric fever.[1]   The complete separation of these three diseases was a matter of gradual development, and his observations were extended by Dr. A. P. Stewart, of Glasgow, and Dr. Gerhard, of Philadelphia, in the following year.   Dr. John Reid, of Edinburgh and St. Andrews, nearly twenty years before had already drawn attention to some of these differences.

---

[1] Murchison : " Continued Fevers," 2nd Edition, 1873, p. 430.

TABLE showing the Teachers in the Medical Schools of Glasgow to the passing of the Medical Act, 1858, and the subjects they respectively taught. (From Duncan: "Memorials of the Faculty of Physicians and Surgeons of Glasgow," Glasgow, 1896, pp. 185 and 186)

Subject	University	Andersonian	Portland Street School
Medicine	1637–46 Robert Maine 1714 John Johnstoun 1751 William Cullen 1756 Robert Hamilton 1757 Joseph Black 1766 Alex. Stevenson 1789 Thos. Chas. Hope 1796 Robert Freer … 1827 Charles Badham … 1841 William Thomson … 1852–62 John Macfarlane …	… … … 1828 Alex. Hannay … 1846–63 Andrew Anderson	1826 Alex. Hannay 1830–42 William Weir
Anatomy	1720 Thomas Brisbane 1742 Robert Hamilton 1756 Joseph Black 1757 Thomas Hamilton 1781 William Hamilton 1790 James Jeffray … 1848–77 Allen Thomson …	1799 John Burns 1818 G. S. Pattison 1819 Wm. MacKenzie … 1828 Robert Hunter … 1841–60 M. S. Buchanan	1826 Robert Hunter 1830 John Stirling 1836 M. S. Buchanan 1841 James Douglas 1844 Robert Knox
Surgery	1815 John Burns 1850 James A. Lawrie … 1860–69 Joseph Lister …	1799 John Burns 1818 G. S. Pattison 1819 Wm. MacKenzie 1829 James A. Lawrie 1850–60 Robert Hunter …	1826 Robert Hunter 1830 Wm. Auchencloss 1840–44 William Lyon
Midwifery	1815 James Towers 1820 John Towers 1833 (Robert Lee) … 1834 William Cummin … 1840–68 John M. Pagan …	1828 James Armour 1831 James Brown 1841–63 James Paterson …	1826 James Armour 1830 James Wilson 1838 Charles Ritchie 1840 Maxwell Adams

SUBJECT	UNIVERSITY	ANDERSONIAN	PORTLAND STREET SCHOOL
Chemistry	*Lecturers:* 1747 William Cullen 1756 Joseph Black 1766 John Robison 1769 William Irvine 1787 Thos. Chas. Hope 1791 Robert Cleghorn *Professor:* 1818 Thomas Thomson ... 1852-74 Thomas Anderson ...	1830 Thomas Graham ... 1837 Wm. Gregory ... 1839-70 Frederick Penny ...	1828 Thomas Graham 1833 James M'Conechy 1836-44 Rob. McGregor
Botany	1818 Robert Graham ... 1821 Sir W. J. Hooker ... 1841 John H. Balfour 1845-68 G. Walker-Arnott	1819 William Cummin ... 1847-63 Joseph Bell ...	1840-42 David Gibson
Materia Medica	*Lecturers:* 1766 William Irvine 1787 Thos. Chas. Hope 1788 Robert Cleghorn 1791 Richard Millar ... *Professors:* 1831 Richard Millar ... 1833 John Couper ... 1855-65 John A. Easton ...	1828 Andrew Buchanan ... 1838 William Hooker ... 1840 John A. Easton 1855-88 James Morton	1827 Wm. MacKenzie 1830 Wm. Davidson 1841-42 J. D. Muter
Physiology	1839-76 Andrew Buchanan ...	1840 Andrew Anderson ... 1846 Maxwell Adams ... 1850-76 Eben. Watson ...	1830 William Weir 1833 William Craig 1836 William Weir 1839-42 Wm. Macdonald
Medical Jurisprudence	1839 Robert Cowan ... 1841-72 Harry Rainy ...	1831 George Watt ... 1842 John Crawford ... 1856-63 J. B. Cowan ...	1826 James Armour 1830 J. M. Pagan 1841-42 H. Cleland 1842-43 John Jackson
Natural History	1807 Lockhart Muirhead 1829 William Couper 1857-66 Henry D. Rogers		

CHAPTER XV

MEDICINE AT EDINBURGH SHORTLY AFTER 1800

DURING the last decade of the 18th century most of the professors in the Medical Faculty were changed. At Cullen's death, in 1790, his place in the Chair of Medicine had been taken by James Gregory, son of John Gregory, an earlier occupant of the Chair. His fame as a teacher lives still, inferior in importance only to that of Cullen. When he walked he carried a stout cane held over his shoulder or at the trail, as if ready for action, and he had the curious habit of wearing

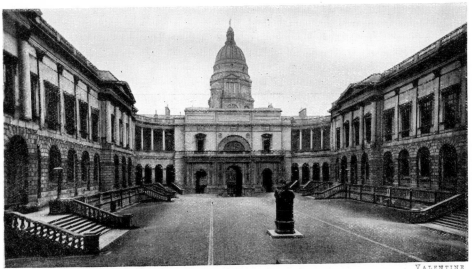

VALENTINE

OLD QUADRANGLE, EDINBURGH UNIVERSITY
(Begun 1789, completed 1828)
Compare this (taken towards the end of the 19th Century) with the views on *page* 30 and *page* 182

his hat throughout his lectures, after an apology to the students for doing so.[1] His most abiding monument in the temple of fame is a powder containing rhubarb, magnesia and ginger, which has been perhaps more universally employed than any other pharmacopœial preparation. He was brilliant and witty as a teacher, and one of the the great polemic writers of his day, so that Lord Cockburn,[2] who admirably sums up the characters of many contemporary worthies in Edinburgh, says of Gregory: " He was a curious and excellent man, a great physician, a

---

[1] " Life of Sir Robert Christison," Edinburgh, 1885, Vol. I, p. 79.
[2] Henry Cockburn : " Memorials of his Time," Chap. II, p. 97.

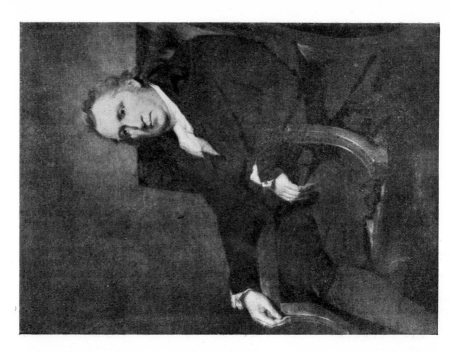

JAMES GREGORY (1753–1821)

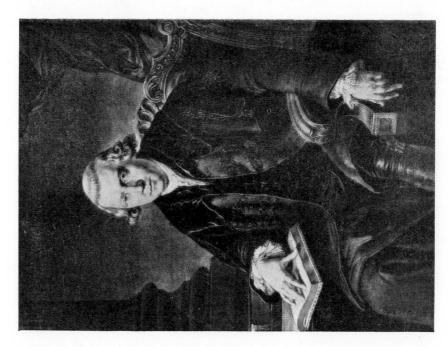

JOHN GREGORY (1725–1773)

great lecturer, a great Latin scholar, and a great talker ; vigorous and generous ; large of stature, and with a strikingly powerful countenance. The popularity due to these qualities was increased by his professional controversies, and the diverting publications by which he used to maintain and enliven them. The controversies were rather too numerous ; but they never were for any selfish end, and he was never entirely wrong. Still, a disposition towards personal attack was his besetting sin."

This disposition got him into trouble with his colleague, Professor James Hamilton. Hamilton was a successful teacher and writer, but he is even better known as one of the most contentious of a singularly pugnacious professoriate. There had appeared anonymously in 1792, " A Guide for Gentlemen Studying Medicine at the University of Edinburgh," which reflected injuriously on a number of the professors. Professor Gregory having charged him with writing it, Hamilton produced a spirited and abusive reply, which provoked Gregory to beat him with his walking-stick. For this, Hamilton brought an action against Professor Gregory, and received £100 by way of damages. Gregory is said, on paying the damages, to have remarked that he would willingly pay double for another opportunity.

Hamilton, however, was a notorious litigant, for he also had lawsuits with Professors Andrew Duncan and Hope, while one with Sir Robert Christison was narrowly averted. In the case of Professor Hope, the cause of the trouble had been that Hope, after a long course of bickering, had used regarding Hamilton the words of Dr. Samuel Johnson on a like occasion : " The fellow lies, and he knows that he lies." Hamilton brought an action against Hope for defamation of character, and, after a prolonged hearing, the jury found a verdict in favour of Hamilton with one farthing damages. The public at large were greatly delighted with the legal proceedings and verdict, and Hope received from his friends a shower of letters enclosing farthings, one of which he sent to Hamilton, demanding a receipt.

Gregory's measures for the cure of disease were sharp and incisive, and there was no question of expectant treatment with him. Disease, according to Gregorian physic, was to be attacked vigorously by free blood-letting, the cold affusion, brisk purging, frequent blisters and vomits of tartar emetic. Since Edinburgh during his régime was frequented by students from all quarters of the British Islands and the Colonies, these measures came to rule medical practice for many years all over the world. His " Conspectus Medicinæ Theoreticæ " was regarded as a model of exactness and completeness in its time, and it remained for long a standard text-book. The rest of his writings are all connected with various disputes about Infirmary management and similar subjects.

Andrew Duncan became Professor of the Institutes of Medicine in 1789. One of his first acts on being made professor was to agitate for the erection of a

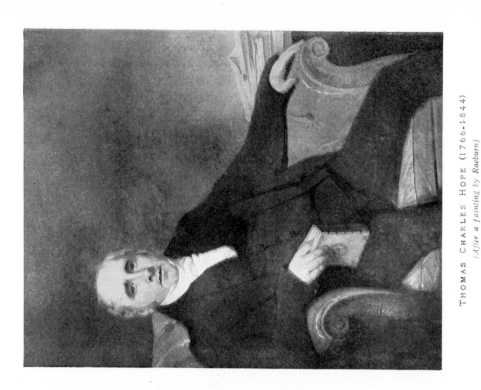

THOMAS CHARLES HOPE (1766-1844)

(After a painting by Raeburn)

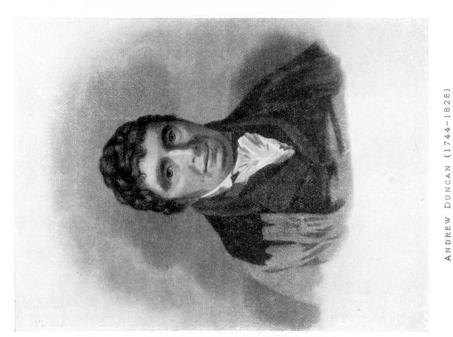

ANDREW DUNCAN (1744-1828)

public lunatic asylum in Edinburgh, which was finally opened in 1813.   He was celebrated for his pleasantness of manner and kindliness of disposition, and he had a hobby for founding convivial societies, of which the Harveian and Æsculapian Societies still exist as dining-clubs.   His activities in obtaining Royal Charters for no fewer than four Societies, and his founding of the Medico-Chirurgical Society of Edinburgh, in 1821, were of more importance in this direction. The four Royal Institutions which owe their Charters largely to him are the Royal Medical Society, the Royal Public Dispensary, the Royal Caledonian Horticultural Society, and the Royal Edinburgh Asylum for the Insane.   He was a great friend of promising young men, among whom his early patronage of the painter, Sir Henry Raeburn, was the most successful.   A singular fatality appears to have overtaken many of his protégés, and an interesting and pathetic spot in Edinburgh is the grave of Andrew Duncan in Buccleuch Burying-ground, where his tombstone is seen within a high-walled enclosure, surrounded by small stones which he erected to the memory of various students who had died under his care, and to whose remains he had accorded this posthumous hospitality.

Thomas Charles Hope had been appointed colleague and successor to Joseph Black in the Chair of Chemistry in 1795, having come like Black from a professorship in the University of Glasgow.   Chemistry, at the beginning of the 19th century, had developed into a very important subject, and his class numbered over 500 students.   Sir Robert Christison records that his lectures were characterised by " uncommon clearness of exposition, and unexampled splendour and success in experimental demonstration," for not a single failure to attain exactly what he announced occurred during all the experiments of a session.[1]   His work in pure chemistry included " An Account of a Mineral from Strontian, and of a Peculiar Species of Earth which it contains," in which he announced the discovery of a new " earth "—strontia.   He is better known by his experiments made about 1800 in connection with the fact that water expands as it freezes, and his determination of its point of maximum density.   His lawsuit with Professor Hamilton has been mentioned.

The Chair of Midwifery was filled from 1800 onwards by Dr. James Hamilton, son and successor of Dr. Alexander Hamilton.   He was reputed to be a man of great energy and alertness, and a powerful lecturer.   His quarrelsomeness has been already noticed.   A three months' course of lectures was given by him thrice annually, and he maintained the lying-in hospital as a school for practical instruction.   A course in this subject was, however, still optional for students, although Hamilton's lectures were almost universally attended.   He was wont to visit his patients in a Sedan chair, a mode of conveyance which he used up to 1830, being the last person in Edinburgh to employ such a vehicle.

---

[1] " Life of Sir Robert Christison," Edinburgh, 1885, Vol. I, p. 57.

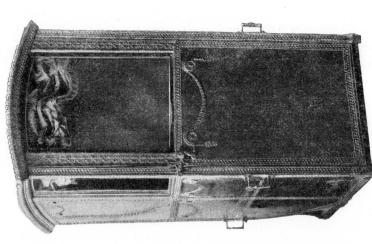

JAMES HAMILTON (The Younger)
Died 1839
(From a silhouette by Edouart, in the Royal
Scottish National Portrait Gallery)

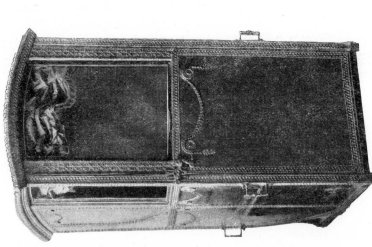

SEDAN-CHAIR OF
PROFESSOR JAMES HAMILTON
The last used in Edinburgh
(Preserved in the Royal Scottish Museum of Antiquities)

The class of midwifery, conducted by James Hamilton (died 1839), son of Professor Alexander Hamilton, after being carried on by him with great success for some years, was made compulsory for the attendance of students after 1833, at the same time that attendance on practical anatomy, clinical surgery, medical jurisprudence and natural history became obligatory classes for all candidates for the degree of Doctor of Medicine. James Hamilton is sometimes known as James Hamilton (*the younger*) to distinguish him from James Hamilton (*senior*) (1749–1835), one of the physicians to the Royal Infirmary. The latter was celebrated for his recourse in treatment to strong purgative medicines, and a pill of aloes and colocynth is still known as " Hamilton's pill." James Hamilton (*senior*) was painted by Raeburn, and he was also known to his intimates as " Cocky " Hamilton, in allusion to the fact that he wore a three-cornered hat long after this article of apparel had ceased to be fashionable.

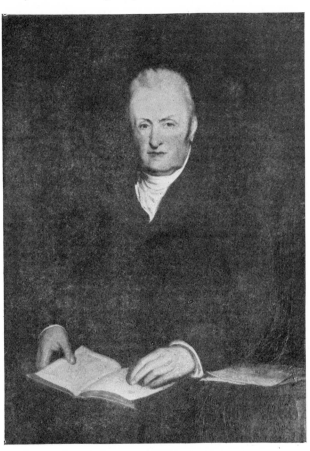

JAMES HOME (1758–1842)

Dr. James Home succeeded his father, Francis Home, in the Chair of Materia Medica in 1798. Christison speaks of him as being so popular as a lecturer that his class-room was crowded every morning in the dark winter session, notwithstanding his early hour of 8 a.m. In 1821, on the death of Professor James Gregory, he was translated to the Chair of Practice of Physic, where, curiously enough, according to the same authority, he failed from the first as a lecturer, his class-room " becoming a scene of negligence, disrespect, noise, and utter confusion, for a few years before his death in 1842." According to Christison, his success in one

Chair and his failure in another was occasioned by the difficulty of following so consummate a professor and so eminent a physician as Dr. Gregory, and also by the error of the Town Council in failing to appoint Dr. Abercrombie, a noted consulting physician of the town, who had given proof by his writings of his high ability.[1]

Towards the end of the year 1798, Monro *secundus* petitioned the Town Council to appoint as his colleague and successor his eldest son, Alexander, then twenty-five years old, afterwards known as Monro *tertius*. The Town Council, after some demur, agreed, and the two Monros held the Chair of Anatomy conjointly for the next ten years, Monro *secundus* retiring in 1808. Monro *tertius* held the Chair till 1846, thus continuing the régime of his family through the long period of 126 years. The experiment of slipping a son in early life into the position of colleague, to become later sole professor, had been very successful as between Monro *primus* and Monro *secundus*, but on the second occasion, as between Monro *secundus* and Monro *tertius*, it proved a lamentable failure.

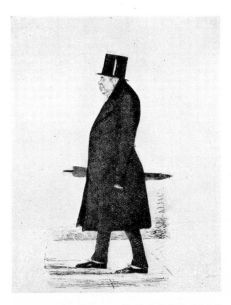

ALEXANDER MONRO *(tertius)* (1773-1859)
(From "Modern Athenians")

Monro *tertius* showed himself an unsuccessful teacher, his students very commonly paying the University fee and getting their instruction from outside teachers, while his voluminous writings are dull and devoid of any initiative or novelty. A recent writer says of him : " He used to read his grandfather's lectures written about a century before ; and even the shower of peas with which the expectant students greeted his annual reference, ' When I was a student in Leyden in 1719,' failed to induce him to alter the dates."[5]   Charles Darwin, who studied medicine at Edinburgh from 1825 to 1827, but afterwards forsook medicine for natural history, in his autobiography gives him the following testimonial, which is amusing as a comment by a student upon his professor : " Dr. ——— made his lectures on human anatomy as dull as he was himself, and the subject disgusted me."[3]   The chief regret about

[1] " Life of Sir Robert Christison," Vol. I, pp. 76–78.
[2] " Edinburgh University : A Sketch of its Life for Three Hundred Years," Edinburgh, 1884.   Quoted in the " Edinburgh School of Surgery before Lister," Miles, London, 1918. p. 84.
[3] " Life and Letters of Charles Darwin," 1887, Vol. I, p. 36.

Monro's appointment is that one or other of two brilliant brothers might have been secured, and if the appointment had been made open, either John or Charles Bell, with the advantages of position and wealth which the Town Council conferred upon Monro *tertius*, would undoubtedly have reflected great lustre upon the Edinburgh Anatomical School.

It has been mentioned that the first two Monros lectured on surgery as a small part of their course on anatomy, and, in 1772, the College of Surgeons had recognised Mr. James Rae as a lecturer on this subject.   In 1776, they had approached the Magistrates to establish a professorship of surgery within the University, but the proposal was so vigorously opposed by Monro *secundus* that it failed, and instead Monro received a new commission in 1777, appointing him professor of medicine, and " particularly of anatomy and surgery."   In 1804, the College of Surgeons decided to take the matter into their own hands, and they accordingly appointed one of their Fellows, John Thomson, to be " professor of surgery of the Royal College of Surgeons."

The University, through the Town Council, opposed the establishment of a professorship outside its own walls, but after all, the word " professor " only means " teacher " and has never been the monopoly of a university, so that Thomson continued to lecture with success as a professor outside the walls, and in spite of the opposition of the University.   Two years later, Thomson was appointed by the Crown professor of military surgery in the University, but he continued, by permission of the College, to perform the extra-mural duties of the professor of surgery.   In 1821, he resigned the College appointment, in which he was succeeded by Mr. John William Turner.   Ten years later, in 1831, the Crown, on the recommendation of the Town Council, decided to establish a Chair of Systematic Surgery within the University, and offered the appointment to Professor J. W. Turner.

The College of Surgeons thus, after a controversy lasting fifty-five years, gained its point.   Mr. John Lizars was now appointed professor of surgery to the College of Surgeons, and held the post for eight years, but on his resigning in 1839, the College decided to discontinue their professorship in view of the fact that the Chair of Surgery within the University had now been established.[1]

It had been decided by the Crown, before 1803, to establish a Chair of Clinical Surgery, which was at first endowed with a stipend of £50 per annum.   The person selected to fill the Chair was James Russell (1755–1836).   His father had been a surgeon-apothecary in Edinburgh, but had relinquished medical practice to become professor of natural philosophy in 1764.   James Russell had been one of the six surgeons selected by the Managers of the Royal Infirmary, in 1800, to take charge of the surgical patients in this institution when the old agreement of 1738, that all the members of the Incorporation of Surgeons should act in turn on

---

[1] Miles : " Edinburgh School of Surgery before Lister," p. 79 *et seq.*

the staff, became unmanageable. All six surgeons were given the power in 1804 to deliver clinical lectures in the Infirmary.

In 1814, Professor Russell retired from the Infirmary, but the Managers granted him a life privilege of delivering clinical lectures on surgery in the hospital.[1] He had thus no hospital beds or cases of his own, but lectured upon the cases of the other surgeons. Under these difficult and somewhat delicate conditions, he appears to have avoided giving offence, and to have conducted well-attended classes. He

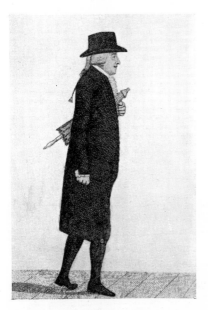

ANDREW DUNCAN (SENIOR)
(1744-1828)
(From Kay's "Portraits")

is described as a tall, thin gentleman of the old school, who wore a red wig, was always dressed in black with a white neckcloth and a broad frill on his shirt breast. He also adopted the style of knee-breeches, silk stockings and shoes.[2] An old pupil says of him : " I must say he was a somnolent lecturer, a quality which was fomented by an evening class-hour, and betrayed by an inveterate habit the professor had of yawning while he spoke, and continuing to speak while he yawned." [3] Russell held the Chair till the age of seventy-eight, and when he resigned in 1833, he made it a condition that his successor should pay him the sum of £300 a year for the period of his lifetime. He was succeeded by James Syme and lived three years after his retirement.

An important adjunct was made to the Edinburgh Medical School with the institution, in 1805, of the *Edinburgh Medical and Surgical Journal*. The full title of this periodical was " The Edinburgh Medical and Surgical Journal: Exhibiting a concise view of the latest and most important discoveries in medicine, surgery and pharmacy." It was issued under the editorship of Andrew Duncan *(junior)*, and continued and embodied four periodicals which had previously appeared in the Edinburgh Medical School. These had been " Edinburgh Medical Essays," first issued in 1731 (six volumes) ; " Essays Physical and Literary," first issued in 1754 (three volumes) ; " Medical and Philosophical Commentaries by a Society in Edinburgh," from 1773 to 1795 (twenty volumes) ; and " Annals of Medicine," which had been issued in 1796 under the editorship of

---

[1] " The Royal Infirmary of Edinburgh : Notes and Excerpts from the Minutes," 1728–1908, p. 7.
[2] Miles : " The Edinburgh School of Surgery before Lister," p. 101.
[3] " Life of Sir Robert Christison," Vol. I, p. 89.

Andrew Duncan *(senior)*, and Andrew Duncan *(junior)*.[1] The last was directly continued by the *Edinburgh Medical and Surgical Journal*, which still survives as the *Edinburgh Medical Journal*.

We must now consider the extra-academical teachers of Anatomy. The teaching of this subject began with the Guild of the Surgeons and Barbers long before the Town's College was founded. The capable brain of Dr. Archibald Pitcairne, about 1680, conceived the idea of founding a medical school in Edinburgh ; he was one of the three Professors of Medicine appointed in 1685 to the Town's College or University as it then began to be called ; and in the combined anatomical demonstrations of the Surgeons' Incorporation after his return from the Leyden professorship, he was, in 1702 and 1704, as we have seen, the guiding spirit.

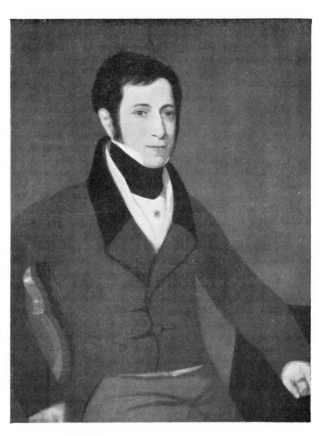

JOHN BELL (1763–1820)

(Original in the Wellcome Historical Medical Museum, London)

During the first sixty years of the Monro régime, the University had a monopoly of anatomical teaching, but it is a significant fact that though the first two Monros lectured on Surgery, neither was an operating surgeon, and the second was a consulting physician with large practice.   Anatomy in their hands, though brilliantly taught, naturally tended to become a formal systematic subject, and in 1786, John Bell, returning to Edinburgh and becoming a Fellow of the College of Surgeons, saw a great chance.   In his " Letters on the Education of a Surgeon," published in 1810, he says : " In Dr. Monro's class, unless there be a fortunate

---

[1] For Index to these publications, see *Edinburgh Medical Journal*," Vol. XX, 1824.

succession of bloody murders, not three subjects are dissected in the year.   On the remains of a subject fished up from the bottom of a tub of spirits, are demonstrated those delicate nerves which are to be avoided or divided in our operations ; and these are demonstrated once at the distance of 100 feet !—nerves and arteries which the surgeon has to dissect, at the peril of his patient's life."[1]

John Bell, therefore, began to lecture, and so successful was he in attracting students that, in 1790, he built an anatomical school adjoining on the east the Hall of the Surgeons in what was later called Surgeons' Square.   He was not only an expert anatomist, but a good classical scholar, a skilful draughtsman and etcher, a ready speaker and a polished writer.   It is no exaggeration to say that he founded the subject of Surgical Anatomy.   The works and atlases of the great anatomists in the 18th century, e.g., Cheselden, Albinus, Haller, Winslow, Scarpa, Soemmering, even the Hunters, all treat the subject from the purely structural point of view.   By these men the various systems and organs are correctly described and often beautifully figured, but the engravings of John Bell, and later of his brother Charles, have a teleological significance, their aim being not so much correctness,   as   utility   to   the   operating surgeon.   This feature is readily seen in John Bell's " Engravings of the Bones, Muscles and Joints," drawn and engraved by himself (1794).

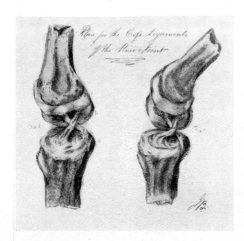

PLATE ENGRAVED BY JOHN BELL
Showing the knee joint

Bell was essentially a surgeon, and his only other anatomical work was the " Anatomy of the Human Body," published Vol. I, 1793 ; Vol. II, 1797 ; Vol. III, 1802.   He taught anatomy for thirteen years and gave it up under peculiar circumstances.   So successful had his anatomical classes proved, that a combination led by Dr. James Gregory, Professor of the Practice of Medicine in the University, was formed against him, and he was pursued in a manner which for audacity, if not for bitterness, would be wellnigh impossible at the present day.   The attack opened with a pamphlet addressed to students warning them against attending Mr. Bell's lectures.   It was followed by a " Review of the Writings of John Bell, Surgeon in Edinburgh, by Jonathan Dawplucker" (Professor Gregory). This malignant attack was, as Bell states, " Stuck up like a Play-Bill in a most conspicuous and unusual manner, on every corner of the city ; on the door of my

---

[1] John Bell : " Letters on the Education of a Surgeon," Edinburgh, 1810, p. 579.

lecture-room, on the gates of the College, where my pupils could not but pass, and on the gates of the Infirmary, where I went to perform my operations."

As an example of the personal abuse to which Gregory descended may be cited : "Any man, if himself or his family were sick, should as soon think of calling in a mad dog, as Mr. John Bell." Bell, at a later period, replied to these attacks

pungently and effectively, in a voluminous collection of "Letters."[1] But Gregory's party having secured his exclusion from the hospital, there was nothing to be gained by Bell from further teaching. He therefore ceased to lecture in 1799, confining himself to surgical practice, in which he was for about twenty years the leading operator and consultant throughout Scotland.

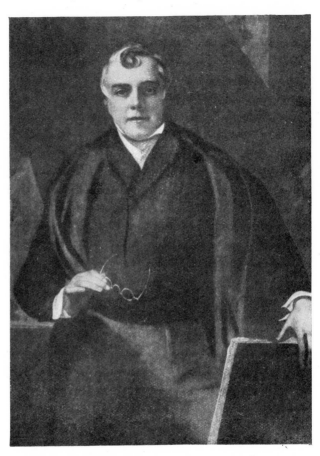

SIR CHARLES BELL (1774–1842)

Charles Bell was younger than his brother John, by eleven years, and was trained by him in anatomy and surgery. In this there is a sort of comparison with the brothers William and John Hunter, half a century earlier. Charles Bell began to assist in the anatomical class while still comparatively a boy, and, like John Bell, he had a genius for anatomical delineation. The same teleological tendency is seen in his drawings, directed in his earlier works, like that of his brother, towards surgery. These earlier works were a "System of Dissections" (published 1792–1803), and "Engravings of the Arteries, of the Nerves, and of the

---

[1] John Bell : "Letters on the Education of a Surgeon," Edinburgh, 1810, pp. ix and 503.

Brain" (published 1801 and 1802), while his "Anatomy of Expression," though not published till 1806 in London, was mainly composed in Edinburgh.   After the withdrawal of John Bell from teaching, Charles took over the anatomy class in 1799, but the opposition to his brother militated against his success and he never attracted more than ninety students.   He determined, therefore, in 1804, to remove to London, where, in 1811, he took over the old Hunterian Anatomical School in Windmill Street, and where he spent thirty-two busy and eventful years. The Edinburgh School made some amends to Bell and to its own reputation by offering him the Chair of Surgery in 1836, when the Gregory faction had passed away.   We are not concerned here with his London period, but one important field of his activities must be mentioned, to which he had been directing attention in the early Edinburgh days, and upon which his fame largely rests.   Since the days of Whytt and Haller, the minute ramifications of the nervous system had been a matter of common knowledge ; but the nerves were regarded as merely exerting some vague influence over the parts to which they were distributed, and effecting a sympathy between different regions of the body.   Whytt, in 1755, was ahead of his time in expressing the opinion that " the power of motion, when stimulated, proceeds from the nerves, or is at least immediately dependent on their influence."[1] Charles Bell was the first to whom it occurred that definite nerves have a definite course from some part of the brain to a certain portion of the periphery, and, further, that different nerves have quite distinct functions.   This led to his " Idea of a New Anatomy of the Brain," printed for distribution in 1811, but often mentioned by him before that time.   This publication included the specific instance of the motor function of the anterior nerve roots, first discovered by him.   It led to the more complete demonstration of motor and sensory nerves by Magendie in 1822, to the localisation of the *nœud vital* by Flourens in 1837, and to the great subsequent developments in mapping out nerve paths and centres in the brain and cord.

Charles Bell, like Harvey, was thus a pioneer in scientific medicine, and it gives no cause for wonder that on one occasion when Bell was visiting Paris, Roux dismissed his class without the lecture for the day with the words : " C'est assez, Messieurs, vous avez vu Charles Bell."[2]

The episode of surgical anatomy in Edinburgh ended for a time when Charles Bell shook off the dust of this city from his feet in 1804, but this branch was revived some twenty years later by a brilliant group of surgeon anatomists, including Lizars, Liston, Syme and Fergusson.

An important place as a teacher of anatomy was filled by John Barclay, who having originally studied for the Church, took the M.D. degree at the somewhat ripe age of thirty-six, and became an assistant to John Bell.   In 1797, he began to teach anatomy on his own account, and, in 1804, when Charles Bell departed

---

[1] " Works of Robert Whytt," 1768, p. 324.
[2] J. Struthers : " The Edinburgh Anatomical School," Edinburgh, 1867, p. 54.

for London, his course of lectures was " recognised " by the College of Surgeons. After the year 1808, the retiral of Monro *secundus* and the ineptitude of the third Monro helped Barclay's class, which gradually rose to 300 students, the University class sinking from 400 under Monro *secundus* to 200 by the year 1821. Barclay had taken a house on the west side of Surgeons' Square (No. 10, next door to the Royal Medical Society's premises), which had been used for lectures by Andrew Duncan, senior, and which he fitted up as an anatomical school.[1] Here he collected a valuable museum of human and comparative anatomy, and lectured twice daily. We have seen that Monro *secundus* took considerable interest in the subject of comparative anatomy, and Barclay now greatly developed it. He also made a considerable reputation by the publication of several valuable works, especially his " New Anatomical Nomenclature " (1803), " The Muscular Motions of the Human Body " (1808), and " Engravings representing the Bones of the Human Skeleton with the Skeletons of some of the Lower Animals " (1819). He had a philosophic conception as well as an extensive knowledge of comparative anatomy, and was one of the first to recognise that all animals have the same general outline of structure, as well as the principle of homology in the two limbs. It was

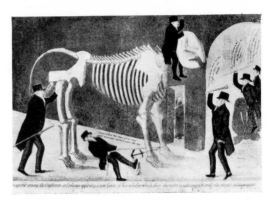

CARICATURE OF "THE CRAFT IN DANGER"
(From Kay's " Portraits ")

John Barclay, mounted on the Elephant, is attempting to enter the University. The other figures, from the left, are Professors James Gregory, T. C. Hope, A. Monro *(tertius)*, Jamieson (Natural History), and Mr. R. Johnston (a member of the Town Council)

proposed indeed to make for him a Chair of Comparative Anatomy in the University, though this was vehemently opposed by Monro and Jamieson, the Professors of Anatomy and Natural History respectively.[2] The proposal, though it never eventuated, gave rise to much discussion, personal, political and scientific, and in Kay's " Edinburgh Portraits " there is a contemporary caricature showing several of the participants, entitled " The Craft in Danger."[3]

Contemporary with Barclay was Dr. John Gordon, who lectured at No. 9, Surgeons' Square, from 1808 to 1818, to a class of about a hundred students. Apart from his activities as a teacher, his best-known work was " Observations on the Structure of the Brain, comprising an Estimate of the Claims of Drs. Gall and Spurzheim to Discovery in the Anatomy of that Organ." This attempt to

[1] C. W. Cathcart : " Some of the Older Schools of Anatomy connected with the Royal College of Surgeons, Edinburgh," *Edinburgh Medical Journal*, March, 1882.
[2] Sir G. Ballingall : " Life of John Barclay," 1827.
[3] John Kay : " A Series of Original Portraits and Caricature Etchings," Edinburgh, 1837, Vol. I, p. 448

show that the claims of these two men to have localised various faculties in different parts of the brain were inadmissible, went far, in this country at least, to discredit the science of Phrenology.

He was succeeded by David Craigie, who wrote the excellent article on " Anatomy " in the seventh and eighth editions of the "Encyclopædia Britannica," and taught Anatomy in No. 3, Surgeons' Square, from 1818 to 1822 ; Dr. Craigie had followed Dr. Smith, of whom little is known, but neither of them had much success as a teacher. Craigie became Inspector of Anatomy for Scotland in 1832 under the new Anatomy Act.

One of Barclay's demonstrators was Robert Liston, who, having disagreed with Barclay, began to teach anatomy on his own account, with James Syme as his demonstrator, to a class of sixty students in the winter session 1818–1819. The class-room was in Surgeons' Square, but at what number I have been unable to discover. Here Liston and Syme carried on the class between them for several years with increasing success, Syme eventually taking over the management. They taught both anatomy and surgery on the lines introduced by the Bells ; and, at a later date, in 1829, William Fergusson, as Knox's demonstrator, began a course on surgical anatomy which proved exceedingly popular with the students.[1]

Another successful lecturer was William Cullen (grand-nephew of the celebrated William Cullen), who lectured in John Bell's old class-room in Surgeons' Square to about a hundred students, moving later (1825) to an anatomical school in " Society," Brown Square, where he succeeded James Syme, who had lectured there for one year on anatomy. Cullen died, after five years as a teacher, in 1828. Mr. Lizars had been teaching anatomy and surgery at No. 1, Surgeons' Square, and on the death of Cullen he moved to the Brown Square School (now the south corner of Chambers Street and George IV. Bridge).

It should be remembered that up to this time the students, as a general rule, did no individual dissection. A few favoured or enthusiastic spirits helped the anatomical teachers to prepare for their demonstrations, but the material available did not permit of universal practical dissection. Instruction was conveyed by lecture-demonstrations, of which one winter's course was compulsory, and of which almost all students took two courses. Preparations ready dissected were also available for reading. To facilitate reading and to supply the dearth of material, there was a great output of plates, tables and coloured illustrations by the various teachers and their assistants. Among these the text-books of John Innes and Andrew Fyfe, who acted successively as prosectors or " dissectors " to Monro *secundus*, were in great demand, and may still be seen occasionally on second-hand bookstalls. There was in them avowedly nothing new, but they frequently displayed considerable merit in draughtsmanship, and the same hands

---

[1] Miles : " Edinburgh School of Surgery before Lister," p. 134.

illustrated the scientific works of Monro *secundus* and other teachers.   Fyfe's
"System of Anatomy" (published in 1800) is especially worthy of note.   It
contained 160 plates and about 700 figures, mostly produced from the works of
Continental anatomists and some from his own dissections, the drawing and
engraving being the work of his own hand and displaying a great degree of skill.
John Aitken, who entered the College of Surgeons as a Fellow in 1770, and
apparently conducted coach-classes on most of the subjects in the medical curriculum
—anatomy, surgery, midwifery, chemistry and practice of physic, had published,
in 1786, an elaborate "System of Anatomical Tables with Explanations."[1]
The works of the Monros, of John and Charles Bell, and of Gordon, have been
already mentioned.   Charles Bell also introduced another form of teaching
apparatus, of which many examples may still be seen in the Museum of the Royal
College of Surgeons.   Clemente Susini and his pupils at Florence had introduced
the making of exquisite wax models of dissections.   Charles Bell copied the
process by making plaster casts, which he covered with a thin layer of variously
coloured wax, moulded as it dripped from candles of the colours required.

Andrew Bell, a professional engraver, produced a number of collections of
plates from 1777 to 1798, under various titles, such as "Bell's Edition of the Plates
of Albinus," "Anatomical Engravings," and "Anatomia Britannica," and he
was extensively employed by the anatomical teachers.   Edward Mitchell, another
engraver, did the plates for Barclay's "Engravings of the Bones, etc." (1819
and 1824) ; he copied largely from Sue and Albinus.   Later editions of this work,
and continuations dealing with the nerves (1829), arteries (1831), muscles (1832),
and ligaments (1834), were published under the superintendence of Robert Knox
(the arteries under that of Wharton Jones), and were generally known as
"Knox's Plates."

Another highly popular "System of Anatomical Plates," in five folio
volumes, was issued by John Lizars from 1823 to 1826.   All these plates by the
various teachers were copied from or based upon the works of Albinus, Haller,
Camper, Scarpa, Soemmering, Walther, Cloquet, Tiedemann, etc., and the great
output in Edinburgh at this time is explained in the preface to Knox's work that
they were to be used as a guide in dissecting, which was now becoming more
prevalent among students, though not compulsory till 1826.   Knox says : "the
experiment was eminently successful ; and it was easy to observe that, by the
use of such delineations and descriptions in the practical rooms, the general
character of the dissections shortly became altogether different."[2]

The College of Surgeons from very early times had been interested in rarities
of natural history, and even in Monteath's time (1694) there had been a semblance
of a museum containing among other things " ane egyle," " three scorpions and

[1] J. Struthers : "The Edinburgh Anatomical School," Edinburgh, 1867, p. 38.
[2] "Engravings of the Arteries, with Explanatory Reference by Dr. Knox," 1831, preface.

a chameleon," " an allegatory or young crocodile," and, later, " a strange creature called ourang-outang." [1]   In 1702, Pitcairne presented to the College a body showing an elaborate dissection of the muscles, still preserved though sadly gnawed by the tooth of time ; and in 1718, Monro *primus* presented a skeleton (still preserved) and other specimens.   Specimens of normal and pathological anatomy gradually accumulated, and at the end of the eighteenth century Barclay commenced his valuable collection of pathological and comparative anatomy, which on his death became the property of the College.

With this nucleus, the College, some time about 1820, conceived an ambitious scheme of purchasing a high-class anatomical museum.   An attempt was first made to secure that of Professor Meckel, of Halle, and on this proving ineffectual Dr. Cullen was sent to Paris in 1823 to secure a steady supply of specimens.   He met with partial success only, and the College finally, in July, 1825, purchased for £3000 the museum of Charles Bell, who was about to retire from teaching anatomy in the Windmill Street School, London.   The arrangements for the transfer were superintended by Dr. Robert Knox, Conservator of the College Museum, and one perceives, from a perusal of the Minute Book of the Curators of the College, that Knox displayed an enormous amount of enthusiasm and labour in the foundation of this anatomical museum, which has become in importance second only to the Hunterian Museum in London.

When Barclay retired in 1824, Knox took over his class and lecture room at No. 10, Surgeons' Square, and quickly became the most popular anatomical teacher in Edinburgh.   When he had been lecturing four years his class numbered over 500—probably the largest anatomical class that has ever assembled in Britain.   Although most of its members were medical students, Knox also attracted to his lectures barristers, scholars, clergymen, noblemen, artists and men of letters.   Probably this very popularity, by associating his name especially with anatomy, was the means of turning against him more than against any of the other teachers the odium of the public, following on the Burke and Hare exposures.

As is generally known, Burke and Hare were two debased Irishmen, resident in Edinburgh, who conceived a scheme of supplying bodies for the dissecting rooms at less trouble and danger to themselves than could be effected by the methods of body-snatching commonly followed by the " Resurrectionists " of the time.   Their method was to entice friendless people into their house in the West Port, stupefy them with drink, and thereafter suffocate them and sell the bodies to the porters of the various anatomy rooms.   At least sixteen people were thus done to death before Burke and Hare were apprehended and tried in December, 1828.   The last of these bodies was found in Knox's rooms, and popular animus was therefore naturally directed first at him.   Yet Lord Cockburn,

---

[1] Miles : " The Edinburgh School of Surgery before Lister," p. 15.

commenting upon the affair, wrote : " All our anatomists incurred a most unjust, and a very alarming, though not an unnatural odium ; Dr. Knox in particular against whom not only the anger of the populace, but the condemnation of more intelligent persons, was specially directed.   But tried in reference to the invariable, and the necessary practice of the profession, our anatomists were spotlessly correct, and Knox the most correct of them all."[1]

Although the students remained by Knox for years, and showed him many examples of their affection and regard, his ability both as a teacher and investigator declined, and in 1844 he left Edinburgh to lecture for a short time in Glasgow and afterwards practice in London.   Teaching·had been Knox's *forte*, and his lectures were studied and rehearsed with the utmost care, even down to his dress and jewellery. He had an extraordinary power of lucid exposition, as one may still perceive from his writings, and he appears to have infused an interest into the dull facts of anatomy, partly by his caustic wit and partly by a constant reference to the structure and functions of the parts he happened to be describing, as they existed in the lower animals. He published numerous short papers on circumscribed anatomical subjects, and longer works, such as " The Races of Men," " A Manual of Artistic Anatomy," " A Manual of Human Anatomy," etc., all of ephemeral interest as regards their subject, but striking for the lucidity and force of their descriptive power.[2]

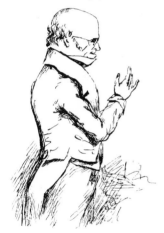

ROBERT KNOX (1791–1862)
(From a sketch made by Edward Forbes, the naturalist, while a member of Knox's class)

The years between 1828 and 1831 mark a definite stage in the history of anatomical instruction. The College of Surgeons had made a course of three months practical anatomy compulsory for its students after March, 1826, and the University followed in the next year. These exactments, by pressure on the already restricted material for dissection, led to an increase of " Resurrectionist " activity, incidentally were indirectly responsible for the Burke and Hare atrocities, and so led ultimately to the Anatomy Act of 1830. This regulation, which made body-snatching unnecessary and useless, had long been craved by teachers in all the medical schools of Britain.

In 1828 the College made attendance on two courses of anatomy compulsory, and in 1829 the practical anatomy course was extended from three to six months, to be again extended to twelve months in 1838. In 1831 the University

[1] Henry Cockburn : " Memorials of his Time," Edinburgh, 1856, p. 257.
[2] Lonsdale : " Life and Writings of Robert ·Knox," London, 1870.

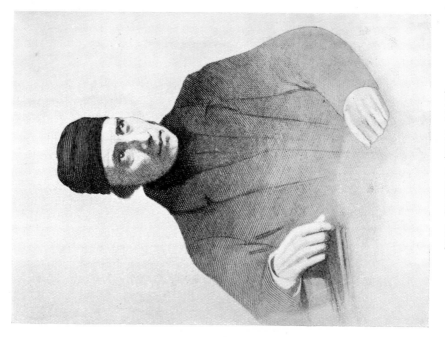

John Goodsir (1814–1867)

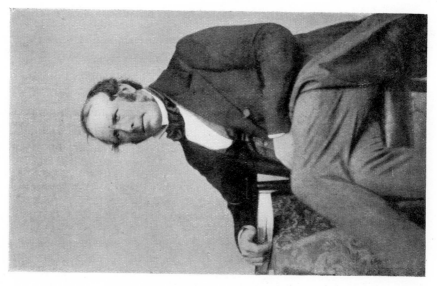

William Sharpey, M.D., F.R.S. (1802-1880)

separated the Chair of Surgery from that of Anatomy, producing a necessary change in the scope of the anatomy lectures.   This had been agitated by the College of Surgeons since 1776, but, being bitterly opposed by Monro *secundus* at that time as an infringement of his rights, the separation could not then be effected.   From this year, 1831, anatomical instruction and surgical teaching entered upon the modern epoch in Edinburgh.

Another extra-academical lecturer of a slightly later period was Dr. William Sharpey, who lectured on anatomy from 1832 to 1836, and who, during his Edinburgh period, discovered the " cilia " possessed by some mucous membranes. Allen Thomson, another extra-academical lecturer on physiology along with Sharpey, and Dr. Martin Barry were two of the earliest inquirers, with the help of the microscope, into the mysteries of the developing ovum, and many fundamental discoveries in embryology were made by them.   In this matter the Edinburgh Medical School kept pace with Joannes Müller and his pupils Henle, Schwann, etc., who at this time were making similar discoveries with the microscope in Berlin.

The Edinburgh School played a notable part in the great movement of the first half of the nineteenth century, which resulted in the recognition of the cell as the morphological unit in vital processes.   This it did through the work of John Goodsir.   Goodsir (1814–1867) acted first as Curator of the College of Surgeons' Museum, then in a similar capacity to the University, and finally, as Professor of Anatomy from 1846 to 1867.   In his early days, like others of the time, he was interested in parasitology, and the *sarcina ventriculi* and the fungus responsible for potato blight were two of his discoveries.   About the period 1842–1845 he published a number of papers dealing with the activities of the cell.   Up to this time it was generally accepted that new cells were developed by a process of precipitation of granules in a fluid exudate. Goodsir, on the contrary, not only advocated the importance of the cell as a centre of nutrition, but considered that the organism was divided up into territories of cells presided over by one central cell.   Virchow recognised his indebtedness to Goodsir by dedicating to him his " Cellular=Pathologie " (1858), in which he calls Goodsir " one of the most acute observers of cell-life."

The cellular doctrines are to be found in Goodsir's " Centres of Nutrition," " Absorption and Ulceration," " Ulceration in Articular Cartilages," " Secreting Structures," " Diseased Conditions of the Intestinal Glands," etc. His treatises on natural history subjects were numerous, as were also those on Morphological and Teleological Anatomy, such, for example, as that " On the Mechanism of the Knee-Joint," " On the Morphological Constitution of Limbs," etc.   He was succeeded by William (later Sir William) Turner in 1867.

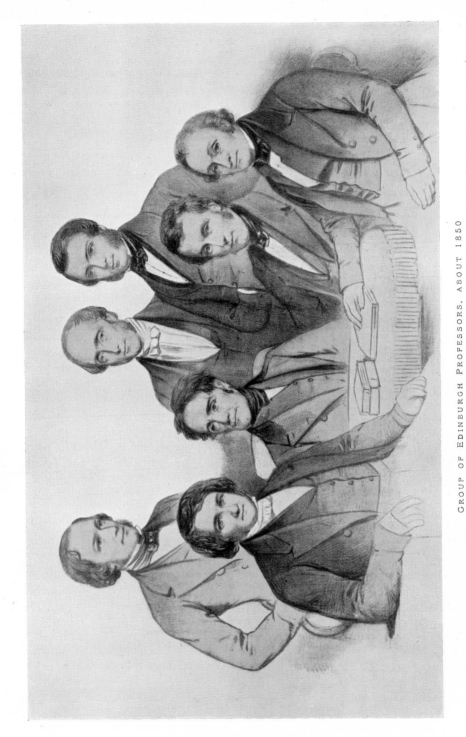

GROUP OF EDINBURGH PROFESSORS, ABOUT 1850

The names, reading from left to right, are.—Back Row: James Miller (surgery), John Hutton Balfour (medicine and botany), John Hughes Bennett (institutes of medicine). Front Row: James Young Simpson (midwifery), Robert Jameson (natural history), William Pulteney Alison (medicine), and Thomas Stewart Traill (medical jurisprudence)

CHAPTER XVI

EDINBURGH MEDICINE TO THE MIDDLE OF THE NINETEENTH CENTURY

UP TO the early years of the 19th century, Edinburgh had been specially distinguished as a school of physic, and had been a resort of students from a distance, who came to hear this side of the healing art expounded by Rutherford, Cullen, Black, Hope and Gregory. It had also become a celebrated school of anatomy under the second Monro, and this aspect of its teaching had been still further improved by the brothers John and Charles Bell, and the surgeon anatomists who followed in their footsteps. Just as the great development of anatomy in London in the hands of the brothers John and William Hunter in the latter half of the 18th century had been followed by a great improvement in surgery with exponents like Sir Astley Cooper and Sir Benjamin Brodie, so in the Edinburgh school, a great development of surgery appeared about the third decade of the 19th century.

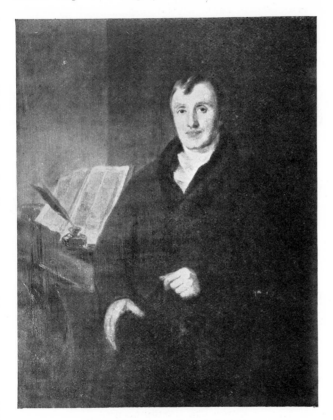

JOHN THOMSON (1765–1846)
(Original in the Royal College of Surgeons, Edinburgh)

A Chair of Military Surgery was founded in 1806 by King George III., who three years earlier had instituted the Chair of Clinical Surgery. The need for teaching military surgery at Edinburgh had first been advocated by John Bell in a memoir to Earl Spencer, then First Lord of the Admiralty. Some years, however, were allowed to elapse, and in 1806 John Thomson (1765 – 1846), was appointed as the first occupant of this Chair.   He had commenced life as an apprentice to his father in the silk-weaving trade, and later had been apprenticed to Dr. White of Paisley, and studied medicine at the Universities of Glasgow and Edinburgh.   He afterwards spent some time in London, working especially under Sir Everard Home, the brother-in-law of John Hunter, and here particularly laid the basis of a sound knowledge of pathology.   Returning to Edinburgh in 1793, he joined the College of Surgeons, and in 1800 was one of the six surgeons selected by the Managers of the Royal Infirmary as its surgical staff.   When the professorship of surgery established by the Royal College of Surgeons was founded in 1804, Thomson was selected as the first professor.   In 1806, he was chosen by the Crown to be the first incumbent of the newly-established Chair of Military Surgery, which he held for sixteen years.   At a later date he was appointed as the first occupant of the Chair of Pathology, established in 1831.

The fact that he was the first holder of no fewer than three professorships led Robert Knox to refer to him with sarcastic humour as " the old chair-maker."[1] Thomson held the Chair of Military Surgery during the important period when the Peninsular War and the other operations which culminated in the battle of Waterloo, were raging.   After the battle of Waterloo he proceeded to Belgium to study the treatment and progress of the wounded.

When he resigned the Chair in 1822, Dr. (afterwards Sir George) Ballingall, was appointed professor.   He had seen considerable service in the East, and threw himself into the duties of the Chair with enthusiasm.   The Royal College of Surgeons of Edinburgh, in 1829, passed a regulation permitting candidates for their diploma to take a course of military surgery in place of one of the two courses of surgery prescribed, and this action of the College was followed by the medical departments of the Army and the Navy for candidates entering these services.   Ballingall published " Outlines of Military Surgery," a work which ran through four editions, and also " Practical Observations on the Diseases of the European Troops in India."   He died in 1855, and, owing to the changed circumstances of the times, the Chair of Military Surgery was abolished in the following year.

In 1807, the Crown decided to establish a Chair of Medical Jurisprudence or Forensic Medicine in the University.   It had been represented by Dr. Andrew Duncan *(senior)* that professorships in this subject existed in many Universities on the Continent, although there was no such Chair at the time in Great Britain. Dr. Andrew Duncan *(junior)* (1773–1832), who has already been mentioned as the first editor of the *Edinburgh Medical Journal*, was the first incumbent of the new Chair.   He was the son of Andrew Duncan *(senior)*, had been apprenticed to Alexander Wood, and had studied in London under Matthew Baillie, as well as at various foreign Universities.   After holding this Chair for twelve years, he

---

[1] Lonsdale : " A Sketch of the Life and Writings of Robert Knox the Anatomist," London, 1870, p. 201.

was appointed Professor of Institutes of Medicine in 1819, and in 1821 became Professor of Materia Medica, holding the latter post till his death in 1832. The Chair of Forensic Medicine was afterwards filled for a year by Dr. William Pulteney Alison, who, in 1821, followed Dr. Andrew Duncan *(junior)* in the Chair of Institutes of Medicine, and held this till 1842, when he was in turn transferred to the Chair of Medicine. The Chair of Forensic Medicine in the first twenty years of its existence seems to have been regarded as a stepping stone to other professorships, and Alison was succeeded in this Chair, in 1822, by Dr. Robert Christison, who in 1832 was transferred to the Chair of Materia Medica.

The latter was then succeeded in the Chair of Forensic Medicine by Dr. Thomas Stewart Traill (1781–1862). Traill had graduated M.D. at Edinburgh in 1802, and immediately settled in practice at Liverpool. He became notable in Liverpool as a lecturer, and, as the first secretary, founded the Literary and Philosophical Society of that city, as well as taking a large part in the foundation of the Royal Institution and Liverpool Mechanics' Institution. He edited the eighth edition of the " Encyclopædia Britannica." After his appointment to the Chair of Medical Jurisprudence in Edinburgh at the age of fifty-one, he prepared the " Outlines of a Course of Lectures on Medical Jurisprudence," which was published in 1836, and went through several editions. He contributed over seventy papers on scientific subjects to various journals, and, on his death in 1862, was succeeded in the Chair by Dr. (later Sir Douglas) Maclagan.

In the Chair of Materia Medica, Andrew Duncan *(junior)* was succeeded by Dr. (later Sir Robert) Christison (1797–1882), who held it till 1877. He was the son of the Professor of Latin in Edinburgh University, and had graduated M.D. at Edinburgh in 1819. Thereafter, he studied in London and in Paris, where he paid especial attention to chemistry under Robiquet, and to toxicology under Orfila. Returning to Edinburgh in 1822, he was immediately appointed Professor of medical jurisprudence, and to this developing subject he applied the scientific principles of Orfila's great work. He speedily attained a reputation as a medical witness of great precision, and in 1829 published his celebrated " Treatise on Poisons."

A contemporary says of him : " As a witness, he was remarkable for a lucid precision of statement, which left no shadow of doubt in the mind of court, counsel, or jury, as to his views. Another noteworthy characteristic was the candour and impartiality he invariably displayed." For many years he was medical adviser to the Crown in almost all important cases. His investigations on bruising of the living body, conducted with reference to the trial of Burke and Hare, and on burns sustained before and after death, belong to the classics of this subject. In this case, his experiments, which showed that bruises cannot be inflicted after death, formed the crucial point for the conviction of the murderers.

R

In toxicology, his work on the effects of oxalic acid, on the action of water on lead, and on cases of arsenic poisoning, was of great value. Christison had spent a period of his early life in study, mainly chemical, at Paris, where Magendie was then introducing the subject of experimental pharmacology and Orfila was busy with toxicology.   His partiality to chemical and toxicological

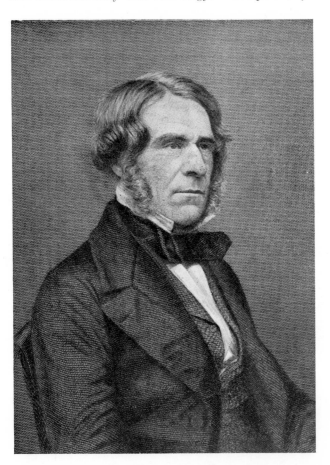

SIR ROBERT CHRISTISON (1797-1882)

science is shown in the "Dispensatory," which he published in 1842 ; this was founded to some extent upon the Dispensatory of his predecessor in the Chair of Materia Medica, Andrew Duncan, and constituted a kind of commentary upon the pharmacopœias of Edinburgh and other places, containing also records of Christison's own experiments and observations. This work prepared the way for the first Pharmacopœia of Great Britain and Ireland, issued in 1864 by a Committee of the General Medical Council, of which Christison acted as Chairman.

Among his best known pharmacological discoveries were that of conine, the active principle of hemlock (1836), of the action of Calabar bean (1855), and of the therapeutic uses of digitalin (1855) ; for though he did not originally isolate this active principle, he was the first in this country to point out its valuable properties, especially as a diuretic.   Christison's work on the action of conine is interesting as being one of the earliest pharmacological experiments to be done in this country.   He showed that it acted by abolishing the functions of the spinal cord, the action being " the counterpart of the action of nux vomica and its alkaloid strychnia." Other active drugs investigated by Christison were Calabar bean, coca leaves, and especially the effects and properties of opium from various sources, and of different kinds of wine. He also made an important contribution to medicine in his work on " Granular Degeneration of the Kidneys " (1839), and his biography forms a valuable source of information regarding the Edinburgh Medical School as it existed in his earlier years.[1]

The Chair of Surgery was founded in the year 1831 under the conditions mentioned in the last chapter. The first incumbent was Dr. John William Turner (1790–1835) who had been assistant to Dr. John Thomson, and had afterwards succeeded him as Professor of Surgery to the Royal College of Surgeons. His tenure of the Chair was short, for he died at the age of forty-six, after a chill contracted in the course of his Infirmary duties. On his death, the Chair was offered to Sir Charles Bell (1774–1842), who had made a great reputation as an anatomist and scientist in London. On Bell's return to Edinburgh, after an absence of thirty-two years, he stepped into a completely new life. His previous work in connection with anatomy has been mentioned on *page* 245.

In 1830, Bell had published his "Nervous System of the Human Body," in which he described his famous researches on the nerves of the face and respiration, and gave the first account of the effects produced by paralysis of the seventh nerve (Bell's palsy) as follows :—

" It appears that whenever the action of any of the muscles of the face is associated with the act of breathing, it is performed through the operation of this respiratory nerve, or *portio dura*. I cut a tumour from before the ear of a coachman. A branch of the nerve which goes to the angle of the mouth was divided. Some time after, he returned to thank me for ridding him of a formidable disease, but complained that he could not whistle to his horses."

Bell acquired a considerable practice among the nobility of Scotland, but he appears at the time to have been in failing health. In 1838, he published his " Institutes of Surgery," and in 1841 a volume of " Practical Essays," and he conducted the routine work of the surgical class and of his wards in the Royal Infirmary. During the spring vacation of 1842, while on the way to pay a visit in London, he was seized with an attack of *angina pectoris*, and died at Worcester.

Sir Charles Bell was succeeded in the Chair of Surgery by James Miller (1812–1864), who had studied at St. Andrews and Edinburgh, taking the licentiate-ship of the Royal College of Surgeons in 1832. He had been assistant to Robert Liston, succeeding to the practice of the latter when he went to London. In addition to his skill as a surgeon, Miller was celebrated as an orator, and at the Disruption of the Scottish Church in 1843, he rendered great service to the Free Church of Scotland both by speech and pen. He was also well known for his speeches as a temperance reformer. The same qualities stood him in good stead

---

[1] " The Life of Sir Robert Christison, Bt.," Edinburgh, 1885.

in his lectures on surgery, which were illustrated by anecdotes and illuminated by flashes of wit.   His most important contributions to surgical literature were his " Principles of Surgery," published in 1844, and " Practice of Surgery," published in 1846, which, after several editions, were amalgamated in 1864 into a " System of Surgery."   This book had a great sale in America as well as in Britain.   When Miller died in 1864, he was succeeded by Mr. James Spence.

The extra-mural teachers, about the third and fourth decades of the 19th century, did much more to develop surgery and to increase the fame of the Edinburgh school than did the University. It has been mentioned that the agitation for a special Chair in Surgery and the first appointment of a Professor of Surgery originated with the College of Surgeons. Several young men followed in the steps of John and Charles Bell as exponents of surgical anatomy. Among these may be specially mentioned John Lizars (1794–1860), William Fergusson (1808–1877), Robert Liston (1794–1847), and James Syme (1799–1870).

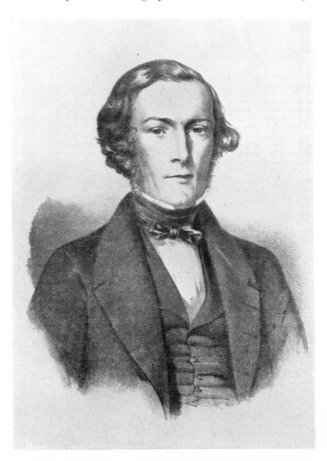

JAMES MILLER (1812-1864)

The deficiencies of Monro *(tertius)* induced most of the medical students in the early years of the century to take out the anatomical classes of John Barclay and his successor, Robert Knox; and their dissecting-rooms in Surgeons' Square formed the training-ground for most of the surgeon-anatomists, who first acted as assistants to Barclay, and afterwards conducted classes of their own in the immediate neighbourhood.   In 1826, the practical study of dissection was made compulsory on all candidates for degrees, so that accommodation and " subjects " had to be provided for about 1000 students in Edinburgh. The Resurrectionist activities to which this gave rise have already been mentioned.

John Lizars was Professor of Surgery to the College of Surgeons from 1831 to 1839, and had also been a popular teacher of anatomy. He was a bold and fearless operator, and enjoys the reputation of having been the first person to ligate the innominate artery for aneurysm, an operation which he performed with the assistance of Fergusson in 1837. His " Observations on Extraction of Diseased Ovaria,"[1] dealing with four cases, was the first description in Britain to place the operation within the bounds of regular surgery, although the operation had been performed and described more than a century earlier by Houston, in Glasgow. He was also the first Scottish surgeon to remove the jawbone for sarcoma.[2] He published a " System of Practical Surgery," and is celebrated for a life-long contention with Syme. His brother, Alexander Jardine Lizars, who had also been a lecturer on anatomy at Edinburgh, became Professor of Anatomy at Marischal College, Aberdeen, in 1841.

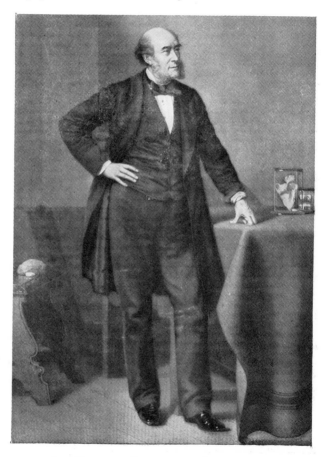

SIR WILLIAM FERGUSSON (1808-1877)

William Fergusson was a pupil and assistant of Knox, and a dissector of extraordinary skill. His dissections of the blood vessels in various parts of the body

---

[1] *Edinburgh Medical and Surgical Journal*, July, 1825.
[2] *Edinburgh Medical and Surgical Journal*, October, 1826.

are still shown among the most valued preparations in the Museum of the Royal College of Surgeons at Edinburgh. Following in the footsteps of John Bell, he began a course of demonstrations on surgical anatomy in 1829, and in 1839 he was appointed a surgeon to the Royal Infirmary in succession to Liston. Although an active teacher and operator in Edinburgh, his professional life in this city was short, for in 1840 the Chair of Surgery at King's College, London, was offered to him, and the greater part of his life's work is associated with London.[1]

Richard James Mackenzie (1821–1854) was another surgeon-anatomist of great promise, who had a short professional life in Edinburgh. He had graduated at Edinburgh and studied surgery in various Continental schools. Returning to Edinburgh in 1844, he became a Fellow of the Royal College of Surgeons, and in 1848 was elected an assistant surgeon to the Royal Infirmary. In the following year he commenced to lecture on surgery at Surgeons' Hall, and he published papers on " A Successful Ligation of the Subclavian Artery," " Excision of the Knee-joint," and " Amputation at the Ankle by an Internal Flap." Having volunteered for service with the Army in the Crimea, he died there of cholera in 1854. His death was regarded as a great loss to the Edinburgh

ROBERT LISTON (1794-1847)

---

[1] Miles : " Edinburgh School of Surgery before Lister," p. 132.

Surgical School of the day,[1] but it virtually made room in Edinburgh for Lister, who succeeded to his lectureship.

Much romance centres around the name of Robert Liston (1794–1847), who is generally associated with his contemporary and relative, James Syme.   He began the study of medicine in Edinburgh at the age of sixteen, as a pupil of John Barclay, under whom he devoted himself enthusiastically to the study of anatomy, and was one of the great Resurrectionist figures of the time.   Later he became a student under Blizard and Abernethy in London, and, in 1818, he became a member of the Royal Colleges of Surgeons both in Edinburgh and in London. In this year he began to lecture upon anatomy, with James Syme as his demonstrator and assistant, to a class of sixty students.   He very quickly became famous as a surgeon possessed of unusual initiative and dexterity in operations.

Partly, no doubt, because of his uncompromising manner and partly by reason of the jealousy of his seniors, he was accused to the Managers of the Royal Infirmary of criticising the practice of the hospital in such a way as to diminish its reputation with the public, and in 1822 the Managers passed a resolution prohibiting Mr. Liston from entering the wards or operation-room of the Royal Infirmary at any time, or on any pretence whatever.   Liston defended himself in an open letter to the Lord Provost,[2] and at the present day the unprejudiced reader almost inevitably takes the side of Liston.   Five years later, however, Liston was appointed one of the surgeons to the Infirmary, and his temporary exclusion from the institution does not appear to have had any great effect in diminishing his reputation or retarding his career.

One of his earliest contributions to surgery was a dissertation read before the Royal Medical Society in 1820, on " Fracture of the Neck of the Femur," and in the same year he published a series of five cases of aneurysm, which are celebrated in surgical annals and which formed the beginning of his great reputation.   About this time he introduced the bone-pliers with which his name is specially associated, and which, though designed to facilitate the cutting of small bones, are said to have been used in Liston's powerful hand for re-section of the femur.   In 1823 (during his period of exclusion from the Royal Infirmary) Liston performed an operation which caused a great sensation at the time.   It was the removal of an enormous tumour of the nature of elephantiasis, weighing 44½ lbs.   The flow of blood during the operation was compared by those present to the discharge of water from a shower-bath, but in three weeks the patient was able to walk about. In this operation Liston says : " I had the valuable assistance of my friend, Mr. Syme, without which the result might have been less favourable." [3]

---

[1] Miles : " Edinburgh School of Surgery before Lister," p. 140.

[2] " Letter to the Rt. Hon. the Lord Provost of Edinburgh," by Robert Liston, Edinburgh, 1822.

[3] *Edinburgh Medical and Surgical Journal*, October, 1823, p. 566.

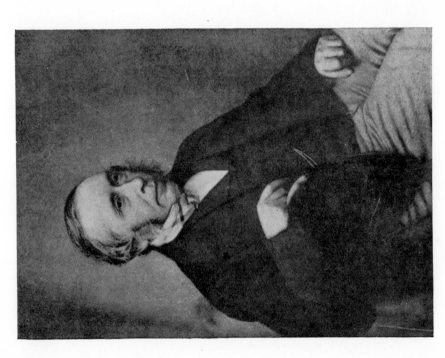

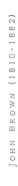

JOHN BROWN (1810-1882)

JAMES SYME (1799-1870)

An idea of the great importance attaching in these pre-anæsthetic days to rapidity of operation, as well as of Liston's great strength and self-confidence, is gained from his " Observations on Amputation."[1]   Referring to the tourniquet, he says that in his opinion it is in many cases worse than useless, and he describes how, when no proper assistance was available, he has repeatedly compressed the femoral artery with one hand while with the other he removed the limb " with the loss of much less blood than if I had followed the ordinary mode."   Another glimpse of his rapidity in operation is obtained from his " Remarks on the Operation of Lithotomy,"[2] in which he says : " Should there be but one or two stones of a moderate size (under the size of a hen's egg), the incisions and extraction should not occupy more than two or three minutes at most."

About the year 1823, Liston and Syme, who up to this time had taught together and had helped one another in their operations, became less cordial. Their differences proceeded to such a height, and they raised so much acrimony between their opposing factions, that when Syme applied for the surgeonship of the Royal Infirmary, the Managers declined to appoint him lest he and Liston should quarrel openly in the institution, and their rival students disturb its peace.   The culmination of their quarrel occurred in 1833, when Syme defeated Liston, after a bitter contest, for the Chair of Clinical Surgery in the University.   Two years later, however, in 1835, Liston was offered the Chair of Clinical Surgery at University College, London, which he accepted.   The remainder of his career, including the first major operation performed under an anæsthetic in England, at University College Hospital, in 1846, belongs to London.

James Syme, who has been called by Miles " the Napoleon of surgery," was born at 56, Princes Street, Edinburgh, in 1799.[3]   As a boy he spent much of his spare time in the company of Robert Christison, working at chemical experiments.   They, and about a dozen fellow-students of Dr. Hope's chemistry class, founded a Chemical Society, which met once a week to repeat the professor's experiments.   Arising out of this, Syme discovered, at the age of eighteen, a solvent for indiarubber, and a process by which cloth might be impregnated with this substance and so attain waterproof properties.   He published his discovery,[4] but he never got the credit for it.   Mr. Macintosh, a manufacturing chemist of Glasgow, heard of the discovery, took out a patent for it and made a fortune, as well as getting his name permanently associated with the useful garment made from the material first prepared by Syme.[5]

Syme spent two years at the Arts classes of the University, and in 1817 began his medical studies by joining the anatomy class of Dr. John Barclay,

[1] *Edinburgh Medical and Surgical Journal*, January, 1824, p. 42.
[2] *Edinburgh Medical and Surgical Journal*, January, 1825, p. 26.
[3] Miles : " Edinburgh School of Surgery before Lister," p. 174.
[4] Thomson's " Annals of Philosophy," 1818, Vol. XII, p. 112.
[5] " Life of Sir Robert Christison," Vol. I, p. 62.

where Liston was at the time the principal demonstrator. In 1818, when Liston commenced lecturing on his own account, Syme joined him as demonstrator and, later, assistant, and in 1823, when Liston gave up teaching anatomy, Syme took over the class, after joining the College of Surgeons as a Fellow. In 1821, he read a dissertation at the Royal Medical Society " On Caries of the Bones," which indicated one of the important lines of his later work. In 1822, along with his friend Sharpey, he visited Paris to attend the clinics of Dupuytren, and to take a course of operative surgery under Lisfranc.

On returning to Edinburgh, one of his earliest major operations was to amputate at the hip-joint the lower limb of a lad, William Fraser, aged 19, who had suffered from necrosis of the thigh-bone for three years. This was the first occasion on which this operation had been performed in Scotland, and Syme was assisted by Liston, who controlled the bleeding in the manner which he favoured, by pressure of his hands. The operation was successfully performed, and did much to establish Syme's reputation as a surgeon. In 1826, he excised the head of the humerus for tuberculous disease of seven years' duration, and in 1828 he published a famous case of excision of the lower jaw for sarcoma. The tumour was of enormous size, and the operation lasted twenty-four minutes, and, at a time when anæsthesia was unknown, must have been a terrible ordeal for the patient. Five weeks later, however, the patient was quite well and thinking of resuming his occupation.

Syme's disappointment in being refused the surgeonship of the Royal Infirmary, in 1829, on account of his quarrel with Liston, has been mentioned. Most of his operations up to this time had been carried out in the homes of patients, often in the most unsuitable surgical surroundings. His reputation, however, had become very great, both with the public and with the students, and he conceived the bold idea of establishing a surgical hospital for himself. In 1829, a surgical hospital was opened by him in Minto House, an old mansion which stood in a position that is now on the north side of Chambers Street. Here patients applied for admission in great numbers, and seventy patients were admitted within the first three months. Very soon this surgical hospital had to be extended, and its reputation came to rival that of the Royal Infirmary.[1] This small hospital has been immortalised by Dr. John Brown in " Rab and his Friends."

One of the landmarks in Syme's career was the publication, in 1831, of his " Treatise on the Excision of Diseased Joints," a type of operation which he was the first to place on a successful basis. In the same year, Syme brought out his " Principles of Surgery." In 1833, Professor Russell vacated the Chair of Clinical Surgery, and, after a sharp contest between Liston and Syme, the latter was appointed his successor and now became one of the surgeons to the Royal

---

[1] Miles : " Edinburgh School of Surgery before Lister," p. 188.

Infirmary. Here he introduced a new method of teaching clinical surgery, instead of the dissertations on allied groups of cases which had been previously delivered by Professor Russell.

His method may be described in his own words :—

" . . . . to bring the cases one by one into a room, where the students are comfortably seated, and if the patients have not been seen previously by the surgeon, so much the better ; then ascertaining the seat and nature of their complaints, and point out their distinctive characters.

" Having done this, so that everyone present knows distinctly the case under consideration, the teacher, either in the presence or absence of the patient, according to circumstances, proceeds to explain the principles of treatment, with his reasons for choosing the method preferred, and, lastly, does what is requisite in the presence of pupils.

" The great advantage of this system is that it makes an impression at the same same time on the eye and ear, which is known from experience to be more indelible than any other, and thus conveys instruction of the most lasting character."[1]

Syme's activites in Edinburgh were interrupted for a time, when on the death of Liston, in 1847, he accepted the professorship of Clinical Surgery at University College, London. Here he remained from February to July, 1848, but found the conditions of tenure unsatisfactory and the surroundings uncongenial, and his Edinburgh Chair being still vacant, he was reinstated in it after an absence of less than six months.

During the thirty-six years through which Syme held the Chair of Clinical Surgery, he became easily first among the surgeons of Edinburgh, and many of his operations and other contributions to surgical practice have become classics of the art of surgery. About one half of this period belonged to the days before anæsthetics, but, fortunately, this great boon to mankind was introduced about the middle of Syme's period of activity. The amputation at the ankle-joint, which goes by his name, was first performed in 1842, and was intended to replace the amputation below the knee in suitable cases. His investigation " On the Power of the Periosteum to form New Bone," in 1837, was an important contribution to surgical pathology. His operation for external urethrotomy, first performed in 1840, gave rise to a great deal of acrimonious discussion among surgeons of the time, which it is difficult now to understand. The treatment of aneurysm, which appears to have been a much more frequent disease in the early 19th century than it is to-day, received a great deal of attention from Syme. Several daring operations were performed by him for the cure of this condition, and greatly increased his already high reputation.

Syme's acrimonious disposition has been mentioned in connection with his bitter quarrel with Liston. Five years after Liston left Edinburgh, he made overtures of friendship to Syme, which, fortunately, were eagerly accepted, and the

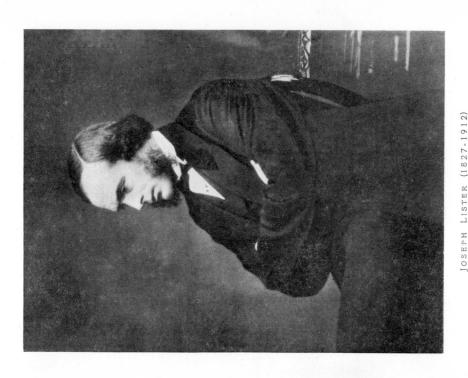

JOSEPH LISTER (1827-1912)

Photograph taken during his first Edinburgh period, 1853-1860, as indicated
by the accompanying letter in his handwriting.

PAGE FROM LETTER BY LORD LISTER

indicating the date of the accompanying photograph

old friendship was renewed and maintained till Liston's death.   Syme's defeat, in 1831, by Lizars for the professorship of Surgery in the College of Surgeons was a cause of perpetual enmity between the two.   Simpson, too, offended him because he, an obstetrician, ventured to recommend acupressure as a means of controlling surgical hæmorrhage, and Syme's adoption of anæsthesia was delayed for a time for the same reason.   Syme's rejection of acupressure was dramatic. Entering the operating-theatre with Simpson's pamphlet, soon after its appearance, he called for an operating-knife, cut the pamphlet to shreds before the assembled students, threw the remains into the sawdust below the operating-table, and remarked to the class : " There, gentlemen, is what acupressure is worth." He also quarrelled with his fellow-members of the General Medical Council, and even on one occasion, in regard to the law of evidence, with the judge who was trying a case in which he was a witness.

In the last year of Syme's tenure of the Clinical Surgery Chair, he spoke of the beginning of the antiseptic principle in surgery, which, he said, " is certainly destined in no small degree to revolutionise the practice of surgery."   In 1868 he had an apoplectic seizure and resigned the Chair, where he was succeeded by his son-in-law, Joseph Lister.

Referring to the year 1853, when Lister arrived in Edinburgh to work under Syme, the following picture of Syme is given by one of his house-surgeons, the late Dr. Joseph Bell : " His hospital life was on this wise,—two clinical lectures a week, operations two days more (perhaps three), a ward visit when he wished to see any special cases ; he spent generally about two hours in the hospital. Driving down in his big yellow chariot, with footman, hammercloth and C-springs, with two big, rather slow and stately white or grey horses, he used to expect his house surgeon to meet him at the door and move upstairs with him to his little room, where he at once took up his post with his back to the fire and his hands under the flaps of his swallow-tail coat.   In this little room he generally held a small *levee* of assistants, old friends, practitioners wanting to arrange a consultation, old pupils home on leave ; and before this select class he examined each new and interesting case that could walk in.   The new cases had been collected, sifted and arranged by the dresser in a little room on the stair, irreverently known as ' the trap,' and Mr. Syme then and there made his diagnosis, which to us young ones seemed magical and intuitional, with certainly the minimum of examination or discussion.   One was sent off with a promise of a letter to his doctor, another was fixed for to-morrow's lecture or next day's operation.   Then, if it was lecture day, a tremendous rush of feet would be heard of the students racing to get the nearest seats in the large operating theatre where the lecture was given. Chairs in the arena were kept for colleagues or distinguished strangers ; first row for dressers on duty ; operating table in centre ; Mr. Syme on a chair on left centre.   In his later days it was a fine cushioned chair called the ' chair of clinical surgery.' (In 1854 it was a meek little wooden chair without arms).   House surgeon a little behind, but nearer the door ; instrument clerk with his well-stocked table under the big window.   He comes in, sits down with a little, a very little, bob of a bow, rubs his trouser legs with both hands open, and signs for the first case.   The four dressers on duty, and in aprons, march in (if possible in step), carrying a rude wicker basket, in which, covered by a rough red blanket, the patient peers up at the great amphitheatre crammed with faces. A brief description, possibly the case had been described at a former lecture, and then the little, neat, round-shouldered, dapper man takes his knife and begins ; and the merest tyro sees at once a master of his craft at work—no show, little elegance, but absolute certainty, ease and determination ; rarely a word to an assistant—they should know their business if the unexpected happens; his plans may change in a moment, but probably only the house-surgeon finds it out ; the patient is sent off, still anæsthetised, and then comes a brief commentary, short, sharp and decisive, worth taking verbatim if you can manage it; yet he has no notes, a very little veiled voice and no eloquence." [1]

Into this atmosphere Joseph Lister stepped in 1853.   Lister's medical education had been gained at University College Hospital, London, where one of his teachers had been William Sharpey, Professor of Physiology.   Sharpey, at an earlier stage of his career, had been an extra-mural lecturer upon anatomy in Edinburgh in association with Allen Thomson, who lectured upon physiology. Both these teachers had been intimate friends of Syme during his student days. Lister had studied under another teacher of Edinburgh origin in the person of Robert Liston, and had been present on the historic occasion when the first operation under ether in England was performed by him in December, 1846, at University College Hospital.

Lister now came to Edinburgh bearing a letter of introduction from Sharpey to Syme, who received him cordially, offered him the chance of assisting with private operations, and set him to work at the hospital. He appears to have been one of the very few of Syme's immediate associates with whom Syme never quarrelled.   Two months after his arrival in Edinburgh, Lister was appointed Syme's supernumerary house-surgeon, and when Dr. Dewar, Syme's house-surgeon, left in December, 1853, Lister took over his duties and continued in this post till February, 1855.

Lister occupied a somewhat unusual position.   He was already a Fellow of the Royal College of Surgeons of England, and Syme apparently gave him to understand that he might consider their mutual relations were those of surgeon and consulting surgeon, so that Lister was allowed the exceptional privilege of deciding as to which of the cases admitted during the night he should himself operate upon.[2]   Syme treated him with

---

[1] " Edinburgh Hospital Reports," 1893, Vol. I, pp. 22 and 23.
[2] Godlee : " Lord Lister," London, 1917, p. 36.

great affection, and Lister became a constant visitor at Syme's house of Millbank, pleasantly situated in the Grange suburb of Edinburgh. This was the period of the Crimean War, and Dr. R. J. Mackenzie, an Edinburgh surgeon of great promise, had volunteered for service in the Crimea as an operating surgeon. He had intended to be back in Edinburgh by November, 1854, to resume his winter course of lectures on surgery, but in October, 1854, he died of cholera, and Lister's friends at once suggested that he should continue Mackenzie's lectures and apply for his post as assistant surgeon at the Infirmary.

With the advice of Syme, Lister took Mackenzie's lecture-room at No. 4, High School Yards, was elected a Fellow of the Royal College of Surgeons of Edinburgh, and took lodgings at No. 3, Rutland Street, in the spring of 1855. At the same time he became engaged to Syme's eldest daughter, Agnes, to whom he was married in April, 1856. He began his course of lectures upon the principles and practice of surgery on 7th November, 1855, to a class of twenty-three students. In the following year, after a tour on which he visited various Continental surgical centres, he returned to Edinburgh in October, 1856, and took the house, No. 11, Rutland Street, being elected in the same month assistant surgeon to the Royal Infirmary.

Before Lister came to Edinburgh, he had done several valuable pieces of research, including his work on the muscular tissue of the iris, and upon the involuntary muscular fibres of the skin. In Edinburgh, although he was busy helping Syme in his operations and in teaching, he was also occupied in writing. During 1855, he sent to *The Lancet* weekly summaries of Syme's lectures, and prepared records of some of Syme's cases for the press. In 1856, a paper was read before the Royal Society of Edinburgh on " The Minute Structure of Involuntary Muscular Fibre."[1] He very soon began his celebrated investigations regarding the nature of inflammation, and, in 1857, read a paper on " The Early Stages of Inflammation " before the Royal Society of London.[2] Two other papers on cognate subjects were also read before the Royal Society of London in the same year : " An Enquiry regarding the Parts of the Nervous System which Regulate the Contraction of the Arteries,"[3] and " On the Cutaneous Pigmentary System of the Frog."[4]

In 1856 he started his experiments upon the coagulation of the blood, a subject which was exciting a considerable amount of controversy at the time, and in 1858 he read a paper on " Spontaneous Gangrene " before the Medico-Chirurgical Society of Edinburgh. During the next year, he was mainly occupied with teaching, hospital work, and the practice which he had been successful in attracting through Syme's influence. In 1860, on the death of Professor James Lawrie, of the Chair of Surgery in Glasgow,

[1] p. 15, [2] p. 209, [3] p. 27, [4] p. 48 : " Lister's Collected Papers," Vol. I.

Lister was nominated by the Crown to this post.   He was inducted to it on 9th March, 1860, and in May of the same year he commenced his summer course of lectures to 182 students.   He was not, however, appointed surgeon to the Glasgow Royal Infirmary till 5th August, 1861.   The later researches on inflammation, and especially those on antiseptics, date from 1864 onwards.

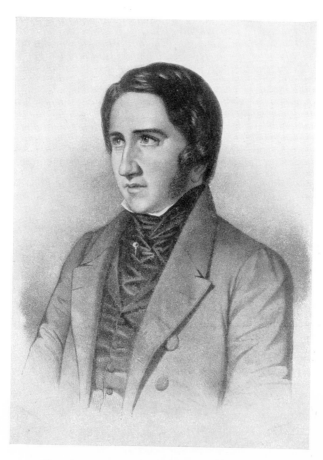

SIR JAMES YOUNG SIMPSON (1811–1870)

The outstanding figure of Edinburgh medicine about the middle of the 19th century was Sir James Young Simpson (1811–1870). He was born at Bathgate, being the youngest of seven sons of a baker in this town, and he went to school at the precocious age of four, being even at this early stage remarkable for the aptitude he showed for lessons.   Entering the University of Edinburgh at the age of fourteen, he graduated M.D. in 1832.   Settling in the Stockbridge district, he quickly attracted a large practice, and in 1840 he was appointed to the Chair of Midwifery in succession to Professor James Hamilton, at the early age of twenty-eight.   His residence in later years was at 52, Queen Street, and here the early experiments on anæsthetics, for which he is especially renowned, were carried out.   In 1846, when news of the first trials of sulphuric ether as an anæsthetic reached Scotland from America, Simpson wrote : " It is a glorious thought, I can think of naught else."   An account of the way in which Simpson conducted his experiments, and of the discovery of the anæsthetic powers possessed by chloroform, a substance of which a small supply had been sent to him by

Mr. Waldie, a chemist of Liverpool, has been given by his colleague, Professor Miller, and may be quoted here :—

" Late one evening—it was the 4th of November, 1847—on returning home after a weary day's labour, Dr. Simpson, with his two friends and assistants, Drs. Keith and Matthews Duncan, sat down to their somewhat hazardous work in Dr. Simpson's dining-room.   Having inhaled several substances, but without much effect, it occurred to Dr. Simpson to try a ponderous material, which he had formerly set aside on a lumber-table, and which, on account of its great weight, he had hitherto regarded as of no likelihood whatever.   That happened to be a small bottle of chloroform.   It was searched for, and recovered from beneath a heap of waste paper.   And, with each tumbler newly charged, the inhalers resumed their vocation.   Immediately an unwonted hilarity seized the party ; they became bright-eyed, very happy and very loquacious—expatiating on the delicious aroma of the new fluid.   The conversation was of unusual intelligence, and quite charmed the listeners—some ladies of the family and a naval officer, brother-in-law of Dr. Simpson.   But suddenly there was a talk of sounds being heard like those of a cotton-mill, louder and louder ; a moment more, then all was quiet, and then—a crash.   On awaking, Dr. Simpson's first perception was mental —' This is far stronger and better than ether,' said he to himself.   His second was to note that he was prostrate on the floor, and that among the friends about him there was both confusion and alarm.   Hearing a noise, he turned round and saw Dr. Duncan beneath a chair ; his jaw dropped, his eyes staring, his head bent half under him ; quite unconscious, and snoring in a most determined and alarming manner.   More noise still, and much motion.   And then his eyes overtook Dr. Keith's feet and legs, making valorous efforts to overturn the supper-table, or more probably to annihilate everything that was on it. . . ."[1]

The various steps in the introduction of the practice of anæsthesia have been much confused, but the matter is clearly stated in a paper by Simpson himself, written just before his death in 1870, as follows :—

" If we try to put into a summarised form the data which we have been discussing regarding the introduction of anæsthesia in America and this country, it appears to me that we might correctly state the whole matter as follows :—

" 1. That on the 11th December 1844, Dr. Wells had, at Hartford, by his own desire and suggestion, one of his upper molar teeth extracted without any pain, in consequence of his having deeply breathed nitrous oxide gas for the purpose, as suggested nearly half-a-century before by Sir Humphry Davy.

" 2. That after having with others proved, in a limited series of cases, the anæsthetic powers of nitrous oxide gas, Dr. Wells proceeded to Boston to lay his

---

[1] James Miller : " The Principles of Surgery," Philadelphia, 1852, p. 701.

discovery before the Medical School and Hospital there, but was unsuccessful in the single attempt which he made, in consequence of the gas-bag being removed too soon, and that he was hooted away by his audience, as if the whole matter were an imposition, and was totally discouraged.

" 3. That Dr. Wells's former pupil and partner, Dr. Morton of Boston, was present with Dr. Wells when he made his experiments there.

" 4. That on the 30th September 1846, Dr. Morton extracted a tooth without any pain, whilst the patient was breathing sulphuric ether, this fact and discovery of itself making a NEW ERA in anæsthetics and in surgery.

" 5. That within a few weeks the vapour of sulphuric ether was tried in a number of instances of surgical operations in Boston—Dr. Morton being generally the administrator—and ether vapour was established as a successful anæsthetic in dentistry and surgery.

" 6. That in January, and the subsequent spring months, 1847, the application of sulphuric ether as an anæsthetic in midwifery was introduced, described in our medical journals, and fully established in Edinburgh, before any case with it was tried in Boston or America.

" 7. That on the 15th November 1847, the anæsthetic effects of chloroform were discovered in Edinburgh, and that it swiftly superseded in Scotland and elsewhere the use of sulphuric ether, and extended rapidly and greatly the practice of anæsthesia in surgery, midwifery, etc."[1]

Apart from the introduction of anæsthesia, which at first met with great opposition, requiring a man of Simpson's prominent position to overcome, his chief work was in the domain of gynæcology and obstetrics. In this department he published many valuable writings upon such subjects as version in deformed pelves, and on puerperal diseases. His teachings included much practical work in regard to the use of obstetric forceps, of which he introduced a new long variety, in the improvement of methods of ovariotomy and similar subjects. He was also distinguished for his writings in regard to general literature, and especially archæology.

His archæological essays, dealing chiefly with subjects bearing on Scottish history, were published after his death, in two volumes. His collected papers include " Obstetric Memoirs and Contributions," published in 1855 ; " Selected Obstetric and Gynæcological Works," published after his death in 1871 ; " Anæsthesia, Hospitalism, and other Essays," in 1871 ; and " Clinical Lectures on the Diseases of Women," published in 1872, under the editorship of his nephew, Professor A. R. Simpson, who succeeded him in 1870.

---

[1] Simpson : " History of Modern Anæsthetics—a second letter to Dr. Jacob Bigelow," Edinburgh, 1870, p. 15.

Simpson appears from the accounts of those who knew him to have possessed a magnetic personality, to have been a great and overpowering controversialist, and a physician who was able to inspire his patients with the highest degree of confidence.

The Chair of Pathology was founded in the University in 1831.   In the early years of the century, the teaching of pathology had been part of the duties of James Russell, Professor of Clinical Surgery, who had duly included information upon this subject in his somewhat systematic " clinical " lectures.   The subject, by 1831, had developed so far as to be one of practical importance, and the Town Council decided to appoint a professor.   Dr. John Thomson, who had studied this subject under Sir Everard Home, in London, and was regarded as a repository of the Hunterian traditions, was the first incumbent of the Chair.   He has already been mentioned as Professor of Military Surgery, and is apt to be confused with his two distinguished sons, Allen Thomson, who was successively professor of anatomy at Aberdeen, professor of physiology at Edinburgh, and professor of anatomy at Glasgow, and William Thomson, who was professor of medicine in Glasgow.   John Thomson also wrote the standard biography of Cullen.

He held the Chair of Pathology till 1842, when he was succeeded by William Henderson (1810–1872). Henderson graduated M.D. at Edinburgh in 1831, and next year was appointed physician to the fever wards and pathologist to the Royal Infirmary.   He was one of the first to apply the microscope to the study of the organs in disease, describing (1841) the minute appearances of the lung in pneumonia, and other pathological conditions. He is credited with the merit of having been the first person to distinguish, in 1843, between typhus and relapsing fevers, both of which were very important diseases of the time.

At the present day, he is chiefly remembered by the storm he raised in 1845, when he announced his adherence to the system of homœopathy by publishing " An Enquiry into the Homœopathic Practice of Medicine."   He resigned his appointment at the Infirmary, and his colleagues, headed by Syme, endeavoured to oust him from the Chair of Pathology, but, failing in this, attempted to make attendance on the class of pathology not obligatory on students.· A long controversy, mainly with Syme and Simpson, who for once were united against a common enemy, lasted until about 1853.   Henderson's pamphlets, in reply to these attacks, are models of reasoning, irony and banter, and although the system is now completely discredited, Henderson certainly, with tact and skill, made out a good argument in its favour.   He resigned the Chair in 1869, when he was succeeded by Professor W. R. Sanders, and died in 1872.

The Chair of Institutes of Medicine was one of the original professorships of the Medical Faculty.   At the beginning of the century it was held by Andrew Duncan *(senior)*, who, in 1819, retired in favour of his son, Andrew Duncan *(junior)*.   He held the Chair for two years, when he was transferred to that of

Materia Medica and was succeeded by William Pulteney Alison.   Alison in turn
held the Chair from 1821 to 1842, when he passed to that of Medicine, and was
succeeded in the professorship of Institutes of Medicine by Allen Thomson.

Allen Thomson (1809–1884) was the son of Professor John Thomson and
brother of Professor William Thomson of Glasgow.   He graduated M.D. at
Edinburgh in 1830, and from 1831 to 1836 conducted a conjoint extra-mural
class at 9, Surgeons' Square with William Sharpey—Thomson lecturing on physiology and Sharpey on anatomy.   In 1837, he left Edinburgh to become private
physician to the Duke of Bedford for two years, and, in 1839, became professor
of anatomy at Marischal College, Aberdeen.

When, in 1842, he came to Edinburgh as Professor of Physiology, he instituted
a celebrated course on microscopic anatomy, which was then quite a new subject.
His researches on embryology, while an extra-mural lecturer, had already made him
famous.   The subject of microscopic anatomy had recently received an enormous
impetus from Johannes Müller, who, working in Berlin with the recently-improved
achromatic microscope, had, along with Henle and Schwann, made many notable
discoveries in the minute structure of the body.   This line of research was taken
up by Allen Thomson in the domain of normal anatomy, and by William Henderson
and Hughes Bennett in the field of pathological anatomy.   Thus a great deal of
credit for extending this aspect of medical knowledge belongs to the Edinburgh
Medical School in the 'forties of last century.   The natural historian of earlier times
came, at this period, to be replaced by the biological teachers of the present day,
and Allen Thomson was one of the leaders of the movement.   He took up the
professorship of anatomy at Glasgow in 1848.

John   Hughes   Bennett   (1812–1875),   who   succeeded   him,   graduated
M.D.   at   Edinburgh   in   1837.   During   his   student   days   his   intimate
associates   had   included   the   Goodsirs,   Edward   Forbes,   John   Hutton   Balfour
and   John   Reid,   all   of   whom   became   distinguished   biologists   of   the   new
school.   After   graduation,   Bennett   spent   two   years   in   Paris   at   clinical
work,   and   two   years   in   Germany   devoted   to   research.   On   his   return   to
Edinburgh, in 1841, he published a treatise on " Cod-Liver Oil as a Therapeutic
Agent."   This   substance   had   long   been   used   by   the   fisher   population   of
Scotland, but following Bennett's advocacy, it now came into general vogue as
a remedy.   In 1845 he published a case of " Hypertrophy of the Spleen and
Liver," the first recorded case of leucocythæmia.   In accordance with the views
of the time, institutes of medicine was regarded as a subject intimately connected
with clinical medicine rather than one of abstruse scientific interest, and Bennett,
like his predecessors, was elected one of the physicians to the Royal Infirmary.

He was a great teacher of clinical physiology.   He taught physiology and
medicine for over a quarter of a century and published a text-book on medicine which
was widely read, but the chief scientific achievements associated with his name

are his original description of the disease leucocythæmia and the great change to which his investigations led in the current treatment of pneumonia. Leucocythæmia was the first disease of the blood to be described (1845), and its recognition opened up an entirely new branch of medicine. (Addison described pernicious anæmia four years later, in 1849.) The question of priority in

the discovery of leuco-cythæmia is sometimes debated, for, like other discoveries in medicine, it was made simultane-ously by different men, three cases of leucocy-thæmia being independ-ently recorded for the first time in the year 1845. Hughes Bennett's history of the matter, given in his treatise on " Leucocythæmia," in 1852, shows that the credit of priority belongs to him.

Bennett's treatise on " The Restorative Treat-ment of Pneumonia," published in 1865, when he was Professor of the Institutes of Medicine, belongs to a type of medical research much more difficult to appraise. The practice of bleeding had come down from the eighteenth century as a moderate method, and had been developed

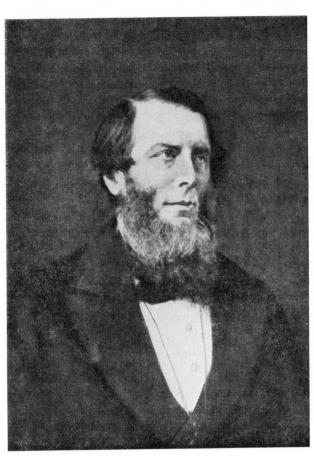

JOHN HUGHES BENNETT (1812–1875)

by the French School of Broussais, by Gregory of Edinburgh, and others, into a powerful weakening or " antiphlogistic " régime, which was supposed to be requisite in order to abort the fever. Hughes Bennett's treatise is a masterly survey of different methods then in vogue for treating pneumonia, which he compares by means of the statistical plan of Louis. By showing that the method of profuse bleeding was followed by death in one case out of three, while of one hundred and twenty-nine cases treated by him on the " restorative " principle, only four had died, he did more than anyone else to banish excessive bleeding as a routine method of treatment.   Bennett was an indefatigable writer, and produced some hundred and five papers.   He was also the author of an " Introduction to Clinical Medicine," of a work on " Outlines of Physiology " (1858), and of a celebrated text-book, " Lectures on Clinical Medicine " (1856), of which many later editions, and various translations into foreign languages, subsequently appeared.   He held the Chair till 1874, when he was succeeded by William Rutherford.

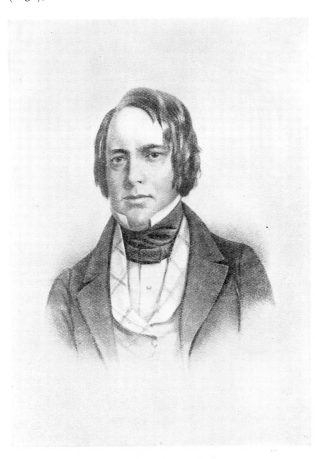

In the Chair of Chemistry, Thomas Charles Hope continued to teach for almost half a century, till he was succeeded in 1844 by William Gregory, the fourth son of James Gregory, the late Professor of Medicine. William Gregory had graduated M.D. at Edinburgh in 1828, and in 1831 made a discovery which has been found of the greatest commercial importance in the manufacture of the active principles of drugs.   In 1816, the Hanoverian, Sertürner, had discovered the alkaline base " mor-

WILLIAM GREGORY (1803-1858)

phium " in opium, and in April, 1831, Dr. Gregory published, in the *Edinburgh Medical and Surgical Journal*, his valuable discovery of the preparation of hydro-chlorate of morphia without the use of alcohol or any other solvent than water.

Morphia, till then used in the form of acetate, had made little progress in Britain, because too expensive, and probably also by no means always pure.   But Gregory's process supplied a soporific dose of morphia at no greater cost than the equivalent dose of laudanum, and in a state of great purity. As is well known, the hydrochlorate, and the subsequently prepared sulphate of morphia, have largely superseded in use the other purified galenical preparations of opium.   As a development of this discovery, Edinburgh has become one of the chief commercial centres in the United Kingdom for the manufacture of the active alkaloidal principles derived from numerous plants.

As a corollary to Gregory's discovery, mention may be made of a minor, though far-reaching, contribution to practical medicine, by a member of the Edinburgh School.   Alexander Wood, an extra-mural lecturer on medicine at Edinburgh, was the first person in Britain to use the hypodermic syringe, though priority of discovery cannot be claimed for him, since Pravaz had already used this form of medication in 1851, and published a description of his syringe in 1853. The idea of administering morphia hypodermically for the relief of pain appears to have occurred independently, in 1853, to Wood, who constructed a small syringe on the plan of the " sting of a bee," for this purpose.   Subsequently he extended its application to the administration of atropine and other substances in his " New Method of Treating Neuralgia by the Direct Application of Opiates to the Painful Points " (1855).   He enjoys, at all events, the merit of having been the first to introduce this now universal method into Great Britain.

William Gregory had successively held the posts of lecturer on chemistry at the Andersonian College in Glasgow, and at Dublin, and of professor of medicine and chemistry at King's College, Aberdeen.   He published his " Outlines of Chemistry " in 1845, and was greatly interested in the subject of animal magnetism, but was better known on account of his translations of German works.   About this time, Liebig had been conducting his celebrated researches upon chemistry in connection with animal bodies, and Gregory translated his " Animal Chemistry " and other works into English.   When Gregory died, his successor, Lyon Playfair, was even more distinguished in the same direction.

Lyon Playfair (1819–1898), had studied at St. Andrews, Glasgow and Edinburgh, and had worked at chemistry with Thomas Graham at University College, London, and with Liebig at Giessen.   He had been influenced by Liebig to turn his attention to the applications of chemistry to agriculture and plant physiology, a subject which at the time became of great social and commercial importance.   In 1845, he had been appointed chemist to the Geological Survey, and had conducted researches into the type of coal best suited for steam navigation.   He was the discoverer of nitro-prussides, and, along with Bunsen, investigated the gases developed in blast furnaces.   His most important activity had been the part he took in 1850 in the organisation of the Great Exhibition promoted by the Prince Consort, and, as a sequel to this, in the development of technical instruction and in the various applications of science to industry.   Even after his appointment to the Chair of Chemistry at Edinburgh, in 1858, he was still occupied on many Royal Commissions and

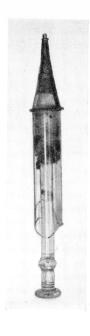

ORIGINAL HYPODERMIC SYRINGE OF

DR. ALEXANDER WOOD

THE FIRST USED IN GREAT BRITAIN

The syringe is 90 mm. in length, and the barrel, which has been broken towards its base, is 10 mm. in diameter. The piston is wrapped round at its extremity with cotton wick to make the plunger fit the barrel. At its apex the barrel is drawn into a conoidal extremity which fits a metal nose cap. The cap is of curious construction and consists of one inner filler-shaped part which fits closely to the diminishing portion of the glass barrel and ends in a pointed extremity, which is threaded externally, to allow a hypodermic needle to be screwed on. The filler-part is grasped by a metal arrangement, whose apex is tightly applied to it at the screw. It is prolonged upwards by two lateral metal strips, bound by a circle round the middle of the inner cap, and prolonged upwards further by the two lateral bands, to end in a ring, which does not touch the barrel, and may have been used to steady the syringe and prevent the metal cap being forced off during administration of a hypodermic injection.

(Preserved in the Museum of the Royal College of Surgeons, Edinburgh)

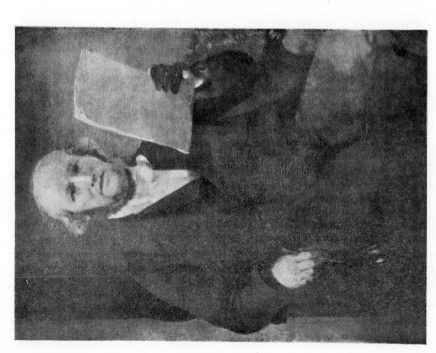

ALEXANDER WOOD (*secundus*) (1817–1884)
(Original in the Royal College of Physicians, Edinburgh)

other forms of public work.   He held the Chair till 1869, when he became Member of Parliament for the University and removed to London. He was succeeded by Alexander Crum Brown.

Despite the fact that by the middle of the 19th century, Edinburgh had become a great surgical school, the fame which had accrued to it through the teaching of Cullen and James Gregory, was still continued in medicine.   James Home, who has been mentioned as a successful professor of materia medica, held the Chair of Medicine from 1821 to 1842, when he was succeeded by Professor Alison, who had previously taught medical jurisprudence and institutes of medicine.

William Pulteney Alison (1790–1859) was a brother of Sir Archibald Alison, the historian, and a grandson of John Gregory. He graduated M.D. at Edinburgh in 1811, and in 1815 was appointed Physician to the New Town Dispensary, where he made a special study of the fevers then prevalent in the city. His quarterly reports,

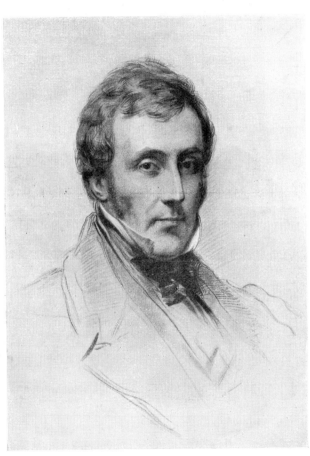

WILLIAM PULTENEY ALISON (1790–1859)

published in the *Edinburgh Medical Journal* from 1817 to 1819, were important contributions to the knowledge of fevers, and especially his description of smallpox as modified by vaccination, which was then a novel mode of treatment.   In 1820, while Professor of Medical Jurisprudence, he also assisted his uncle, James Gregory.

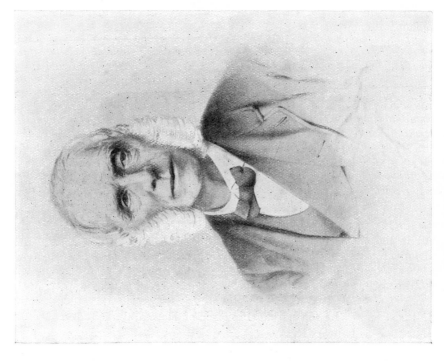

THOMAS LAYCOCK (1812-1876)

SIR DOUGLAS MACLAGAN (1812-1900)

From his early experience among the poor, he had been impressed by the manner in which poverty and unfavourable social conditions assisted the spread of disease, and in 1840 he published an important pamphlet entitled " Observations on the Management of the Poor in Scotland, and its Effects on the Health of the Great Towns." The poor in Scotland were at that time largely dependent on charity administered through the Kirk Sessions, and Alison advocated an approach to the English system, with relief for the poor on a basis of assessment. A Royal Commission was appointed to investigate the subject in 1844, and the Poor Law passed in 1845 embodied much that Alison had recommended. He was celebrated for benevolence and kindliness of manner, and the social work which he did in this respect has been of enormous advantage up to the present day.

In 1831, Alison had published " Outlines of Physiology," a work which included much of his philosophy in regard to the vital attraction and repulsion which he considered to be characteristics of life as exhibited by the tissues. He wrote various articles dealing with subjects such as vital affinity and inflammation. Although he conducted a large consulting practice, he found time for much public activity, especially on subjects connected with the amelioration of the conditions under which the poorer classes lived. He acted as President of the British Medical Association when it met in Edinburgh in 1858, and he died in the following year.

He was succeeded in the Chair of Medicine by Thomas Laycock (1812–1876). Laycock was an Englishman, had qualified as M.R.C.S. in 1835, and had graduated M.D. at Göttingen in 1839, and studied under Lisfranc and Velpeau at Paris. In 1840 he had published " A Treatise on Nervous Diseases of Women, comprising an Enquiry into the Nature, Causes and Treatment of Spinal and Hysterical Disorders." This was the result of much profound observation, and to a great extent it anticipated the similar work done by Charcot and other French observers. In 1844, in a paper read before the British Association at York, he had formulated the theory of reflex action of the brain, by which he accounted for the phenomena of delirium, dreams and somnambulism. In 1855 he succeeded William Pulteney Alison in the Chair of Medicine at Edinburgh, and in 1856 published his " Lectures on the Principles and Methods of Medical Observation and Research." His " Mind and Brain " (1859) prepared the way for the study of unconscious cerebration, to which he afterwards chiefly devoted himself, and in which he described mental phenomena that have received due recognition only in the last few years, in connection with the great numbers of nervous cases arising out of the War. He was a prolific writer, and some three hundred papers on medical subjects emanated from his pen. He died in 1876, and was succeeded by Sir Thomas Grainger Stewart.

In addition to those who held professorial Chairs during the earlier half of the 19th century, many of the well-known Edinburgh physicians and surgeons acted for some years as extra-mural lecturers connected either with the College of Physicians or College of Surgeons, while others became celebrated for the development at an early stage of certain special branches in medicine or surgery.

Dr. John Roberton, who practised in St. James's Street, Edinburgh, at the beginning of the century, published a " Treatise on Medical Police," in 1809. This was the first notable treatise in English upon the subject of public health. Johann Peter Frank had directed attention to the importance of this subject in his " Complete System of Medical Polity," published at Mannheim in 1777, and Roberton was the next writer after him to pursue this subject. He devotes one book to discussing the causes of diseases in Edinburgh, and another to those in London. The subject of public health came to be regarded as part of the duties of the professorship of medical jurisprudence, founded in 1807 at Edinburgh.

The practical side of public health was greatly developed at a later date by Dr. Henry Duncan (later Sir Henry) Littlejohn. Graduating M.D. in 1847 at Edinburgh, he began, in 1855, to lecture on medical jurisprudence in the Extra-Mural School, and took much interest in matters affecting the health of the city. He was later appointed Medical Officer of Health for Edinburgh, and many of the early improvements dealing with drainage, water-supply, and overcrowded localities were suggested by him. He succeeded Sir Douglas Maclagan as professor in 1897, the Chair being now known as Forensic Medicine, and Public Health being erected into a separate professorship in 1898.

Dr. John Abercrombie (1780–1844) was one of the most eminent among the Scottish physicians of the first quarter of the 19th century. He laboured hard at pathological anatomy in its connection with clinical research, but it is a singular fact that he remained to the last unconnected officially with any hospital or even with the Medical School. He was, however, constantly surrounded by pupils in dispensary practice, and conducted what is known in Germany as a " poliklinic " long before this method of teaching was introduced in the latter country.[1] He was a voluminous writer on clinical and pathological subjects, especially in connection with diseases of the nervous system. His general eminence in medicine was recognised by his election, in 1835, as Lord Rector of the University of Marischal College, Aberdeen. On this occasion he delivered an address upon " The Culture and Discipline of the Mind," which has been often reprinted.[2]

The subject of midwifery had been greatly developed in the previous century by Professors Gibson and Young, and in the early years of the 19th century by Professor James Hamilton, while Sir James Y. Simpson made the Edinburgh

---

[1] " Life of Sir Robert Christison," Vol. II, p. 121.
[2] " Fasti Academiae Mariscallanae Aberdonensis," Vol. II, p. 22.

School specially distinguished in regard to this department of practice.   While Simpson was lecturing in the University, Dr. William Campbell founded a school of obstetrics known as Queen's College, connected with the Royal College of Surgeons.   This was largely attended by students, to whom Campbell issued diplomas after examination, in which he was assisted by Dr. Robert Knox. Dr. Campbell was also the first person in Edinburgh, for some years before and after 1840, to give a full course of lectures upon diseases of children. Partly in consequence of the interest created by these lectures, the idea of founding a hospital for sick children came into being about 1856.   Dr. Campbell was assisted and, later, succeeded by his son, Dr. Alexander Dewar Campbell, and he in turn was succeeded, in 1853, as lecturer in midwifery at the Royal College of Surgeons, by Dr. Alexander Keiller (1811–1892).

In 1851, Dr. Keiller was elected one of the ordinary physicians to the Royal Infirmary, and, during the fifteen years for which he held this post, he arranged with Dr. W. T. Gairdner and Dr. J. Warburton Begbie, who were physicians to the hospital, that he should institute a course of clinical teaching on the diseases of women.   Some years after this, an extra ward was set apart for Keiller's course on the subject, and this was the beginning of gynæcological teaching in the Edinburgh Medical School.

James Matthews Duncan (1826–1890), after taking the Fellowship of the Royal College of Surgeons in 1851, became a lecturer in midwifery in the Extra-Mural School, and was appointed physician for diseases of women to the Royal Infirmary in 1861.   His connection with Simpson in the discovery of the anæsthetic properties of chloroform has been mentioned.   He afterwards went to London and became attached to St. Bartholomew's Hospital in 1877. During his Edinburgh period a considerable number of papers dealing with obstetric subjects, and with the advancement of education in midwifery in Scotland emanated from his pen.

Thomas Keith (1827–1895) was apprenticed to Professor James Y. Simpson in 1845, and afterwards was house surgeon to Syme.   He conducted a large practice along with his brother, Dr. George Skene Keith, but was particularly attracted to obstetrics and the developing subject of gynæcology.   His first operation for ovariotomy was performed in 1862, and his celebrated series of 136 operations with 81 per cent. of recoveries was performed in the next ten years. He formed one of the famous chloroform party in Simpson's dining-room already mentioned.   His successful results appear to have been obtained in part by a scrupulous attention to cleanliness in all the surroundings of his operations, but they began before the antiseptic era, and he found that antiseptics, as used in the early days of their employment, interfered with the success of his results.

Among the early physicians to the Infirmary may be mentioned the following : Dr. Thomas Spens, son of Dr. Nathaniel Spens, whose portrait in the uniform of

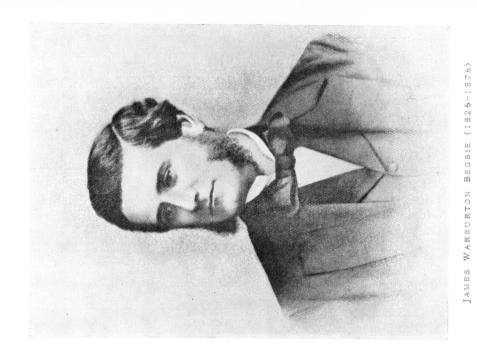

James Warburton Begbie (1826–1876)

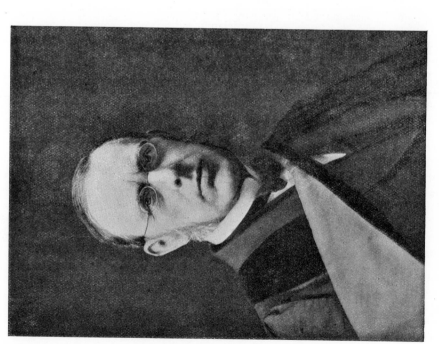

William Tennant Gairdner (1824–1907)

a Royal Archer is generally regarded as Raeburn's chief masterpiece, translated Richter's " Medical and Surgical Observations," in 1794.

Dr. David Craigie, another of the physicians to the Infirmary, who was a great linguist and a voluminous writer upon clinical and pathological subjects, has been already mentioned in connection with the subject of anatomy, which he taught for several years.

Dr. Robert Spittall (1804–1852) was one of the earliest physicians to introduce the methods of Laennec to Edinburgh practice, and, in 1830, issued " A Treatise on Auscultation, illustrated by cases and dissections."

Dr. J. R. Cormack (1815–1882) graduated at Edinburgh in 1837, and became one of the physicians to the Infirmary, but in later life practised in London and in Paris, eventually becoming Sir John Rose Cormack.

Sir William Tennant Gairdner (1824–1907) was one of the most distinguished of the younger physicians to the Royal Infirmary about the middle of the 19th century.   As pathologist to the Royal Infirmary in 1848, he entered upon a career of great scientific energy, and in 1853 became physician to the Royal Infirmary, at the same time lecturing upon medicine in the Extra-Mural School. Meanwhile, he was engaged on the preparation of his classic work on clinical medicine, and his notable volume on " Public Health in Relation to Air and Water," which were published after he had gone to Glasgow as professor of medicine.   In a series of early papers, " Contributions to the Pathology of the Kidney " (1848), he supplied an early description of waxy disease, and in the " Pathological Anatomy of Bronchitis and Diseases of the Lung connected with Bronchial Obstruction " (1850), he was one of the earliest observers to describe the condition of bronchiectasis.

James Warburton Begbie (1826–1876) was the son of Dr. James Begbie, also an Edinburgh physician.   About 1852 he settled in Edinburgh, becoming in 1854 physician of the (temporary) Cholera Hospital, and in 1855 physician to the Royal Infirmary, and lecturer on medicine in the Extra-Mural School.   Here also he gave a short annual course of lectures on the history of medicine.   In middle life he was generally regarded as the most popular and highly esteemed physician in Scotland, and it has been said that for some years no one could die happy in Scotland without having been seen by Begbie in consultation.   He wrote numerous short memoirs, but his best-known work was " A Handy Book of Medical Information and Advice by a Physician," published anonymously in 1860.

Among the surgeons of this period were the two brothers Lizars, both of whom lectured upon anatomy in the College of Surgeons.   The work of John Lizars (1794–1860) has been mentioned in connection with the teaching of anatomy.   He was also a surgeon to the Royal Infirmary.   Alexander Jardine Lizars has been mentioned as professor of anatomy at Marischal College from 1841.   He was succeeded as professor of anatomy in the University of Aberdeen in 1863 by John Struthers, who had been a lecturer on anatomy in Edinburgh from 1847, and surgeon to the Royal Infirmary for a year before he went to Aberdeen.   During his Edinburgh period, Struthers published important anatomical and physiological observations, and he had taken a considerable part in the agitation for improving the teaching in the Scottish Universities.   His " Historical Sketch of the Edinburgh Anatomical School " forms a valuable account of the teachers in anatomy before his time.

Alexander Watson was surgeon to the Royal Infirmary in 1837, and devoted a good deal of attention to diseases of the eye, having published a treatise on this subject in 1830.   He afterwards, on succeeding to a property, changed his name to Watson Wemyss.

John Argyll Robertson, a lecturer on surgery in the Extra-Mural School, had at an early date, devoted himself chiefly to ophthalmic surgery.   He died in 1855, but his work in this special department was continued by his son, D. M. C. L. Argyll Robertson, who was the first to describe the phenomenon connected with the pupil, which now goes by his name.   The subject of ophthalmology, in consequence of the new operations introduced by von Graefe and the invention of the ophthalmoscope by Helmholtz, developed into an important specialty shortly after the year 1850.   This new development was speedily recognised by the management of the Royal Infirmary, and William Walker, a surgeon who had given much attention to ophthalmology, was the first ophthalmic surgeon on the staff of this institution, elected in July, 1855, to take office on the 1st September following.   He was succeeded by D. M. C. L. Argyll Robertson.

Peter David Handyside (1808–1881) was one of the surgeons to the Royal Infirmary about 1840, but was better known as a teacher of anatomy, a subject on which he lectured for many years, and in regard to which he published a large number of contributions.   James Duncan (1812–1866) was a pupil of Liston, and later surgeon to the Infirmary.

Andrew Douglas Maclagan (1812–1900) was for some years, about 1848, surgeon to the Royal Infirmary.   Afterwards he was a lecturer on materia medica in the Extra-Mural School, and in 1862 was elected professor of medical jurisprudence in the University of Edinburgh, later becoming Sir Douglas Maclagan.

James Spence (1812–1882) became surgeon to the Royal Infirmary in 1854 in the absence of Mr. R. J. Mackenzie in the Crimea.   He also lectured on surgery, and in 1864 became professor of surgery in the University, in succession to James Miller.   He was known to a later generation of students as " dismal Jimmy," and is best remembered by his " Lectures on Surgery " (1868), which formed one of the chief text-books on this subject for some twenty years.

CHAPTER XVII

MEDICAL LEGISLATIVE CHANGES IN 1860

FOR some years prior to 1860 considerable dissatisfaction had been felt with regard to the qualifications and instruction of members of the medical profession, not only in Scotland, but in other parts of Great Britain. In consequence, there had been much writing and lecturing in regard to suggested improvements in medical education.

Up to the year 1858, eight bodies in Scotland had had power to grant medical degrees or qualifications, *viz.*, the Universities of Edinburgh, Glasgow, Marischal College Aberdeen, King's College Aberdeen, and St. Andrews, as well as the Royal College of Physicians of Edinburgh, the Royal College of Surgeons of Edinburgh, and the Faculty of Physicians and Surgeons of Glasgow. In order to obtain a degree or licence to practise, the intending practitioner had to engage in a course of study lasting three years, and to pass an examination held by one or other of these bodies. Unless, however, he intended to practise either in or near Edinburgh or Glasgow, it was quite unnecessary for him to obtain any degree or qualification whatever. Almost up to the middle of the nineteenth century, the M.D. degree of Scottish Universities, other than Edinburgh, was not held in much favour. This was due to the practice, mentioned in previous chapters, of conferring this degree at some Universities, after an examination which was merely perfunctory, or even without any examination.

For practice in other parts of the country it was customary for a young man to indenture himself as apprentice to some person already in medical practice, and in this way to learn the practical side of medicine and surgery. Those, who desired to occupy a position of good standing in the profession and with the public, invariably took a degree or obtained a licence, although there was no compulsion on them to do so except for practice within the jurisdiction of one or other of the three Scottish Medical Corporations.

This state of affairs had the unfortunate effect of failing to establish a definite line between those who were worthy to enjoy the confidence of the public, and those who were quite incompetent, or who in some instances preyed upon the community to its detriment. Further, there was no form of control to regulate professional conduct.

In 1858, two important Acts of Parliament were passed. One was " An Act to Regulate the Qualifications of Practitioners in Medicine and Surgery," better known as " The Medical Act," which took effect from the 1st of October, 1858. This Act set up a General Council of Medical Education and Registration

for the United Kingdom, which was to be elected partly by the licensing bodies
and partly by the Crown.   One of the most important duties of this General
Medical Council was to prepare a " Register " of medical practitioners, and to
arrange for this to be correctly kept.   Admission to the Register was in future
to be obtained on presentation to the Registrar of a diploma of one or other of the
recognised examining bodies, or a diploma granted by two or more of these bodies
in combination.   Powers were also given to the General Medical Council, after
due enquiry, to remove from the Register the name of any practitioner in Scotland
found guilty of any crime or offence or adjudged by the General Medical Council
to have been guilty of infamous conduct in any professional respect.   At the
same time, every person registered under the Act was entitled to practice in any
part of Her Majesty's dominions and to recover in any court of law reasonable
charges for professional aid, advice and visits.   The General Medical Council
was also charged with the duty of publishing a book containing a list of medicines
and compounds and the manner of preparing them, to be called the " British
Pharmacopœia."   An amending Medical Act, containing further provisions,
was passed in 1886.

As a result of these regulations, in 1859 important arrangements were made
by the Royal College of Physicians in Edinburgh with the Royal College of
Surgeons of Edinburgh and with the Faculty of Physicians and Surgeons of
Glasgow.   Both the latter bodies had the right to license in surgery, and in
combination with each of these bodies the College of Physicians granted a Double
Qualification, conferring upon the holder the right to practise after registration
all branches of the profession in every part of Her Majesty's dominions.   At
a later date, in 1884, the three bodies united to grant a Triple Qualification
instead of the two Double Qualifications as previously.

In the year 1858, another Act of Parliament of great importance for Scotland
was passed.   This was " An Act to make provision for the better government
and discipline of the Universities of Scotland, and improving and regulating the
course of study therein ; and for the union of the two Universities and Colleges
of Aberdeen."   This Act applied to the Universities of St. Andrews, Glasgow,
Aberdeen and Edinburgh.   At Aberdeen, King's College and Marischal College
were to be united from a date to be specified by the Commissioners appointed
under the Act as one University, under the style and title of the University of
Aberdeen.   The actual union took place in the year 1860.

The Senatus Academicus for each of the Universities was to consist of the
Principal and Professors in each University, and was especially to regulate the
teaching and discipline of the University.   A General Council was set up in each
University.   A University Court was also established in each University for
the purpose of reviewing the actions of the Senatus Academicus, effecting improvements in the University, requiring due attention on the part of the professors to

teaching and other duties imposed upon them, with power of suspending professors or depriving them of office, and for the purpose of controlling and reviewing administration of the property and revenues of each University.

The Commissioners appointed under this Act drew up ordinances for the management of the various Universities, which took effect in and after the year 1860. In regard to medicine, one of the principal ordinances instituted degrees of Bachelor of Medicine and Master of Surgery to be conferred after successful examination at the end of four years of professional study, for which a definite course was laid down. The M.D. degree thereafter became a higher qualification. By subsequent ordinances of the Scottish Universities' Commissioners the medical course was extended, in 1893, to five years.

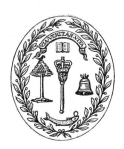

SEAL
GLASGOW UNIVERSITY

INDEX

Illustrations are indexed with antique (heavy-faced) figures

T *

BOOKS ON THE HISTORY OF MEDICINE

WELLCOME HISTORICAL MEDICAL MUSEUM
RESEARCH STUDIES IN MEDICAL HISTORY

Crown Quarto Size.   Cloth Binding.

THE authors of these unique volumes have rescued from the oblivion of the past much mediæval medical history which, otherwise, would have been unavailable, or accessible only with difficulty.

The contents of these volumes are fascinating to all interested directly or indirectly in medicine, and are of outstanding value to students and research workers in medical history.

The quality of production is in harmony with the excellence of the subject matter, and each book is abundantly illustrated.

De Arte Phisicali et de Cirurgia of Master John Arderne, Surgeon of Newark, dated 1412.   Translated by Sir D'Arcy Power, K.B.E., from a transcript made by Eric Millar.   (Wellcome Historical Medical Museum, Research Studies in Medical History, No. 1.)   London, John Bale, Sons & Danielsson, Ltd.   1922.

60 pages.   14 plates in colour and monochrome.

10s. 6d. net ;   post free, 11s. 3d.

" Mr. Henry S. Wellcome has increased the already heavy debt of gratitude owed
" him by historical students by causing to be published a translation of the old
" Newark practitioner's De Arte Phisicali et de Cirurgia.   The editor and
" translator is Sir D'Arcy Power, which is a concise way of saying that text, notes
" and introduction leave nothing to be desired.   The translation is of an illuminated
" MS. from an early fifteenth century hand, preserved in the Royal Library, Stockholm.
" The editor says that it ' omits much, adds something, and takes out entirely the
" personal element and quaint touches which make the original manuscript such
" excellent reading.'   Sir D'Arcy Power is much too modest in the appraisement
" of his literary wares ; indeed, any one of the thirteen beautiful plates with which
" the volume is embellished established a better claim to be called picturesque than
" most historical monographs."—*British Medical Journal.*

" This translation has been carried out by Sir D'Arcy Power, K.B.E., F.R.C.S.,
" from a transcript made by Mr. Eric Millar, M.A., from a replica of the Stockholm
" manuscript in the Wellcome Historical Medical Museum.   Born in 1307, Arderne
" practised in Newark from 1349 until 1370, when he came to London.   He was
" essentially an operating surgeon whose practice lay amongst the nobility, wealthy
" landlords and higher clergy.   He was evidently a sound practical surgeon and

" well abreast of knowledge of surgical craft in his days. The manuscript, which
" is here given, is an epitome in Latin made some years after Arderne's death. The
" present volume contains thirteen plates and a coloured frontispiece, and the
" numerous and unique illustrations mirror well the quaint ingenuity of those
" responsible for art in the fourteenth century. The book will afford fascinating
" reading, and will assuredly stimulate interest in the study of medical and surgical
" lore of bygone days."—*Medical Times.*

" This excellent rendering of the text into modern English makes this volume
" a most convenient peep-hole into mediæval medicine."—*Times.*

Magistri Salernitani Nondum Cogniti. A Contribution to the
History of the Medical School of Salerno by Doctor Pietro Capparoni,
General Secretary of the "Instituto Storico Italiano dell' Arte Sanitaria,"
Counsellor of the "Società Italiana di Storia delle Scienze mediche
e naturali." With a foreword by Sir D'Arcy Power, K.B.E. (Wellcome
Historical Medical Museum, Research Studies in Medical History, No. 2.)
London, John Bale, Sons & Danielsson, Ltd. 1923.

68 pages. 28 plates in colour and monochrome.

15s. net ; post free, 15s. 9d.

" This book constitutes a valuable contribution to the history and diplomatics
" of the Medical School of Salerno. When on military duty in Salerno in 1916,
" Dr. Capparoni had an opportunity of studying a very rare manuscript belonging to
" the Library of St. Matthew's Cathedral, and from this was gleaned much information
" not hitherto known relating to this medical school, which has been incorporated
" in the present volume. Sir D'Arcy Power points out that a medical school was
" founded at Salerno in the twelfth century. This school increased until the
" fourteenth century, after which it gradually diminished in importance until it was
" summarily suppressed by Napoleon in 1811. This book, which is the second
" volume of Research Studies in Medical History issued by the Wellcome Historical
" Medical Museum, is illustrated by a coloured frontispiece and twenty-seven unique
" and exquisitely executed plates, and cannot fail to attract the attention of keen
" students of medical history, all the more so if they are interested in medical
" archæology."—*Medical Times.*

" Everything connected with Salerno is of interest to the medical profession,
" and we congratulate Dr. Capparoni on having made some notable additions to
" the already published and valuable researches of De Renzi and Piero Giacose, the
" fruit of his study of a MS. belonging to the Library of the Cathedral of Salerno.
" Before entering on a description of the MS. and his researches therein, Dr. Capparoni
" gives a most interesting historical review of Salerno and its medical school, which
" probably began somewhere about the eleventh century, though there had been
" a hospital as early as the year 820. He gives his readers a number of illustrations,
" reproduced from photographs of various leaves of the MS. and of other documents
" in the Cathedral of St. Matthew. Dr. Capparoni has conferred a real benefit
" upon all those interested in the history of medicine, and altogether the book is a
" joy both to read and to look at."—*Lancet.*

The Iconography of Andreas Vesalius (André Vésale), Anatomist and Physician. 1514–1564. Paintings—pictures—engravings—illustrations —sculpture—medals. With notes, critical, literary and bibliographical, by M. H. Spielmann, F.S.A. (Wellcome Historical Medical Museum, Research Studies in Medical History, No. 3.) London, John Bale, Sons & Danielsson, Ltd. 1925.

244 pages.   68 plates in addition to text illustrations.

30s. net, post free.

The Iconography of Vesalius was for many years a mixed question of debate in artistic and medical circles, and everyone, except perhaps the owners of certain of the " portraits," will welcome the critical and authoritative contributions to the question which Mr. M. H. Spielmann has now made.   Vesalius, by the publication of his " De humani corporis fabrica," in 1543, laid the foundation of genuine anatomy and freed medicine from the trammels of authority.   The general opinion of men of science was voiced by Sir Arthur Keith when he wrote that " in the quality of his work Vesalius is akin to Shakespeare."   In characteristic fashion he continues :   " Now and again there is born into the world a man who, turning his back on the lore of his forefathers, seeks for his information direct from the book of nature.   Vesalius was one of these ; he read and translated for his fellows the text of the human body from the original imprint.   He studied the dead body to learn how the living body moved and had its being.   Vesalius breathed life into the dead human body ; in this act he still stands supreme."

" The work is in every way worthy of the distinguished anatomist ; we doubt " whether so complete an iconography of any one individual has ever before been " compiled.   Mr. Spielmann has omitted nothing which can throw light on his " subject.   He deals with portraits in oils, pictures, engravings, illustrations, " sculpture and medals ; there are numberless illustrations, most admirably " reproduced, and an iconographic bibliography which is a model of what such " things should be, while Mr. Spielmann's critical and literary notes are of " extreme interest."—*Lancet.*

" Mr. Spielmann's iconography is a large and admirably produced volume, a " credit to all concerned.   It represents a world's tribute, which under the " direction of Prof. Paul Heger, of Brussels, would have appeared earlier but for the " war, with contributions from other writers.   These contributors, still identified " with it, have left the work in Mr. Spielmann's hands, and hence it appears a critical, " biographical, bibliographical and artistic volume on a subject of front-rank " importance."—*Graphic.*

" We have here illustrated and critically described some twenty-nine portraits " of Vesalius in oil, a number of pictures in which he figures, reproductions of title- " pages of his works now so rare, about fifty engravings, illustrations of sculptures " and portrait medals.   There is also a bibliography and a list of artists.   The " work is altogether a most interesting as well as valuable monograph that should " find a place in every public and medical library."—*Glasgow Herald.*